SOUTHEAST
MEDICINAL
PLANTS

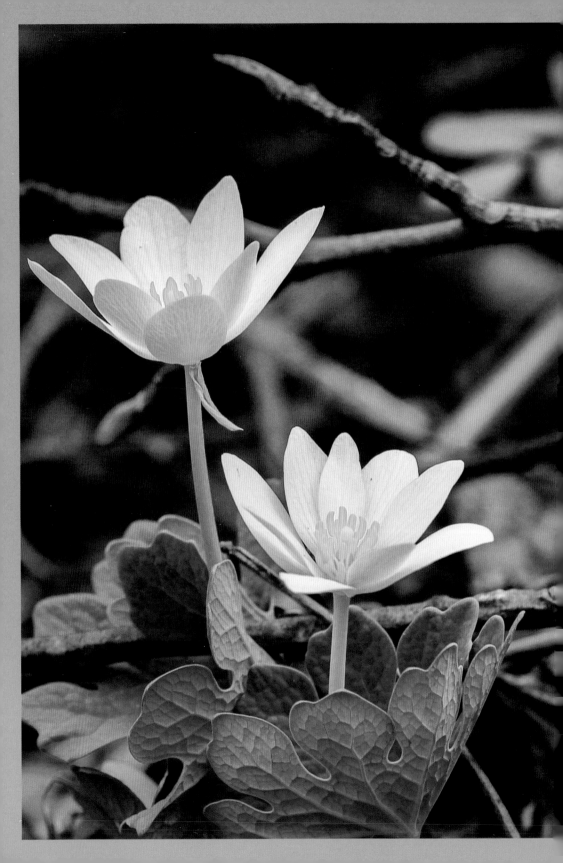

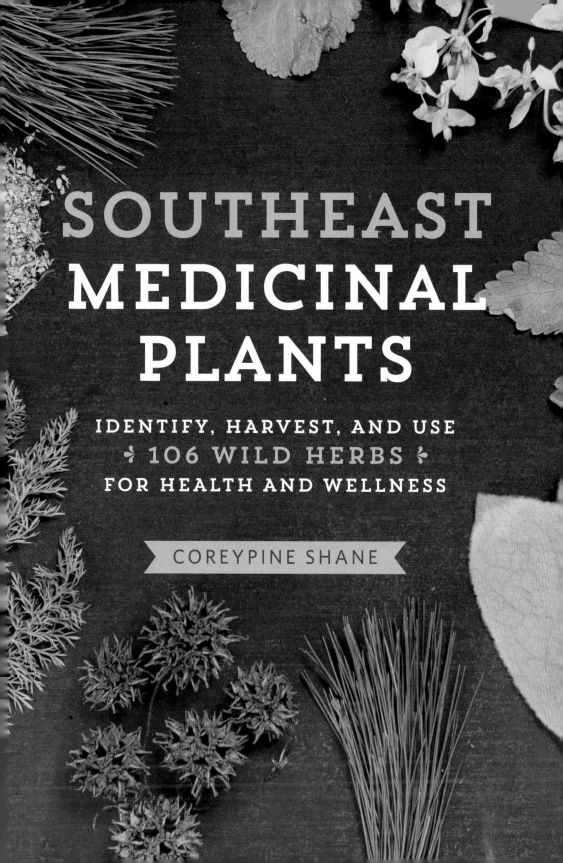

SOUTHEAST
MEDICINAL
PLANTS

IDENTIFY, HARVEST, AND USE
❦ 106 WILD HERBS ❦
FOR HEALTH AND WELLNESS

COREYPINE SHANE

The information in this book is true and complete to the best of our knowledge. All recommendations are made without guarantee on the part of the author or Timber Press. The author and publisher disclaim any liability in connection with the use of this information. In particular, ingesting wild plants is inherently risky. Plants can be easily mistaken, and individuals vary in their physiological reactions to plants that are touched or consumed. Please do not attempt self-treatment of a medical problem without consulting a qualified health practitioner.

Frontispiece: Bloodroot (*Sanguinaria canadenis*).

All photos are by the author, with the exception of those on pages 3, 5–7 by Sarah Milhollin, page 9 by Taylor C. Johnson, pages 134, 235 by Paul Rothrock, page 245 by Mike Masek, page 252 by Steven Foster, and pages 32–33, 46, 47, 61, 65 (lower right), 66, 90, 91, 95, 96, 137, 147, 148, 187, 188, 215, 216, 253, 281, 282 by 7Song.

Published in 2021 by Timber Press, Inc.,
a subsidiary of Workman Publishing Co., Inc.,
a subsidiary of Hachette Book Group, Inc.
1290 Avenue of the Americas
New York, NY 10104
timberpress.com

Printed in China on responsibly sourced paper
Third printing 2023
Text design by Mary Velgos
Cover design by Vincent James, based on a series design by Adrianna Sutton

The publisher is not responsible for websites (or their content)
that are not owned by the publisher.

The Hachette Speakers Bureau provides a wide range of authors for
speaking events. To find out more, go to hachettespeakersbureau.com or
email HachetteSpeakers@hbgusa.com.

ISBN 978-1-64326-007-5
A catalog record for this book is available from the Library of Congress.

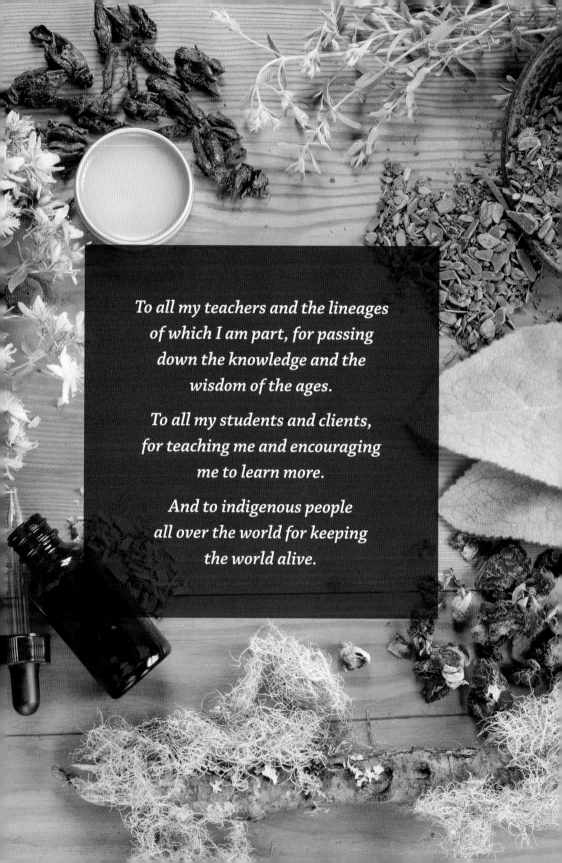

*To all my teachers and the lineages
of which I am part, for passing
down the knowledge and the
wisdom of the ages.*

*To all my students and clients,
for teaching me and encouraging
me to learn more.*

*And to indigenous people
all over the world for keeping
the world alive.*

CONTENTS

Preface: Making Friends with the Plants • 8

IDENTIFYING AND HARVESTING IN THE SOUTHEAST • 11
FROM PLANT TO MEDICINE • 25

MEDICINAL PLANTS OF THE SOUTHEAST • 33

agrimony • 34
anemone • 36
angelica • 39
bacopa • 43
balm of Gilead • 46
baptisia • 49
barberry • 51
bayberry • 54
bearsfoot • 56
beggar ticks • 59
blackberry • 61
black cohosh • 64
black haw • 68
black walnut • 70
bloodroot • 72
blue cohosh • 74
blue vervain • 76
boarhog • 79
boneset • 81
buckeye • 83
bugleweed • 85
burdock • 87
calamus • 90
catnip • 93
cleavers • 95

clematis • 98
cotton • 100
cow parsnip • 102
crossvine • 104
dandelion • 106
elder • 110
figwort • 113
fringe tree • 115
gentian • 117
ghost pipe • 119
ginkgo • 121
ginseng • 124
goldenrod • 127
goldenseal • 130
gotu kola • 132
gravel root • 134
hawthorn • 136
honeysuckle • 139
horsetail • 141
Japanese knotweed • 143
juniper • 145
kudzu • 147
liferoot • 149
linden • 151
lion's mane • 153

lobelia • 155
mimosa • 158
motherwort • 161
mountain mint • 163
mullein • 165
nettle • 167
oat • 170
partridgeberry • 173
passionflower • 175
peach • 178
pipsissewa • 180
plantain • 182
pleurisy root • 184
poke • 187
prickly ash • 189
ragweed • 192
raspberry • 194
red clover • 197
red root • 199
reishi • 202
sarsaparilla • 205
sassafras • 208
saw palmetto • 210
self heal • 213
shepherd's purse • 215
skullcap • 217
skunk cabbage • 220
slippery elm • 222

Solomon's seal • 224
spicebush • 226
spikenard • 229
St. John's wort • 232
stone root • 235
sumac • 237
sweet gum • 240
teasel • 243
usnea • 245
violet • 247
white cedar • 250
white oak • 252
white pine • 254
white pond lily • 257
wild cherry • 259
wild geranium • 261
wild ginger • 263
wild hydrangea • 265
wild sarsaparilla • 268
wild yam • 270
willow • 272
witch hazel • 274
wood betony • 276
yarrow • 278
yellow dock • 281
yellowroot • 284
yellow sweet clover • 286
yucca • 288

Bibliography • 291
Index • 292

✤ PREFACE ✤

MAKING FRIENDS
WITH THE PLANTS

As a socially awkward adolescent, I felt more at home in the woods than with people, and thankfully my mom encouraged me to spend time outdoors. I still feel a profound sense of belonging when I spend the day in the wild—I can drop my mental chatter and come back to myself. I feel that I'm a part of something so much bigger and older than my small life, and it realigns my problems into a healthier perspective.

Learning that there were things I could eat out there was a revelation, and I started getting to know the individual plants. And when I learned they could also help me when I'm sick, I was even more fascinated. It drew me into learning specific plants, their names, and their uses.

As a college student I became friends with 7Song, a local herbalist, and started informally apprenticing with him, coming by his cabin to chop roots and walk around the land and talk about the plants there. When he opened a school, I was in his first class. But the funny thing is, I never thought about becoming an herbalist, let alone a clinician or a teacher,

until school was almost over—I just studied it because I was following my passion. Looking back, I realize that without even knowing it I was searching for a way to get back to my roots, to remember what my great-grandparents once knew. When I started learning this, I found I wanted to share it with others.

More and more people feel this way, hearing a calling to get away from screens and virtual interactions, and to re-engage with the natural world. This connection is our birthright. It is how humans lived for as long as there have been humans, up until pretty recently. No matter where you come from, you have indigenous ancestors—maybe not

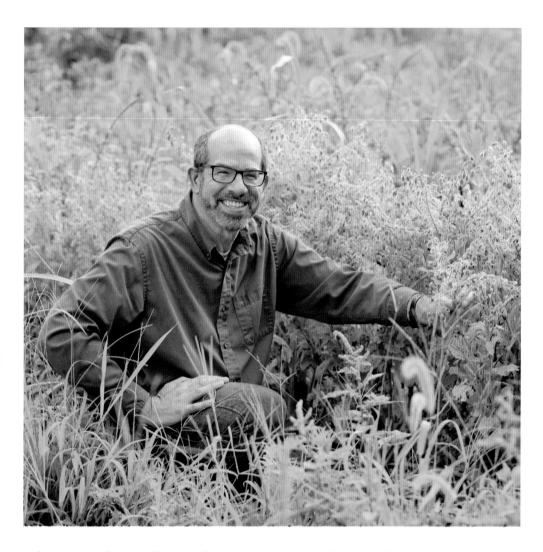

indigenous to where you live now, but they were native to somewhere. They knew their land, the plants that grew there and how to use them. It's safe to say that without some form of plant medicine, your ancestors wouldn't have survived and you wouldn't be here today. Maybe we're trying to find the magic and the wisdom that our ancestors knew.

Herbal medicine is about so much more than healing diseases with plants. It's about relating to the world around us in a more connected way, it's about recognizing how everything is related, seeing ourselves not as separate but as a strand woven into the complex nature from which we came. The deepest healing of herbal medicine is not the specific remedies we take but the connection we experience when we remember that we live among our food and our medicine. Whether you're in the city, the suburbs, or out in the woods, there are plants growing all around you just waiting for you to learn and remember them.

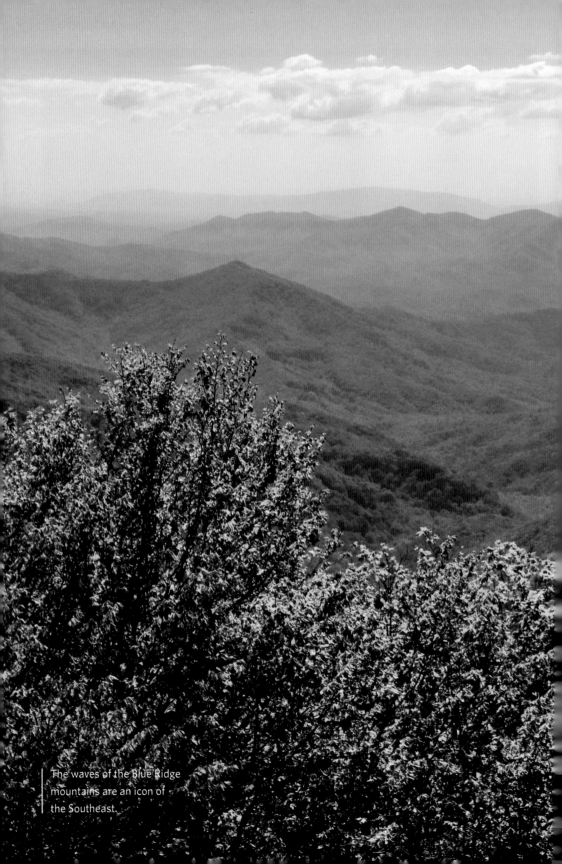

The waves of the Blue Ridge
mountains are an icon of
the Southeast.

IDENTIFYING AND HARVESTING IN THE SOUTHEAST

This book is a travel guide to a land we're already living in but haven't fully discovered. By learning how to find medicine and food in the wild, we change our relationship to forests and front yards alike. We reconnect with everything outside of our front door. And then, by understanding how to use these same plants for healing, we learn and grow and deepen our relationship with our own body. More than a guide about how to identify the occasional plant, this is ultimately an introduction to a different way of seeing the world, both internal and external.

Herbalist and friend Frank Cook talked about how we need to get past the "green wall" in order to see the plant world. When most modern humans look at the woods or even a meadow, what we see is an imposing wall of undifferentiated green things. But then as we learn the individual plants, trees, and ferns, we start to get more of a three-dimensional picture of what's around us. We begin to feel more at home outdoors, more in our element. What was once a flat picture gains depth and nuance. The plants that were once strangers at a party become our friends.

In this book, you'll meet some of the medicinal plants that live and thrive in the southeastern United States. You'll find the weeds of Raleigh and Birmingham, the deep-woods plants of the Blue Ridge and Ozark mountains, and the low-country plants of the Mississippi's floodplain and Georgia's Golden Isles.

It should be noted that, as many plants as I have covered here, they are still only a small part of the many plants that grow in this vast region. Not every plant has a known medicinal use, and some plants are medicinal but are seldom used or have uses that are easily replicated by more common plants. Instead, I have focused on the ones that I or other herbalists use most.

In doing so, I have excluded some plants that are part of the southern folk tradition that I don't know from personal experience. Among them are some plants that have a long history of use but little written about them—trees like dogwood, magnolia, and tulip poplar; herbs like bee balm, Indian pink, and senega snakeroot. All these and more deserve attention, research, and integration into modern herbal practice.

I have also excluded some plants that are not abundant enough to harvest—there's no pink lady's slipper, Virginia snakeroot, or false unicorn root for instance. But I do cover ginseng and goldenseal, two at-risk herbs that should very rarely if ever be harvested from the wild. But they are good well-known medicines that can be cultivated in the woods. I trust the reader to know when not to harvest these endangered plants.

Overall, I have done my best to include so-called mainstream herbs along with herbs from the many folk traditions of the South. We know about these plants from Native American, Black, Afro-Caribbean, Spanish, Latin, and Scotch-Irish traditions. It is important to recognize the many influences in modern herbalism—it is the product of thousands of years of indigenous peoples' direct experience with the plants; it has been and continues to be adopted and adapted by colonizers.

Some of the invasive weeds are also great medicine and are used in the Chinese herbal tradition. Some of these plants are routinely found on the shelves of U.S. and European herb stores, and some are lesser known but essential nonetheless. It's hard to know why some herbs are popular and others are obscure—sometimes there's a good reason not to use a plant anymore, and sometimes the use has just been forgotten.

This book was inspired by the work of one of my teachers, herbalist Michael Moore, who wrote and taught extensively about the plants of the American West. He was a champion of bioregionalism before that word was even coined. He used local analogues to closely related plants among the classic canon of Western herbalism; and he learned about other native plants from the local people who had been living on the land for centuries. His work helped to bring such plants back into use in mainstream herbalism.

Like Michael, I want to share the indispensable specifics of where and when to find a medicinal plant, what species to use, how to make the best preparation from it, and of course, how to use it to help people heal. My goal is to uncover the genius of each plant, when is the best time to use it, and for whom. Understanding what the plant really does—its "personality"—gives us the flexibility to use it for conditions well beyond what any book tells us. And therein lies the depth of herbal medicine.

FINDING YOURSELF AND YOUR PLANTS IN THE SOUTHEAST

The Southeast is an incredibly diverse area with a wide variety of elevations, rainfall, soil geology, and habitats. It would be almost impossible to cover every medicinal plant in this area, and I have done my best to avoid prioritizing plants of Southern Appalachia (where I live), which already have a lot written about them. And by the way, it is pronounced ap-uh-LAH-chuh (not ap-uh-LAY-chuh) down here. Just so you know.

This book covers the medicinal plants that grow from the Maryland–Pennsylvania border south to Florida and west through West Virginia and Kentucky, down through Arkansas and the Ozark mountains south to the Gulf Coast, including Alabama, Mississippi, Louisiana, and even eastern Texas.

Within this range, we can define some broad regions, each of which can be further broken down into more subtypes and ecotypes. Starting from the east there is the coastal plain, extending from eastern Maryland south through Virginia, North Carolina, South Carolina, and southern Georgia, all of Florida, and then across the southern parts of Alabama, Mississippi, and Louisiana as well as eastern Texas. Then moving west there's the rolling hills of the Piedmont, then the Southern Appalachians, which include both the Blue Ridge and Smoky mountain ranges, before the land falls back into the Cumberland Plateau of middle Tennessee and Kentucky and then changes to the inner coastal plain of the Mississippi River Basin. Crossing the great Mississippi, we cover the Ozarks of southern Missouri and northern Arkansas, and southern Arkansas, Louisiana, and eastern Texas contain some plants possibly washed down the river over time that are present further north but less common among the other Gulf Coast states.

THE HOW-TO OF HARVESTING

Wildcrafting, a name for harvesting plants that you didn't grow yourself, has recently become much more popular, as has herbal medicine in general. As exciting as it is to see this once marginalized activity become more mainstream, it's also led to problems of over-harvesting, native ecosystems being damaged, and inexperienced harvesters collecting the wrong plants. It's also led to illegal and unethical poaching on private and public land.

There is nothing like wildcrafting—going out and harvesting the plants to make your own food, tea, and medicine might be one of the most empowering feelings. Instead of tending a garden all year, planting and weeding and watering, we just go out and pick what nature offers us. No need to visit a pharmacist, doctor, or even health food store. Just a few basic supplies, some money for alcohol, glycerin, and/or vinegar, and you're good to go! There is no more direct way to connect to nature and plants.

But it's not always so easy or so fun. There is a cost, not in money but in our time, our attention, and above all, the responsibility it incurs to those plants and places we visit. We didn't plant these plants, but once we start harvesting them we take some responsibility for the health of that plant and for the health of the area where we harvest. We take on the role of a gardener, not in the sense that the location is "ours," but that some of the responsibility for tending that area now falls to us. I highly encourage everyone harvesting from the wild to read about the "honorable harvest" in *Braiding Sweetgrass* (Kimmerer 2015).

There are some things you need to know before harvesting wild plants to protect both yourself and the places you harvest from. The first thing you need to learn is how to harvest ethically and sustainably. I've seen too many stands get decimated by well-meaning harvesters who aren't aware of some of these basics. People generally don't mean to do harm, they just haven't learned how to harvest with the forest in mind yet. Here are the basic rules for wildcrafting:

• Harvest like you want your grandkids (or friends' grandkids) to be able to harvest from the same place.
• Don't harvest when you're feeling angry, rushed, greedy, or out of sorts. It will throw off your decision making and affect the medicine.
• Harvest only from abundance and take only what you need.
• Ask permission and leave a little something.
• Know what plants not to harvest and leave those plants be.

Though many plants in this book are common weeds that can be easily picked without much concern for the sustainability of the plant (hello dandelion, ragweed, and honeysuckle!), it takes careful consideration to harvest from the woods in a sustainable way. We need to remember that even when plants are available to us on public land, they are not "ours." Our attitude has to be less of a colonial mindset of coming in and taking what we think we deserve and more about creating a relationship with the wild plants. Growing into this relationship earns the respect of the plants as well as fellow wildcrafters and herbalists. And every time I harvest plants from this place of respect, I always come away feeling like I know the plant better.

The first thing to do when you find a stand of plants is to do a stand count. After hours spent looking for a plant, it can be tempting to harvest the first one you find, but take the time to walk around first and see how many plants are there and what impacts them. Ask questions. Is there agricultural runoff nearby? Are there wildlife that feed on this plant? Are other people potentially harvesting here? Do pollinators depend on this plant? You might not be able to answer all these questions, but observe as much as you can, counting the number of plants while you assess the area. A good rule of thumb is to never harvest more than one out of four plants—though in practice I usually harvest much less than even that. If you start harvesting before you know there's enough, you might end up taking the only plants in that area and then not even have enough plants to make a cup of tea.

Once you've found a big enough stand in a good location, ask the plant's permission. Maybe this sounds woo-woo, but trust me when I say it makes a difference. If you, like me, have a more science-y mind, think about it as quieting your mind and tuning in to your intuition, which is really just the sum of all the factors you've already unconsciously noticed but can't put into words. Find the largest, most robust plant, or maybe just the first plant you saw, sit down and quiet your mind, then introduce yourself to the plant and ask permission. Next, and most importantly, stop and listen.

Now I should say that plants don't exactly talk to me, or at least not like humans do, and I'm a little jealous of those who do have conversations with plants. I get more of a felt sense—if it's the right place to harvest then I feel a peaceful sense of rightness, and if it's not then I feel a sense of unease, like it's not quite the right fit. Here's a thought: if every time you ask, the answer is yes, then you're probably not listening enough.

Next, make an offering as a token of appreciation. I've heard a lot of people say that Native American peoples leave tobacco as a thank-you gift. Personally, I don't think it matters what you leave—it's the thought that counts (as they say). Tobacco is not a plant I use or interact with, so I don't have a sacred connection to it. I like to leave a bit of whatever precious snack I have in my backpack, like a small piece of dried mango or a square of chocolate. It's just about creating some energy exchange, some appreciation.

I like to leave the biggest and healthiest plant in the stand to propagate and spread its good genes, but I do like to harvest larger plants because then I can harvest fewer of them. As you're harvesting, ask yourself what you can do to make the stand healthier. If you're digging roots, can you dig a plant that's growing so close to another that they are competing, like thinning carrots? If harvesting flowers and leaves, can you pinch off upper parts so that the plant will branch out and produce more, like picking basil? If you're harvesting branches, can you prune the plant like a fruit tree to encourage healthy growth? This is a holistic approach to harvesting.

As for when to harvest, generally it is better to harvest leaves and flowers on sunny days after the dew has dried. Aromatic herbs are best picked when the sun warms up the aromatics and it hasn't rained in a day or two. Sun and rain matter less with roots and barks, and I've dug roots on cool rainy days. Some subscribe to the idea that upper plant parts are better picked closer to the full moon when the energy is more upward, and roots are best dug closer to the new moon when the energy is more down and in.

Then there's time of year. Generally, roots are best harvested in the fall after the flowers have finished and the leaves are starting to look a bit rough. Some plants (blue cohosh,

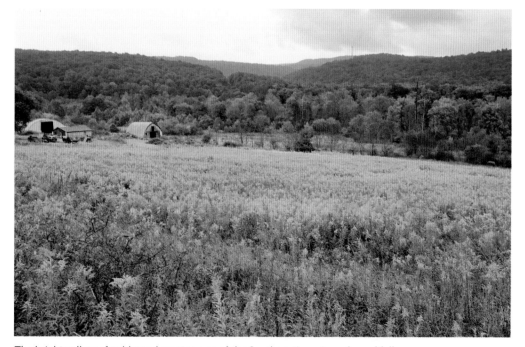

The bright yellow of goldenrod creates one of the Southeast's major colors of fall.

bloodroot, Solomon's seal) come up early in the spring and die back early, and their roots need to be dug in August. Some plants (pleurisy root, red root) are almost impossible to find if they're not in flower, and so even though they are best harvested after flowering, I sometimes harvest them early because that's when I can find them. Most barks are best harvested in spring and early summer as the sap is rising and the new bark is slipping, forming its new ring.

Our medicine can only be as good as the plants we harvest, though the energy we harvest with also affects our final product. Harvest carefully and with intention. Tune in to the woods to be more present, whatever that looks like for you. Choose healthy plants growing in a good location. Though there are better and worse times to harvest a plant, sometimes the best time to harvest is when you are there and the plant is there. Sometimes it's better to have some tincture from not-the-ideal-time than to have no tincture at all because you were waiting for the moon to rise and the stars to align.

And finally, scouting for plants is a big part of wildcrafting—getting to know where plants grow, where they are abundant and where they are few, and how things change over time. This means getting to know your area and making more than one trip to the same place, and it may mean years of careful observation to get to know your area and what grows where.

WHERE TO GO AND WHERE NOT TO GO

Since most of us do not live in a pristine wilderness with access to every plant we want, where can we go to harvest?

The first thing to know is that many plants are already growing as weeds in your yard or in your neighborhood. If you have friends with gardens or farms, you can ask them about their weeds, and you can check local parks for weeds. Just make sure you choose places that haven't been sprayed with pesticides or herbicides because you don't want those chemicals contaminating your medicine. So that is an important question to ask, and always ask permission if you are on private land.

Some commonly sprayed places where you can't necessarily ask about pesticide use include the sides of railroad tracks and underneath power lines. Furthermore, avoid harvesting from or near non-organic farms, along busy roads, or even within 10 feet or so of side roads; they are not only sprayed but also contaminated with exhaust and other environmental pollutants from traffic. I don't usually harvest on the sides of trails, not because they are sprayed but because most people won't go off the trail and I want to give them the chance to see this plant too.

If you live near public land, you can expect some general guidelines but always check with your local office because rules change from area to area. In national parks, you can only pick fruits or harvest mushrooms; other types of harvesting, such as digging roots, are strictly prohibited. State forests, Bureau of Land Management land, and game lands are usually OK, and state parks are generally not. National forests are usually fine to harvest in, but they require you to get a permit for anything beyond limited personal use. Some plants that are highly impacted by harvesting, like ginseng and goldenseal, require a special permit—harvesting ginseng without a permit or in the wrong season can result in a $5,000 fine or up to 6 months in jail, so take this seriously.

And then of course there's always the option of finding plants on private land. Sometimes this means making friends out

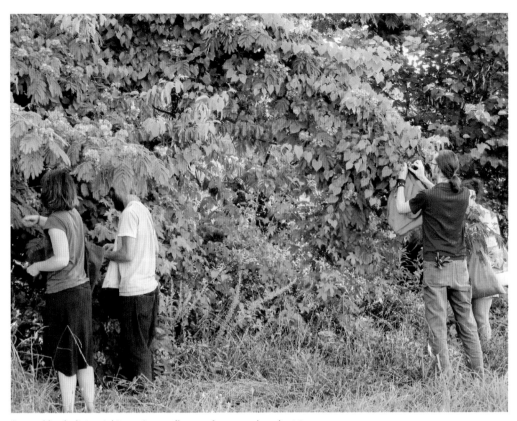

Several herbalists picking mimosa flowers from an abundant tree.

in the country and asking around about specific plants. Sometimes it means seeing plants in someone's field and mustering up the courage to go knock on the front door. I've had some very interesting and almost always positive conversations this way. Sometimes I offer to give them a bottle of the finished product if it seems appropriate, but often people are just satisfied asking a few questions.

PLANT IDENTIFICATION TERMINOLOGY

In this book I have done my best to avoid technical botanical language. This language has its place—knowing the 14 different words for "hairy" can help tell the difference between two very similar plants—but it can

be more confusing when we're just beginning. I recommend you carry at least one other identification guide with you in the field, as cross-referencing is the best way to be sure of proper ID. And please, don't ever harvest anything unless you are 100% sure that you have the right plant.

Even though this books steers away from technical botany lingo, there are still some basic botany terms we should be aware of. Begin with careful observation, because so much of identification comes down to specific details. But how do we even know what to look for? Here are some steps to get you started for proper botanical ID; they are arranged in a common-sense order to notice things. Some plants may require you to work through the whole list; for others, one particular characteristic might make the correct ID.

- Is the plant an herb, vine, shrub, or tree?
- Are the leaves simple or compound? If compound, are they pinnate or palmate?
- Are the leaves alternate, opposite, whorled, or basal?
- Is the margin of the leaves entire, toothed, or lobed?
- Are the flowers regular (radially symmetrical) or irregular?
- How many petals does the flower have? How may sepals? Are they separate or united?
- Are the flowers individual or in some kind of head or cluster?

To start at the beginning, whether or not a plant is a tree might seem obvious—but you'd be surprised! I had a challenging time identifying red root when I first met it because I didn't realize it was a small shrub, not an herb! And sometimes a "stumper" that a student brings to me is actually a sapling tree that's only a few feet high.

The word "herb" can mean different things in different contexts, but in botany it means a plant that's not woody and whose aerial parts die to the ground each year. What's confusing is that it is not size-dependent, so a 6-foot-tall spikenard is still an herb because the aboveground plant dies back each fall, whereas a 2-foot-tall red root is actually a shrub because the woody stems stay alive and regrow leaves each spring. The easiest way to tell is to check for a tough and woody stem (without breaking the stem accidentally).

The second question in the list is a little more complicated, as compound leaves aren't always perfectly straightforward. A compound leaf is when one leaf is made up of several leaflets, which may at first resemble separate leaves. So how do we tell the difference?

The strictly botanical way is to look for buds or new growth: one leaf comes from one bud—so there will never be buds within a compound leaf, only one at the base of the whole leaf. An easier and more intuitive way is to look for numerical consistency; a plant that always has 7–9 leaves per branch is probably compound and not just lucky. Though there can be some variation in the exact number, there's a general feeling of every leaf being composed of a similar number of leaflets. And finally, new growth at the tip will be of the same age, unlike a simple leaf, where separate leaves will more clearly be of different ages.

Compound leaves can be either palmately compound, meaning the leaflets come from a single point like fingers from a palm, or pinnately compound, meaning the leaflets branch out from a central stalk like a feather. Examples of pinnately compound leaves include agrimony, elder, black walnut, mimosa, and raspberry. Examples of palmately compound leaves include buckeye, blackberry, and cannabis. Examples of trifoliate leaves, those that have only three leaflets, include red clover, kudzu, and poison ivy.

With time and experience, this distinction starts to become second nature and can be made even from a distance; but it does throw people when first identifying plants, which is why it's a good thing to practice noticing.

Now that you know whether the leaves are simple or compound, check to see how the leaves (not leaflets!) are arranged on the main stem. If there is only one leaf attached at each place along the stem, the leaves are alternate, and if there are two leaves attached at the same place on the stem, they're opposite. If there are three or more attached at the same place, then you're looking at whorled leaves. If the leaves all come directly from the ground, they are basal, that is, they come from the base of the plant.

Next check the margin of the leaves. If the edges are smooth like a plantain leaf, then they are entire; if they are cut like a saw edge (like a birch leaf), then that's toothed. And if the indentations are deeper, maybe a third to halfway toward the midrib (like an oak or maple leaf), then that leaf is lobed.

And finally we get to the flower. There needs to be a flower present for positive botanical identification, except for trees. So, first: is the flower regular or irregular? A regular flower can be cut through the middle in any direction and there will be two equal parts—think of a starfish or a lily. If it is irregular then it may be two-lipped with different top and bottom parts, or one of the petals may be larger and will only make two equal parts if cut through the middle along one line. Mints, orchids, and peas are examples of plants with irregular flowers.

Now count the number of petals, or, if the petals are fused together, count the number of lobes. Beneath the petals are the sepals, the part that encloses the flower in bud— these might be brightly colored and look like petals (as with some plants in the buttercup family), but they are usually plain green. Count the number of sepals.

Do the flowers grow one per stalk or are they growing in heads or some other kind of formation? There are many different names for the structure of a flower head; for example, if all the flower stalks come from one place on the stem like spokes of an umbrella then it is called an umbel (think of Queen Anne's lace, angelica, or elder). If the flowers are attached to a central stalk then it is called a spike, but if each individual flower has a stalk where it attaches to that central stalk then it is called a raceme. There are more terms, but those are a few to get you started.

Finally, getting geeky: inside the flower are the stamens, which produce pollen, and then inside of that is the pistil or pistils, which produce the seeds. Look for both types, and note whether there are just a few or many.

POISONOUS PLANTS

The first things to learn are the very poisonous plants so you can at least know that you aren't inadvertently harvesting one of them. The first plant I teach students on plant walks is poison ivy (*Toxicodendron radicans*) because it is widespread and common, and it can cause severe, long-lasting symptoms for many people. Some call it "sister ivy" as a way of respecting the plant's important role of keeping people away from disturbed areas that are trying to regrow.

The old summer camp adage "leaves of three, let it be" applies here. But if we did this, we would also miss out on strawberries and red clover. So to be more specific, poison ivy's middle leaflet has a longer petiole (leaf stalk), and there is a red dot where the three leaflets meet. Every leaf seems to be differently wavy-margined, but usually the bottom leaflets are wavier facing away from the central leaflet.

This vine can run along the ground and even climb up trees with hairy aerial roots, a behavior that is more common in the southern than the northern states. There are times I look up to identify a tree by its leaves and find that the first 15 feet of leaves are actually poison ivy! Please be aware that the vines can cause more irritation than the leaves, and the roots even worse. So be sure there's no poison ivy within ten feet when you're digging roots to be on the safe side.

Less common though far more dangerous are the deadly poisonous plants water hemlock and poison hemlock, both in the parsley family (Apiaceae) and not at all related to the hemlock tree, which is a conifer and not poisonous at all. These plants are particularly dangerous because the parsley family has a lot of edibles and medicinals that one might want to harvest. So be extra careful when harvesting parsley family plants with flowers in an umbel like angelica, boarhog, or cow parsnip, to name a few.

Although many people warn about poison sumac, this is actually an uncommon plant. It does cause a much worse rash than poison ivy or poison oak, but most of us are unlikely to encounter it, as it is found only in swampy areas. Most of the common sumacs, on the other hand, grow in meadows and on roadsides and are not poisonous. Poison sumac can be differentiated from other sumacs by its white or yellow berries. All other sumac species have red berries.

A few plants in the lily family with long parallel veins are quite dangerous if misidentified; false hellebore (*Veratrum viride*) and lily of the valley (*Convallaria majuscula*) are deadly poisonous and can be mistaken for ramps, a commonly foraged and delicious edible.

Jimson weed (*Datura stramonium*) doesn't look like any medicinal in this book, but despite its reputation as a potent psychedelic, it too is deadly poisonous. Some of those who have physically survived ingesting the plant did not necessarily survive mentally, never quite coming back from their trip.

Other poisonous plants are out there, but these are the ones most commonly encountered in the Southeast and therefore most likely to be confused with (or grow near) medicinal plants.

TOOLS OF THE TRADE

Let's get down to brass tacks: what do you need to bring with you when you harvest? The first thing to think about is taking care of yourself. Wear pants that can get dirty, bring a rain jacket even if there's no rain in the forecast, and bring sun protection, like a hat and a loose long-sleeved shirt. I always wear long pants to harvest because you never know when there's going to be poison ivy, wild roses, blackberries, or greenbriers around. Boots will help protect your feet from snakes and stinging insects. Always carry a bandana because you just never know—it can be a sweat band on your forehead, sun protection on your neck, an impromptu basket for carrying berries or mushrooms, a small towel, or a host of other uses, including first aid. And, it may seem obvious, but don't forget to carry water!

Speaking of insects, it can be helpful to bring insect repellant. Rose geranium essential oil is particularly effective for repelling ticks, as is tucking your shirt into your pants and your pants into your socks. Although chiggers (aka red bugs) aren't common up in the mountains, they are certainly found in the rest of the Southeast. Rubbing some sulphur powder into your socks, around the bottoms of your pants, and in your waistband can help prevent them from digging in and causing an itch that can last 2–3 weeks. If you do get bitten, then putting a drop of propolis tincture on each bite and letting it dry for a minute can help shorten the intensity and duration of the itching.

As far as actual tools go, the hand tools are going to be your most important and most used tools—specifically, pruners and a soil knife, though you should always have a pocketknife on you too, just in case. Larger tools to have on hand include a digging fork, a nursery or trenching spade, loppers, and a folding saw. And of course you'll need some bags to put your harvest into.

When it comes to the basics, it's the hand tools you'll use the most. Spend the money

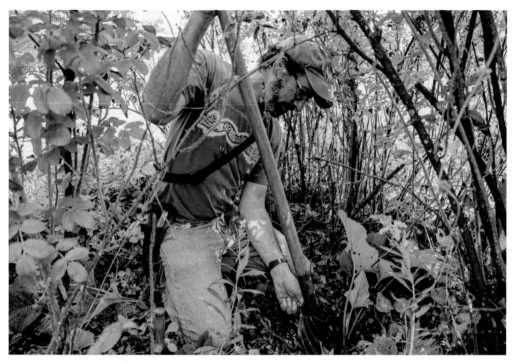
Yours truly, using a digging fork to dig up some tough burdock root.

and get a nice pair of bypass pruners—it might seem extravagant for clipping thin stems of mint or skullcap, but you can also use it to harvest small branches of witch hazel or wild cherry, and for processing tough roots that a knife won't be able to get through. My pruners are always in a holster on my belt.

The next most important tool is a soil knife, or a hori hori if it comes from Japan. Unlike trowels that can break where the digging part attaches to the handle, soil knives are more or less one piece, are flatter so they're easier to direct, and often come with a cool holster so you can also wear this on your belt. A soil knife can be used for digging down to find taproots or for trailing along a root that's running laterally. It also has a sharp edge on one side, so if you can't dig any deeper and the root won't yank out, you can cut it and run.

As for long-handled tools, I rarely use a wide shovel unless I'm trying to dig a hole. Mostly I use a digging fork on each side of a root to loosen the soil so I can get in there with a soil knife. This looks like a pitch fork, but instead of the many thin tines, a digging fork has a few strong tines that don't bend so easily.

The shovel that I use is a long thin one sometimes called a nursery or trenching spade. I really only use this when digging roots that grow in fields and meadows, where roots have to compete with grass and other surface plants. Think of dandelion, burdock, or yellow dock: all have strong deep taproots that go straight down. You won't need a shovel in the woods.

Loppers are like pruners but with a long handle. This is the ideal tool for harvesting branches from trees, but I use it just as often to cut tough, stubborn roots like red root, wild hydrangea, or stone root, preferably with a trusting friend holding the root so both my hands are free to use the handles. Please be careful with these as they could do some serious harm.

When you're finished for the day, make sure to wash all the dirt off your tools, and wash your pruners with soap and water before drying them right away. Any dirt on there will cause rust. You can get a steel-bristle brush to remove crusted-on mud. Some harvesters also carry with them a length of pipe to help bend back digging fork tines that get bent.

Finally, you need a place to put those plants as you're harvesting them! I usually use cloth shopping bags, which I seem to keep acquiring. Burlap bags also work great,

especially for roots; they are tough and durable, don't fall apart when wet, and won't let dirt through. Often, you can find these used at coffee roasters or other bulk suppliers. Paper bags can be useful sometimes, as long as things aren't too wet, and can also be used to dry herbs. Plastic shopping bags are convenient and compact but will cause the herbs to "sweat" because the moist respiration from the plants can't escape.

PROCESSING HERBS

Wildcrafting takes time, and processing takes even more time—more time than you would think. Always plan at least twice as much time to process as to harvest, and three times as much time as you think for both! Each plant has its own challenges: black cohosh

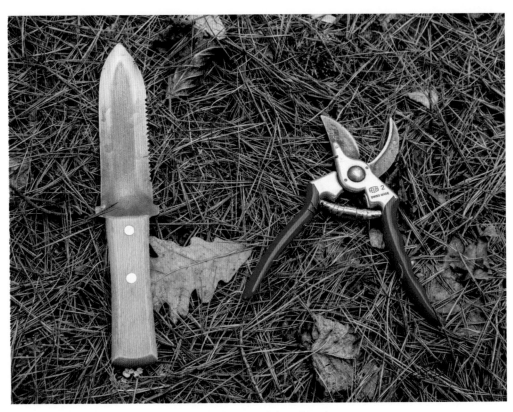

A soil knife and a nice pair of pruners are the harvester's best friends.

is easy to harvest, but it takes a long time to clean its convoluted roots; red root and wild hydrangea are notoriously tough to chop up; and stripping the bark off any harvested limbs can take hours. So remember to always give yourself plenty of time so you don't cramp your time.

The first step in processing aboveground (aerial) plant parts is to garble them. Lay down butcher paper, packing paper, or newspaper on a table and lay out the herbs a little bit at a time. Pick out any other plants that might have snuck in there while you were harvesting, and pick out any leaves that look diseased or badly bug-eaten. Also pick out the bugs at this point—no one wants a ladybug or (heaven forbid) a stink bug in their finished product.

When processing roots, less garbling is usually needed if you've made sure to harvest the right plants in the field, but keep an eye out as you're processing to be sure another plant's roots didn't cross yours and make its way into your harvest bag. Washing and chopping is what really takes the most time with root harvests.

If it's warm enough, I like to lay my roots down on a tarp outside and use a garden hose to get off the first thick layer of dirt with a gentle spray (too hard a spray might damage the root). Some folks like to put their roots in a steel utility tub and soak them in cold water for a little while to loosen the dirt up a bit before spraying them down. My favorite way is to knock as much dirt as possible back into the hole I dug from, and then wash that next layer off in a creek near where I've harvested, allowing the rest of the dirt to stay in that ecosystem. Make sure the creek is big enough that you're not disturbing salamanders.

Whatever way you do it, leaving most of the dirt outside makes the next step of scrubbing the roots much easier and will mean fewer clogged sinks. Use a natural-bristle vegetable brush and scrub hard enough to get the majority of the dirt off without scratching the root surface. A few specks of dirt aren't going to harm the tincture, but you definitely don't want your tincture tasting like dirt!

Once they're washed, chop each root into half-inch chunks with a sharp knife, like you're cutting carrots up for a stir fry. A heavy meat cleaver is useful for getting through thick roots and saving some wear and tear on your arms, but sometimes a solid set of pruners are what's really needed to get through extra-tough roots. For the hardest roots, loppers might be indicated, and I have even used a hatchet to chunk up red root.

It's a good idea to wear gloves when harvesting potentially toxic roots so that the chemicals don't absorb through the skin. As far as herbs covered in this book, I'm referring specifically to poke, because I have heard of people getting nausea, diarrhea, and headaches just from processing a lot of its root.

Barks are easy to harvest in abundance with a healthy set of pruners or even better, loppers. But what takes 10 minutes to harvest in the field might take 3 hours to strip. Never ever harvest bark off a living tree—trim off the limbs and then harvest the bark from them. Or if you're lucky and observant, harvest bark from recently downed limbs or trees.

Barks are best harvested in the spring and early summer when the new bark is slipping, meaning that the new cambium is forming and is not yet firmly attached to the tree. Though bark can be harvested year-round, this is by far the easiest time to process it. It's also much easier to process bark on the day you harvest; waiting even a day will make your job much harder.

The easiest way to debark a limb is to score a circle with a sharp knife, score another circle maybe 8–12 inches away, then cut a line between these two circles. This is the place your knife is most likely to slip so don't prop it up on your leg. Next, slide the tip of your knife under that long line and slide it up from one circle to the next. If the bark pops up nicely, then you can use either fingers or a knife to pry off the rest of it, making a nice cylindrical quill of bark. Score another circle up the limb and repeat. This method would, of course, kill a live limb, which is why it's better to take it off the tree first.

DRYING PLANTS

Plants that are dried well—both completely and quickly—make better medicine and store for longer. Since the Southeast has a humid climate, it's even more challenging and more important to get this right. The most important things needed to dry any herb are heat and air circulation, and always make sure to avoid direct sun for both drying and for storage.

Roots need to be washed and chopped first, but leaves, flowers, and seeds can be dried whole. All plants should be garbled when fresh and labeled on the drying rack because all dried plant material looks the same. You'll know that the plant is dry when it snaps instead of bending.

There are many ways to dry plants: maybe the easiest and fastest is a dehydrator set to between 95°F (for delicate parts like flowers) to 105°F (for tougher parts like roots). But most of us start out by just laying out the plants on newspaper or a clean window screen. I emphasize clean and preferably food grade because screens gather a lot of dust. The screen can be set between two pieces of furniture so that there's at least a foot of space underneath for air circulation.

Another method requires a hanging mesh drying rack, with screens that can be clipped on or taken off as needed, and this is what I've been using around my house recently. Some people just put their plants in paper bags and leave them in a hot car, but I worry that it will get too hot.

And then there's another method for long-stalked plants like nettle or goldenrod: bundle several stalks together with a rubber band, then unfold a paper clip and put one hook through the rubber band and hang the other on a length of twine. If you have an extra room in your house, you can put a fan and a dehumidifier in there and close the door for a few days to make an impromptu drying room.

FROM PLANT TO MEDICINE

Whole books are dedicated to making herbal medicine preparations, but there are only three main techniques home herbalists use: tea preparations (infusions and decoctions), concentrated liquid extracts using either alcohol or glycerin (maceration tinctures or glycerites), and oil extracts for topical applications (infused oils). There are at least a dozen other methods, but start simple and check out the books in the bibliography for more ideas.

MAKING YOUR OWN MEDICINE

Tea versus tincture is a common debate in the herb world, and each has its advantages. People have been using herbal tea as medicine for tens of thousands of years, and it is the most traditional way of taking herbs besides just eating them. Making tea is in itself a calming, healing ritual, and it also happens to be the best method for getting nutrients and minerals out of a plant: hot water extracts all the water-soluble constituents.

Tinctures, on the other hand, are definitely more convenient—you can fit a week's dose in your pocket. Alcohol and glycerin both powerfully extract the chemistry of the plant and preserve it for years. They can pull out resins and other constituents that don't dissolve well in water, but they don't do a good job of extracting protein or minerals. Furthermore, the taste can be off-putting—either the harshness of alcohol or the cloying sweetness of glycerin. Tinctures are best taken in a few ounces of water to dilute that strong flavor.

MAKING TEA

Strictly speaking, "tea" refers to the tea plant (*Camellia sinensis*), but it also colloquially refers to a technique using water to extract the medicine from plants—yielding either an infusion, which is made by steeping a plant, or a decoction, which is made by simmering.

You don't need anything fancy to make herbal teas, never mind the overwhelming variety of tea accoutrements on the market—tea connoisseurs would be aghast to see that my canning jar is a stand-in for an actual tea pot! That said, there are two things that have helped my clients ease into making tea for themselves: electric kettles and a French press.

An electric kettle boils water rapidly and shuts off when it reaches the boiling point, so it's ideal for scattered people who have burned too many pots in the past, get annoyed by a piercing whistle, or are tired of using their saucepan to boil tea water. Be sure to get one that is metal or glass because plastic and hot water don't mix.

A French press is usually found in the coffee section of most stores, but it's also a very effective way to brew bulk tea. To use a French press for tea, just toss the herbs in the carafe, pour the hot water over them, and put the lid on, leaving the plunger up. When it is time to pour the tea, just push slowly down on the plunger, which pushes a screen down over the brewing herbs, forcing them to the bottom of the carafe. Now you can pour your tea just like from a tea pot! Personally, I'm low-tech and just pour herbs and boiling water into a canning jar, close the lid loosely, wait and then pour through a strainer into my cup.

A French press is perfect for a hot infusion, a method used to extract leaves, flowers, and aromatic roots. It is similar to how we think of "real" tea being made—dried plant material is put into a cup and boiling water is poured over. But there are three things going on here that make this a more medicinal brew and not your average cup of tea: more plant matter is used, it is steeped for longer, and it is covered while steeping.

To make an infusion, use 1 ounce by weight of herb to 16 ounces by volume of just-boiled water poured over the herb, cover, and let steep for 10–15 minutes. Since not everybody has a scale in their kitchen, that's around 2 teaspoons to a tablespoon of loose herb to every cup of water, adjusting if the herbs are lighter or denser than average.

Then there are long infusions, following the same basic process but letting the herbs steep for 4–8 hours. This is great for mineral-rich herbs like nettle, but steeping peppermint (*Mentha ×piperita*, for example) this long will make a bitter and astringent tea, so know which herbs do better with this process. All infusions are good for about 24 hours if refrigerated.

And finally, a simmered tea is called a decoction. This method is best for roots and barks—plant material that is tougher to extract. To make a decoction, place an ounce of dried root into a quart of room-temperature water. Bring the water to a light boil, and then gently simmer for 20 minutes. Take it off the heat and strain. This tea will be good for up to 3 days if refrigerated, and one cup at a time can be reheated before drinking.

MAKING TINCTURES AND GLYCERITES

Tinctures and glycerites are both made using the same method, with the only difference being alcohol vs. glycerin; both may also be referred to as macerations because the herb sits and macerates in the fluid for 2–4 weeks. Though one can dive into details and get complex, the basic process is simple: put plants in a jar and cover them with liquid, let sit for a while, then strain. If you ever get overwhelmed by the following information, just remember that the basics are that easy.

Whenever you make an extract, the liquid you use is called a menstruum, whether that's alcohol or glycerin in a maceration, water to make a tea, or vinegar to make an acetic extract. We sometimes combine these to make a specific menstruum. For example, when you see a percentage of alcohol or glycerin in a formula, that means the rest is assumed to be water that was mixed in to give the desired ratio. If you read that an herb is best extracted in 75% alcohol that means your menstruum is going to be 75% pure alcohol and 25% water. Keep in mind that most of the alcohol you buy is already part water, so you would need to buy a 150-proof spirit to achieve a 75% alcohol menstruum.

The easiest way to get the percentage correct is to start with the highest-proof alcohol you can get and dilute it down from there. The highest that is shelf-stable is 95% alcohol (190 proof), but the liquor store in your state might not sell anything higher than 150. It is often cheaper and better quality to order from a bulk distiller and have it shipped. If not, don't get discouraged; 150-proof, or even 100-proof in some cases, will do just fine.

The next thing you'll see in directions for macerations is a specific weight to volume ratio, meaning weight of the herb to volume of the menstruum. So if you read that you should make black cohosh tincture at 1:2, that means for every 1 ounce by weight of root you should use 2 fluid ounces of menstruum. The same goes for metric, where for every 1 gram by weight you would use

2 milliliters of menstruum. With me so far? Let's put this into practice looking at fresh and dried herbs.

The typical ratio for fresh herbs is 1:2 and for most dried herbs it's 1:5. The reason for the difference is that fresh herbs have a lot of water weight in them, so you don't need to add as much fluid. To get a proper 1:2 ratio you really need to pack the herbs in tightly, even getting something to tamp them down with. The easiest way to get it all to fit is to find the exact right-size jar; for now, a half pint or a pint canning jar will be about the right size. When you are first making tinctures it's easy to make more than you'll ever use, so start with these sizes at first.

Sometimes it's challenging to get all the herb covered by liquid, so make sure to pack the herb tightly and pour the menstruum on slowly to allow time for air bubbles to come up; you may even want to poke it around with a chopstick. And if all else fails and the liquid is still not covering the herb, you can just add a bit more to make sure it's covered. And even if a bit is sticking up, it will get washed with antiseptic alcohol when you shake it.

OK, now we have our ratio all set. What should our menstruum be? For fresh herbs I typically use straight 95% alcohol, like cane or grain alcohol, or 100% glycerin. This is because there is already water in the plants, so the final product has the plant water in it, which means it will be a lower alcohol concentration than you started off with. (The alcohol is basically dehydrating the plant material through osmosis, and when the water gets sucked out, all those beautiful chemicals do too!)

For dry plants, the alcohol percentage can be anywhere from 25% to 95% depending upon whether you are trying to extract more alcohol-soluble or more water-soluble

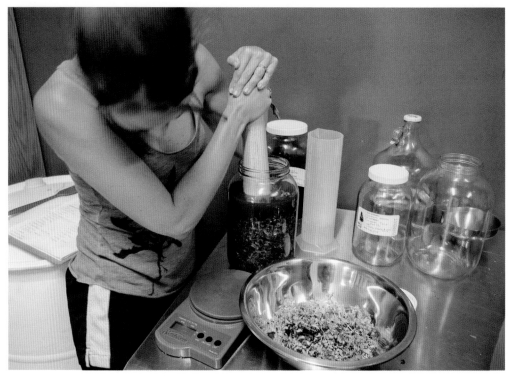

Herbalist Anna Claire Lotti is working hard and using a sauerkraut pounder to pack all that St. John's wort herb into the tincture.

constituents. This book will let you know what percentage to use for each plant, but an easy default is to do 50% alcohol or 50% glycerin, because then you can extract both the alcohol- or glycerin-soluble constituents and the water-soluble ones.

After all this, the actual process of making the tincture is remarkably easy. Just weigh out the herb, stuff it into a canning jar—I'm a big fan of canning jars cause the lids are super tight—and then cover it with the correct amount of menstruum. Always blend the different parts of a menstruum (water and alcohol, for example) first before pouring it over the herb.

Let this sit for at least 2 weeks (though there is a tradition of letting it sit for a month to get a whole lunar cycle) and strain it out. Cheesecloth is the easiest way to

strain tinctures and can easily be wrung out to get the most out of your plant material. You can also use a heavy-duty potato ricer, which looks like a giant garlic press, to press out any remaining liquid from the marc (leftover spent herb). Or if you want to get really fancy, there are tincture presses available online that use hydraulic jacks or the equivalent to physically press the herb and get every last drop out of the plants you've harvested. If you start making a lot of tinctures, the cost is definitely worth it in the end.

Most importantly, label your tincture. It might seem obvious what is in the jar at the time, but please do yourself a favor and label every bottle every single time. You won't regret it. On the label, put the common name and scientific name of the plant, the part(s) used, whether it was fresh or dried, where you got it from, when you made the medicine, and any other details you want to add. It can be fun and rewarding to notice when different locations or times of year make a difference in the strength of your final product.

And there's your tincture! Store it in a cool, dark place where it won't get exposed to sunlight, and it should last 5–10 years, or maybe even longer.

INFUSING OILS

Infused oils are made much the same way a tincture is made: by soaking the herb in a fixed oil for a certain period of time. These are very different from essential oils, where a more complex distillation process extracts just the volatile oils from the plants. Infused oils are easier to make at home and are only used topically, not internally. You can use many types of fixed oils, but the most commonly used these days is extra-virgin olive oil. You can also use raw sesame oil for a penetrating and warming muscle rub, almond oil for a massage oil, etc. Back in the old days, most infused oils were made with lard, probably because that's what was available on a homestead.

I don't typically use a certain ratio with oils, and I never add water. In fact, it's best to harvest plants for oil when it hasn't rained in a day or two and the dew has dried off the plant. Water and oil don't mix and can lead to stinky fermentation, so some folks will make oils only with dried plants; but I like the feeling of fresh plant oils, so I just let my plants wilt for 12–24 hours to lose some water weight before infusing.

There are two basic ways to make an infused oil: the time method and the heat method. The time method is just like making a tincture, in that the herbs are stuffed into a jar and the menstruum is poured over; and

in this case, the oil is poured on until it is covering the herb. You might need to poke around with a chopstick or a butter knife to get the oil in there and the air out, as it is so much thicker than water or alcohol. Cover the jar tightly and let it sit for 2–4 weeks before straining. Don't use a press with an oil because it can also press out the water that was in the fresh herb.

In the heat method, the process is hurried along by warming the oil. This has the advantage of making an infused oil more quickly with much less chance of fermentation. The downside is that if the oil gets too hot, then it changes consistency and you'll have deep-fried plantain chips instead of infused medicinal oil. In general, you don't want to heat oil over 120°F when making this medicine, though some books say you can go as high as 140°F.

One way to do this is to set an oven on the lowest temperature possible and keep it around 120°F by turning it on and off, and opening and closing the oven door for a period of about 12 hours. Other methods include a double boiler, hot water bath, bain-marie, crock pot on its lowest setting, yogurt maker, sous vide cooker, or even an electric turkey roaster. Any of these methods will allow you to monitor and maintain a more consistent temperature than the low-tech oven technique. These can also be done for 12 hours or at a lower temperature for a longer time, up to a few days.

When you're finished and the herb is fairly dead-looking, strain out the marc and keep the oil. Let it sit for a few days, and when there's a layer of water and debris at the bottom of the jar, decant it off and either dispose of that layer or use it within a week. Keep the rest of the oil in a closed container in a cool, dark place. Refrigeration is not necessary.

EXTRACTING MUSHROOMS

There's a trick to extracting mushrooms because many mushrooms have both water- and alcohol-soluble components. This two-step extraction process gets out both by making a strong decoction, then that decoction is used as the water portion of the menstruum to make a 1:5 tincture (weight to volume) at 25% alcohol.

If the mushrooms are tough (like reishi), it's best to chop them up into chunks when fresh, then dry. Weigh the dried mushrooms, then put them in a good amount of water and decoct for 2–4 hours. Strain—*but retain the mushroom*—then check the volume of tea.

The volume you want is 75% of the volume of your finished tincture. So multiply the weight of the dried mushroom you started out with × 5 to get the total tincture volume. Divide this by ¾, and that's the final volume of your decoction.

If the volume is still too high after boiling, you can then put the tea back on low heat with the lid off to evaporate some water and to concentrate the water extract. This might take a few hours, so leave your windows open as the scent can be strong. When you reach the right amount of fluid, turn off heat and let cool. Be careful not to scorch the concentrated decoction.

Once close to room temperature, add 1 part pure alcohol (95%) to every 3 parts decoction so that final alcohol content is just about 24%, and you now have a preserved decoction. Since most medicinal mushrooms were traditionally used as decoctions, you can call it good here, or instead of adding alcohol you could just freeze the concentrated tea in ice cube trays and then pop those containers when frozen. Then just drop an ice cube in hot water to make instant mushroom tea.

Or to make the double extraction, put the mushroom pieces into a jar, cover with the preserved decoction and let sit for a month. After this maceration time, strain off and compost the spent mushroom marc to get a final 1:5 tincture at approximately 25%.

Here's an example using numbers. Let's say you weigh out 200 grams of dry mushroom, then at 1:5 you want to end up with 1000 ml of finished tincture. So, your final reduced decoction will be 750 ml, and you will add 250 ml of straight alcohol (190 proof) to make the menstruum about 24% alcohol by volume.

Before You Head Out: Tools and Supplies

Harvesting

- pruners
- soil knife or hori hori
- gloves
- digging fork
- nursery or trenching spade
- loppers
- folding saw
- mattock
- canvas or burlap bags
- pocketknife
- drinking water

Making medicine

- pure alcohol
- water
- extra-virgin olive oil
- glycerin
- canning jars
- scale with tare
- measuring cup
- cutting boards
- cleaver or sharp knife
- electric kettle
- French press
- potato ricer
- cheesecloth
- funnels
- labels
- waterproof marker

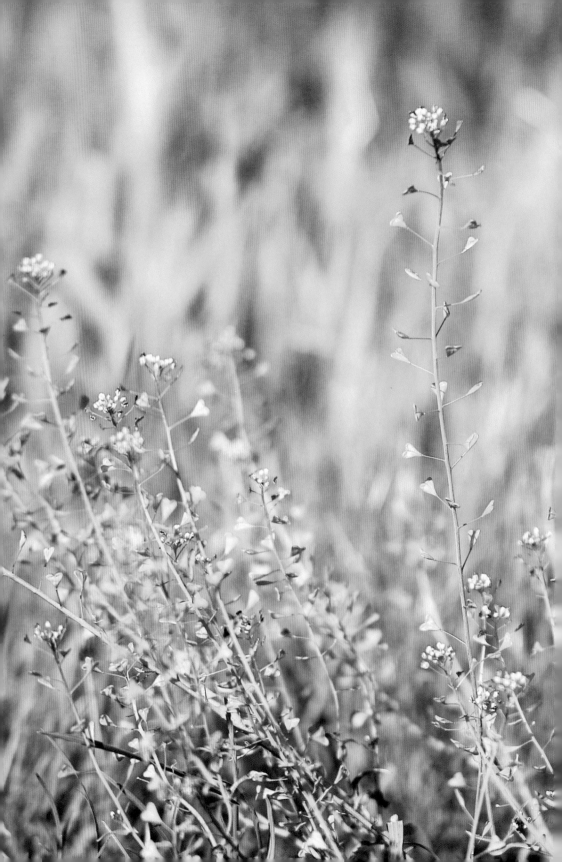

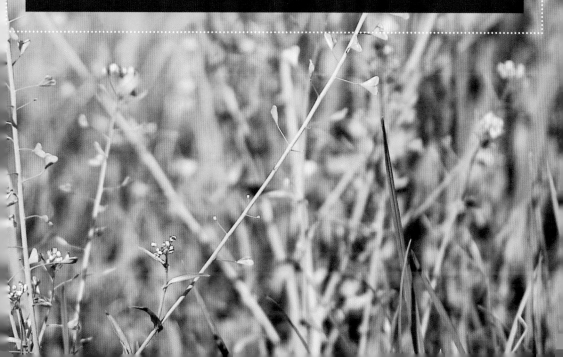

MEDICINAL PLANTS OF THE SOUTHEAST

agrimony

Agrimonia parviflora, A. pubescens, A. gryposepala
PARTS USED aerial

A useful astringent wound-healing herb that is also a diuretic.

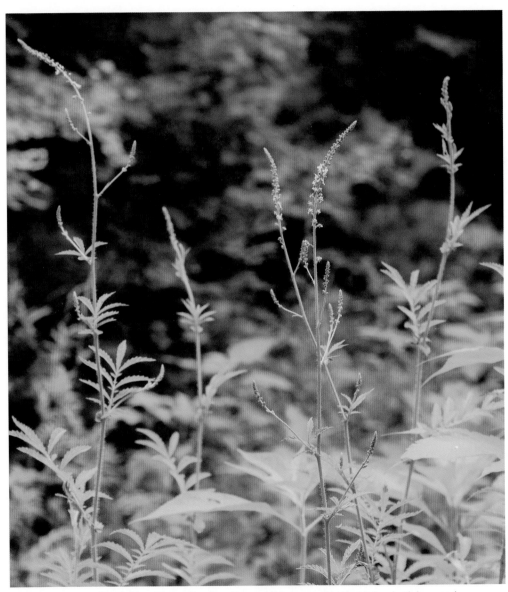

Agrimony grows tall and thin with small yellow flowers. It is unusual in that it has both long and short leaflets.

How to identify

Agrimony is a fairly common herb, growing 3–5 feet tall. The stem is densely hairy, and the most noticeable characteristic of the plant is the way the leaves alternate between short and long leaflets. The only other similar-looking plant that does this is the related meadowsweet (*Filipendula ulmaria*), but that plant has a larger and broader leaflet at the tip, where the terminal leaflet in agrimony is the same size as the other large leaflets.

Agrimony has an abundance of tiny yellow flowers in long clusters starting in July that turn into small burs, which then can and will get stuck in dog hair, jeans, sweaters, and whatever else they come into contact with. It's a great strategy for spreading seeds, but a pain in the butt after you've taken your dog for a walk in the woods.

Where, when, and how to wildcraft

Agrimony is found in meadows, along trailsides, and in places that are only cut once or twice a year. It is common throughout much of the Southeast from Virginia to South Carolina and west to Missouri, Arkansas, and Louisiana but is scarce in Georgia, Alabama, and Mississippi.

Harvest the whole plant in full flower, typically in July or August, and tincture leaves, flowers, and flexible stems.

Medicinal uses

Though some list many possible uses for agrimony, I think of it as a simple and useful astringent. Astringents are herbs that feel drying in the mouth and tighten and tone tissue. Most of agrimony's traditional uses are based on this astringent effect, including topical use to help slow-healing wounds, or as an eyewash for sore and irritated eyes.

It is most commonly used for incontinence and has a long tradition of use for toning the lining of the urethra and the urinary tract. I've used it in formulas for people with urge incontinence after pelvic surgery, but it would also be useful for the incontinence of age. It tightens up the lining (mucosa) and sphincters of the urinary tract, but it is also somewhat anti-inflammatory. It can be used for blood in the urine, though this can be a sign of something more serious and should be checked by a medical professional.

Just as it tones the lining of the urinary tract, agrimony can tone the lining of the digestive tract. This makes it useful for mild or chronic diarrhea, poor assimilation, or even, according to some sources, appendicitis. It is also mildly bitter, so tasting the herb can stimulate digestive secretions and movement.

Future harvests

This is a fairly common and abundant native plant. Just make sure to leave plenty for the pollinators.

HERBAL PREPARATIONS

The whole aboveground plant can be used, fresh or dry, as a tincture or a tea. The tea can be used as a wash on open wounds or diluted as an eyewash.

anemone

Anemone virginiana, A. quinquefolia

PARTS USED aerial

A potent herb that is grounding for anxiety, panic attacks, and shock.

How to identify

Most of what we know about the medicinal use of *Anemone* species comes from the use of either the European pulsatilla or its relatives out west. But there are two species in the east that are potentially medicinal, though they look very different and even bloom at different times. Wood anemone (*Anemone quinquefolia*) is a spring ephemeral, low-growing—not higher than 8 inches high—with leaves that split it into 3 or 5, cut deeply and palmately almost to the base.

The flowers bloom in early spring and have 5 regular white sepals that look like petals. Hepaticas flower around the same time and are about the same height, but their leaves are not deeply cut and have 3 rounded lobes at the tip.

Thimbleweed or tall anemone (*Anemone virginiana*) blooms in early summer and is tall and slender, 2–3 feet high. The plant is mostly stalk with a whorl of divided leaves like a skirt around the middle from which shoot up a few stalks, each topped by a flower

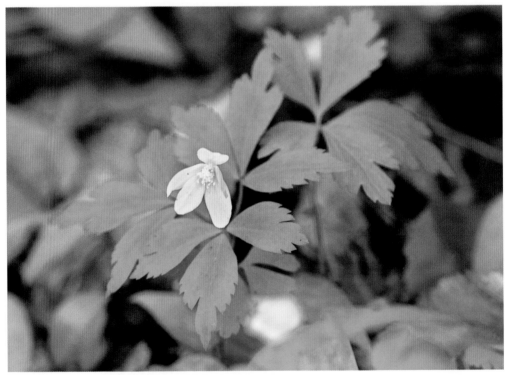

Wood anemone is a small plant growing close to the ground early in the spring, dying back by May.

with 5 white petal-like sepals.
The fruits that follow are oblong
inch-long spiked cylinders that
somewhat resemble thimbles.
Anemone caroliniana is a rare
species that should not be
picked. It has only one flower
per plant, with 5–15 pale blue
to white sepals.

Where, when, and how to wildcraft

Wood anemone can be found
in the woods, as one might
guess from the name, in early
to mid-spring before trees leaf
out, around the same time that
many of the spring ephem-
erals bloom. They are fairly
plentiful where they grow in
the mountains and adjacent
Piedmont of Virginia, West
Virginia, Kentucky, North
Carolina, northern Georgia
and west into the Cumberland
Plateau of Tennessee. Because
each individual plant is small,
gather only when there are a
lot of them, clipping the whole
aboveground plant and tincturing the same day.

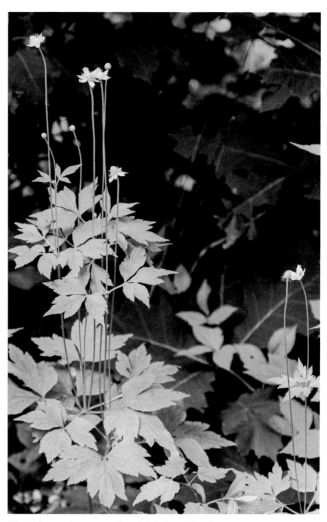

Thimbleweed grows tall and thin in mid to late summer.

Thimbleweed grows throughout the
Northeast south to South Carolina and
mid-Georgia and further east than wood
anemone, then west to southern Arkansas
and mid-Mississippi. It's usually found in
fields and meadows, roadsides and trailsides, and I've got it coming up in the weeds
along the side of my driveway. It can be
found growing individually, but sometimes
a decent-sized group can be found and that's
the best time to harvest. Clip the whole aboveground plant and use the tincture fresh.

Medicinal uses

This herb has the unique character of helping
people come back into their body. The genus
name comes from the Greek word for wind,
which is very appropriate since anemone is
the perfect remedy when someone feels like
their mind is all up in the air, disconnected
from their body, and that their emotions are
as changeable as the wind. It can be used for
anxiety or panic attacks, emotional shock,
bad drug trips, or PMS with fast-changing
emotions. It's like an herbal "rescue remedy"

that works with almost any kind of triggered state.

Anemone is my go-to herb for when someone is not behind their eyes, whether from a recent or past trauma, or from other causes. I use it when someone has just had a physical trauma and is experiencing psychogenic (emotional) shock, and I also use it when past traumas come up and create anxiety. It is not a sedative and doesn't numb someone out. It helps people stay present without being overwhelmed by intense emotions—they feel like they are able to swim instead of drowning in the emotional response, so that the trauma can actually be processed. Just a few drops can stop a panic attack or anxiety attack.

Ithaca herbalist 7Song uses it to help someone on a bad trip, or to help bring someone back who's gone out just a bit too far. Though this is the opposite energetic of ghost pipe, which helps when people are feeling too much in their body, both can be used for bad acid trips and for trauma—anemone to help ground and stop dissociating, and ghost pipe when people are too stuck in a loop, too focused in, and they need to let go and zoom out.

Finally, anemone can be surprisingly effective for certain kinds of migraine headaches. Migraines can be tricky and very individual, but as a vasodilator anemone can help with migraines that have the classic visual aura and feel like a band is being tightened around the head. The person is more pale and chilly, not hot and irritated. Like any migraine remedy, the earlier it is taken the better the chances, because full-blown migraines are very difficult to turn around.

Its ability to relax pressure in the cerebro-spinal fluid could be why anemone is effective for migraines, and it has also been used to reduce pressure in the eyes, such as in glaucoma.

Though this plant was popular in the 19th and early 20th century, I learned about it from one of my teachers, Michael Moore, who brought back the use of this herb and others that had been forgotten in herbal medicine. He only used the species that grow in the western half of the United States, saying that the East Coast species weren't as potent. This is a low-dose botanical; the East Coast species do work, just at a slightly higher dose.

Future harvests
While both these plants are common, neither is very large nor found in great abundance, so harvest with appropriate care for the environment and remember that you don't need much.

 Caution
Anemone is a low-dose botanical; do not exceed the recommended dose. Taking too much causes stomach irritation and excess vasodilation, which could manifest as feeling spaced out and the skin becoming cold and clammy.

HERBAL PREPARATIONS

Tincture the whole fresh plant in flower 1:4 at 95% alcohol. It can be made this dilute because both species are lightweight plants and very potent. Dose is 5–10 drops for these species, but always start low and work up. Don't overdo it—these are potent plants!

Angelica triquinata
PARTS USED root, seeds

An aromatic herb that breaks up congestion in the lungs, stimulates digestion, and helps with arthritis.

How to identify

This is a plant to be 100% sure you have identified correctly. Plants in the parsley family (Apiaceae) can be tricky to identify, and though this family contains edible and medicinal plants, it also contains some of the deadliest plants in North America, namely poison hemlock (*Conium maculatum*) and water hemlock (*Cicuta maculata*). This family holds other toxic members, but these two plants are deadly. Harvesting your own medicine is not worth dying over.

Both toxic hemlocks mentioned here have purple-splotched (maculate) stems and flowers in compound umbels. Poison hemlock has finely divided leaves, looking more like parsley or carrot greens, and can be mistaken for Queen Anne's lace; water hemlock has leaves divided into larger segments that more closely resemble angelica. People have reportedly been hospitalized for mistaking water hemlock for *Angelica* species. Use a second book or a botanist to make sure you have the correct identification.

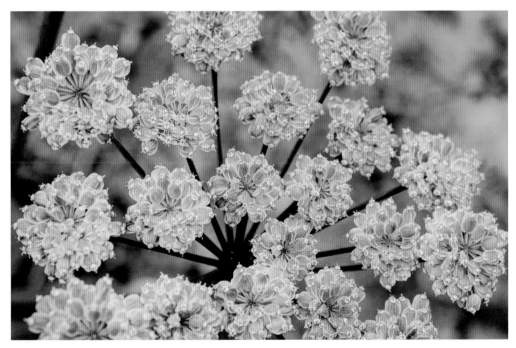

The unripe seed heads of angelica make a beautiful mandala of medicine—as they are turning maroon is the perfect time to harvest. The winged seeds help tell it apart from similar-looking plants.

The easiest way to differentiate angelica is the way that the leaf stalk becomes flat and wide enough at the base to actually wrap around the main stalk. Cow parsnip also has leaf wings but has only 3 leaflets instead of many pinnately divided leaflets. Water hemlock also has flattened petioles, but they are not as wide as angelica, and the leaflets and leaves are more widely spaced apart with sharper teeth. If you follow the veins in the leaflets, water hemlock has leaf veins ending in between the teeth and angelica veins end at the tip of the leaf.

Water hemlock also has white flowers as compared to yellow-green of mountain angelica, and stems that have streaks or splotches of purple, where angelica stems are more of a solid purple—though they can be more greenish growing in the shade. And when they go to seed, angelica has seeds that are more oval with 2 or 3 prominent wings on each side.

Purplestem or great angelica (*Angelica atropurpurea*) is the more commonly used native angelica, but that mostly grows from Pennsylvania and Ohio north, only rarely appearing further south. It has more rounded flower clusters than mountain angelica but still has those uniquely winged petioles. The ominously named deadly angelica

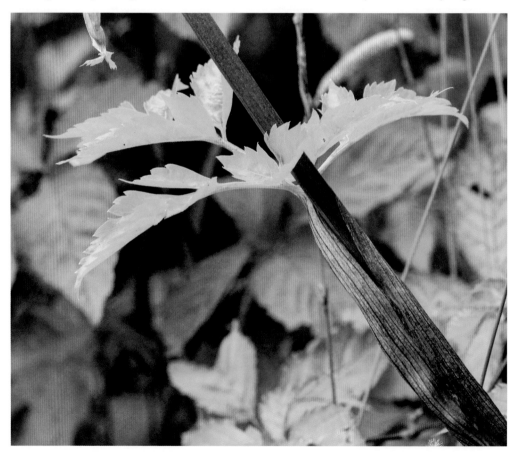

Look for the way the leaf stalk flattens out like a wing to distinguish angelica from other plants; there are poisonous look-alikes, so never harvest unless you are 100% sure of your ID.

(*A. venenosa*), so called because it looks the most like water hemlock, is listed as a folk remedy in some places and as a poison in others, so I don't suggest using it for medicine.

Mountain angelica (*Angelica triquinata*) is the most common one in the Southeast, and grows up to 5 feet high, with flowers and then seeds in a few umbels 3–6 inches across. The individual flowers are a nondescript greenish yellow that still somehow manage to attract an abundance of pollinators. It has smooth stems, and the flower heads themselves are also smooth or barely hairy, whereas deadly angelica is hairy.

Where, when, and how to wildcraft

This plant grows in great abundance at elevations over 4,000 feet along the North Carolina–Tennessee border north along the mountain ridge following the Virginia–West Virginia border up into Pennsylvania. The other species on the East Coast, *Angelica atropurpurea*, runs from very northern West Virginia north into Pennsylvania, Ohio, and New England, and also north and west as far as Minnesota, only sporadically further south. It can be used the same way as the mountain angelica.

Dig roots in the spring or in the fall after they go to seed. The roots are not very big so make sure there are a lot of plants before you start harvesting. The seeds are abundant and easy to harvest in August and September, and they are best picked when maroon to green-brown and slightly unripe—they taste more aromatic and have more of a numbing taste on the tongue than when they turn totally brown. Harvest only when you see large stands of it, which you often will at certain places in the high mountains.

Interesting naturalist note: the nectar is both strongly attractive and very intoxicating to yellow jackets and hornets (Weakley 2019).

Medicinal uses

The roots of related angelicas have a long history of use in both the European and the Chinese herbal traditions. *Angelica archangelica* is one of the most highly regarded herbs in the European tradition, as can be told from the name, and Chinese medicine uses several different species. Our angelica is used similarly to the European angelica and one of the Chinese angelicas, but it is very different medicinally from dong quai (*A. sinensis*), which is more building and less stimulating.

This herb does so many different things that it's good to remember that most of what angelica does can be summed up by its taste and energetic—it is warming and moving. It is aromatic and bitter, which stimulates digestion and the liver; the oils and resins penetrate into the bronchioles and help break up mucus in the lungs; and its blood-moving and detoxifying properties make it useful for arthritis and other types of long-term joint issues. This is a great plant to have on hand for all the reasons just named.

Just the digestive action shouldn't be underestimated. Herbalists often use plants that are either aromatic (fennel, peppermint, ginger) or herbs that taste bitter (dandelion, gentian, yellow dock) to stimulate digestion. Angelica, having both these properties, can stimulate digestive secretions like other bitters and also stimulate peristalsis like other aromatic digestive herbs. This makes it a great stand-alone herb for poor digestion in someone who feels bloated and heavy after meals or who has very little appetite. It can also be used before or after a meal to help anyone digest their food better.

As an herb for the respiratory system, angelica is great for when a simple cold has progressed into bronchitis or pneumonia and there's a lot of thick phlegm. It seems to penetrate deeper into the lungs than other herbs and has some traditional use for both dry and psychogenic asthma.

Finally, angelica has long been used for chronic joint pain and stiffness. In many systems of traditional medicine, arthritis or rheumatism was thought of as toxins accumulating in the joints, so the herbs used are those that move the blood (circulatory stimulants) and cleanse the blood (alteratives). Angelica has the distinct advantage of being both a blood cleanser and a blood mover. Think of angelica for the type of arthritis that's worse in cold and damp weather, or someone with generally cold hands and feet and/or a pale complexion.

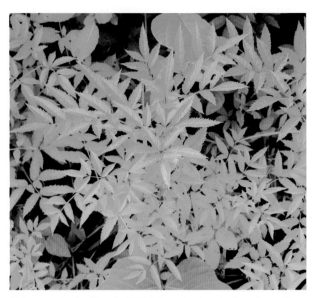
Poisonous look-alike alert! This is water hemlock, *not* angelica. It is deadly.

Though mountain angelica might not be quite as strong as the European angelica, it is a useful plant that grows abundantly in some places and is worthy of more attention. All the aforementioned uses refer to the root, with the seed being stronger as a digestive stimulant and also somewhat numbing for tooth pain but weaker for the other uses.

Future harvests

These plants seem to grow only in specific areas at high elevation, so harvest only when there is an incredible abundance of them. If there is any question of quantity, the seeds are a more sustainable way to harvest than the root.

⚠ Caution

Angelica contains furanocoumarins, chemicals that can cause skin to sunburn quickly after touching. Though I haven't seen it with this species, there are reports of people brushing up against angelica leaves then getting a sunburn in that area.

HERBAL PREPARATIONS

Fresh root can be tinctured 1:2 at 95% alcohol and the dry root 1:5 at 65% alcohol. The dry root can be made into a decoction. Seeds can be chewed for digestive issues, made into an infusion, or tinctured at the same ratios and percentages as the root.

Bacopa monnieri

PARTS USED aerial

A powerful brain tonic that improves memory, concentration, and focus.

How to identify

Bacopa is a low-growing plant that creeps along the ground, sending down small roots as it runs. The leaves are opposite, mostly entire, and fairly small, about a third of an inch long. They are oval, are slightly wider toward the tip, lack a petiole, and are thick like a succulent.

The most noticeable part of the plant is actually the long green stems that snake around and form thick mats. The flower is tiny, hardly any bigger than the leaves, with 5 equal white petals. It is borne where the leaf meets the stem.

Carolina water-hyssop (*Bacopa caroliniana*) looks similar but has a blue flower and when

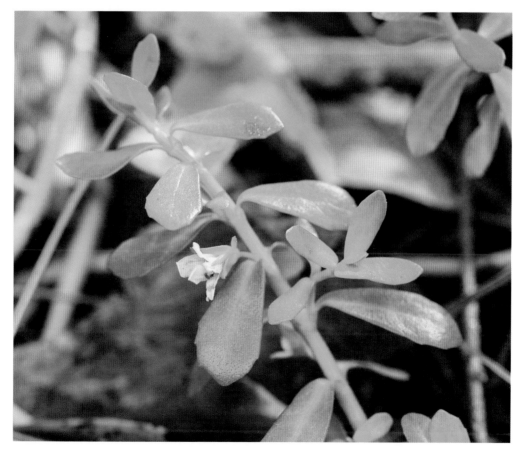

A sprig of bacopa, an herb that helps rejuvenate the mind and increase memory and focus.

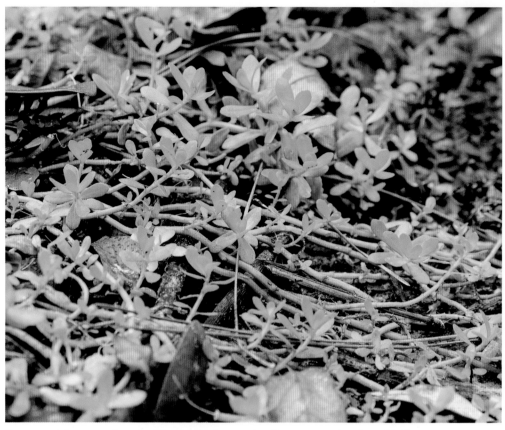
Some coastal area ponds and wetland areas have mats of bacopa growing alongside them.

crushed smells strongly like lemon. This doesn't seem to have the same medicine as other *Bacopa* species.

Where, when, and how to wildcraft

Bacopa is found all along the coast from the Virginia–North Carolina border down through Florida, where it marches across the state and across the Gulf Coast deep into Texas. It is always found either growing in shallow water or right next to it, on the edges of ponds and marshes, for example.

Herein lies the challenge of harvesting. Because it's usually found either in a pond or in a place where the pond overflows, how do you know how clean the pond is? The short answer is, you don't really. So it might be

better to take cuttings, bring them home, replant them, and then use what grows from that as your medicine—unless you happen to find bacopa growing in a beautiful pristine natural area, which is hard to find along the developed coast.

Bacopa is not frost tolerant and grows throughout the year, so any time is good to harvest. Trim the stems and use the whole aboveground plant—stems, leaves, flowers, and all.

Medicinal uses

Bacopa is up there as one of the best herbs for the brain. Originally used in Ayurveda, bacopa has gotten more popular in the states over the last few years. This herb is incredibly nourishing for the whole nervous system as well as the brain. It has the paradoxical quality of being generally calming while also stimulating the brain and increasing cognitive ability, a nootropic if you will. Many studies have been done recently on its ability to improve memory and even possibly prevent Alzheimer's and senile dementia. This has made a lot of news and probably accounts for the popularity of this herb in the United States in the past few years.

Because it calms the brain while enhancing cognition and memory, it is an excellent herb to increase focus. It has a long history of use to enhance meditation, and many modern herbalists use it for ADHD as a regular tonic.

In addition, its ability to nourish the brain and nervous system make it useful for recovery after a brain injury—anything from a concussion to a stroke. Bacopa can be used for this purpose along with milky oat seed, lion's mane, skullcap, and other nourishing nervines.

In these modern times, it seems like we all should be growing a bit of bacopa in a pot somewhere!

Future harvests

Harvest from areas with good-sized populations and just trim stems here and there. It is fairly abundant in places, but it is a native plant that helps prevent erosion so don't harvest too aggressively.

 Caution

The only side effect noted is occasional temporary digestive upset in some people.

> **HERBAL PREPARATIONS**
>
> Traditionally bacopa is used as an infusion made from the dried herb, but my favorite preparation is the fresh plant tincture. It's fairly bitter and not the tastiest herb, but you get used to it when you take it for a while.

balm of Gilead

Populus ×jackii, P. balsamifera
PARTS USED buds (leaf and flower)

*A powerful pain-relieving herb for muscle and joint
pain throughout the body, both internally and topically.*

How to identify

Balm of Gilead (aka bam'a'gil, bamgilly), a
hybrid involving balsam poplar (*Populus balsamifera*), is just one of the handful of species
of the genus *Populus* around the Southeast,
variously called cottonwood, aspen, or poplar
(not to be confused with the unrelated tulip
poplar). All have light-colored bark and triangular leaves.

    Populus species are notoriously difficult to
tell apart as they hybridize easily, so a good
book on tree identification is recommended
for accurate identification, though all the
poplars are more or less medicinal and the
more resinous and sticky, the more medicinal
it is. Note that the balm of Gilead in the Bible
is a totally different plant that's more closely
related to myrrh.

Where, when, and how to wildcraft

The best time to harvest is in late winter or
early spring before the tree leafs out. This

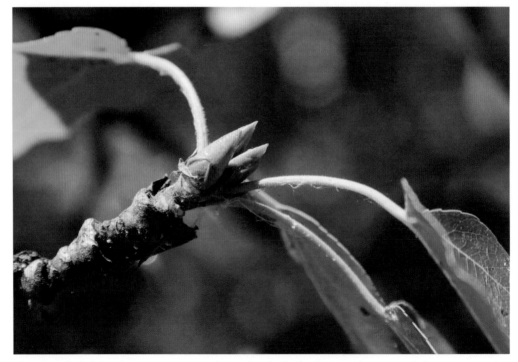

Though not related to the more common tulip poplar, the buds of any poplar tree, including aspens and
cottonwoods, can be used for medicine.

means you need to identify the tree and find the stands the year before you harvest unless you have really good winter tree ID skills.

Like willows, which are in the same family, it likes a good amount of sun and often grows near water, though water isn't as necessary as it is for willow. But you won't find it in a forest—more likely to see it in a cleared meadow that hasn't been tended in a few years.

The easiest and most ethical way to harvest the buds is to have a stand in mind that you can visit after a good windstorm, as the branches break off easily. Another option, if you're lucky, is to find a farmer who has to take some trees down because they are shading crops, then walk around the downed trees picking off buds. The second option is of course much easier and more abundant. Either way, just use your fingers to pinch off the buds. If harvesting from a live tree, pick only a third of the buds on any branch and never pick the terminal bud. This is less desirable, of course, as you can pick to your heart's content on the downed branches without harming any tree.

Many books recommend using the leaf buds, which are slightly larger, but what I see in commerce is a mixture of leaf and flower buds, and it doesn't seem to make any difference in medicinal use. They are both incredibly sticky and resinous, so harvest into a clean paper bag, yogurt container, or basket that is OK getting sticky. That resin only seems to come off with something like isopropyl (rubbing) alcohol—much more effective than soap and water.

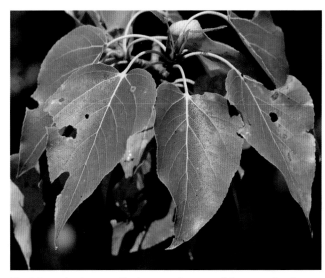

The triangular leaves of balsam poplar, one of the parents of balm of Gilead.

Medicinal uses

This relative of willow also contains the salicylic acid that makes both analgesic and anti-inflammatory. But these trees also have a significant amount of pain-relieving and antiseptic resin. This combination of pain-relieving, anti-inflammatory, and antiseptic actions makes for an amazing all-purpose remedy. And it has a long history of use across the continent for muscle and joint pains. Balm of Gilead is primarily used topically as an oil or salve on inflamed or painful joints. The tincture can also be used internally, but it tastes horrible.

It's interesting to note that resins are used differently in Western and in Chinese herbalism. In Western herbalism, resinous plants like myrrh or frankincense (aka boswellia) are primarily used as antiseptic herbs, whereas in Chinese medicine they are primarily used as pain-relieving remedies. This plant is interesting because historically it was used for both, but more for pain relief since both the resins and the salicylic acid help with pain and are anti-inflammatory.

The other traditional use for resinous plants is as an expectorant, like in the use of white pine bark. Balm of Gilead tincture can be taken internally to help break up sticky phlegm and help expectorate it out of the lungs. The salve can also be rubbed on the chest for similar effect.

This highly useful plant has a long history in both the indigenous and settler populations of southern Appalachia; it deserves to be known better.

Future harvests

As balm of Gilead forms abundant stands where it grows, and it's easiest to harvest from downed branches and trees, your harvests won't affect the trees very much. Don't pick the buds from live trees unless there is an abundance of trees and you harvest very selectively. Pick only one of three buds and never the bud at the end of the branch.

 Caution

Those who are allergic to salicylates should probably avoid this.

HERBAL PREPARATIONS

The buds can be tinctured 1:2 fresh at 95%, or 1:5 dry at 75% alcohol. This high alcohol content is because the resins are much more soluble in alcohol than in water. The salve can be made by infusing buds in olive oil, sesame oil, or what have you, straining, then warming and adding beeswax. An even better way to make the oil is to use the alcohol intermediary method. To do this, mix the dry buds with just enough alcohol to moisten them, then let sit for a few hours to a day. Then add the oil and warm it up for a few hours with the lid off but keeping the temperature under 130°F. Then strain out the buds and add the beeswax to make the salve.

baptisia

Baptisia tinctoria

PARTS USED root

A powerful antiseptic medicine that can be applied topically or used internally with caution.

How to identify

This medium-tall perennial in the pea family looks like yellow sweet clover or some of the bush clovers (*Lespedeza* spp.) with its leaflets of three. There is a bluish green color to the leaves, though, and they have very little leaf stalk, the middle leaflet having no stalk at all. The stems are stiff, yellow, and tough, giving it a shrubby appearance rather than the tall willowy look of those just mentioned. It has numerous yellow pea flowers in mid to late summer; these mature into black capsules.

Where, when, and how to wildcraft

You'll find baptisia in sandy acidic soils in company with oaks, hickories, and blueberry bushes. Why it grows in some places and not others is a mystery to me, but usually when I find some in one area I find a good amount. For some reason it seems to like growing under power lines, but make sure it's not chemically sprayed there. It is found from Maryland and Delaware south through South Carolina and west somewhat into Tennessee and Kentucky.

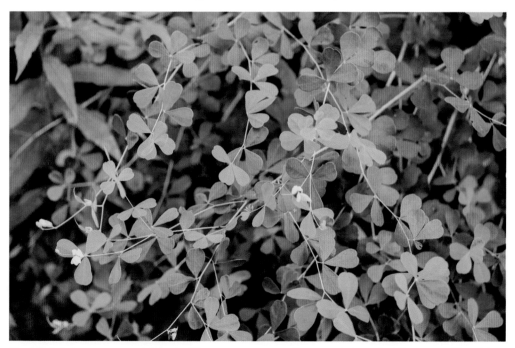

The trifoliate leaves are reminiscent of the more common yellow sweet clover, but the stems of baptisia are tough and woody.

Dig the root in the fall after the flowers have passed but the plant is still green and recognizable. It is a thick tough root, so be prepared to spend some time with it.

Medicinal uses

A powerful immune stimulant and lymph mover, this is a strong plant that needs to be used with respect. This is a bit of a niche herb—not broadly useful, but when you need it, it can really kick ass.

This is the herb the 19th-century Eclectic physicians used for sepsis and poorly healing wounds. Not something you would use for an ordinary cold, but for when a condition lingers on and on and there's not enough local blood flow to bring fresh white blood cells. This lingering condition shows up as a blue-black or dusky hue on wounds or on the face. This color is mentioned in almost every account of this herb, and it is also the color that the leaves turn when they dry.

The immune-stimulating property makes baptisia very useful for entrenched infections that are just not going away, even if you are already using antibiotics. It has been used for everything from tonsillitis to gangrene to septicemia (not that herbalists should be treating these). I've also seen it help in the aftermath of rattlesnake and brown recluse bites where the tissues are blue or black a few days after the bite. It helps stop the tissue death caused by the toxins in the venom, specifically when there is that blue-black color to the skin.

Future harvests

It's a native perennial and the root is the part that's used, so harvest no more than one out of every four plants, and preferably less. You don't need much anyhow—a few roots might last you for years.

Caution

Excess dose can cause nausea, discomfort, and possibly vomiting or diarrhea in very high doses. Not for use during pregnancy.

HERBAL PREPARATIONS

Make a tincture of the fresh root, 1:2 at 95% alcohol. Dose is 3–10 drops, 3 times a day. I've also made a wash or compress of the dried root for external use by making a strong decoction and then soaking a washcloth and wrapping it on. The Eclectics mostly used this as an external remedy, but modern herbalists also use it internally.

---

barberry

Berberis thunbergii, B. canadensis, B. vulgaris

PARTS USED root

A great antimicrobial herb, especially for gut infections.

How to identify

Of the several species in our area, Japanese barberry (*Berberis thunbergii*) is the most common and the easiest to find and harvest. This is especially true because it is an exotic invasive, and people are often glad to have it removed. Be sure to differentiate this from our less common native species, American barberry (*B. canadensis*).

Barberry is first and foremost a small shrub, about the height and shape of multiflora rose and easy to mistake at a distance. But once close to the plant the difference is obvious—barberries have simple leaves, not pinnate like the roses, and the thorns are small and straight, not curved. The individual leaves of barberry are simple and wider toward the tip. In the spring there are many yellow flowers that turn into oval, red, sour-tasting berries by the fall. The "barb" in the name refers to its thorniness.

Japanese barberry has simple thorns, leaves with a smooth edge, and flowers that are solitary or up to 4 in a cluster. American barberry and European barberry (*Berberis vulgaris*) both have small bristles on the

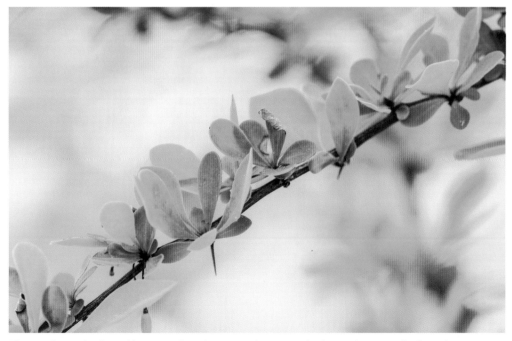

The small spatula-shaped leaves and single spines of Japanese barberry; American barberry has 3-parted spines.

edge of the leaves and branching thorns. American barberry has 5–10 flowers/berries in a cluster; European barberry has 10–20 flowers/berries in a cluster. The root of all three species is intensely yellow, and all three are medicinally interchangeable.

Where, when, and how to wildcraft

Like all roots, barberry is best harvested in the fall when the plant is storing up energy for the winter, or in the spring before it uses up some of that stored energy to grow more.

It is a shrub, and the roots are appropriately large. Get out your digging fork and shovel, maybe a mattock, and start digging in. Find the main root crown and figure out in which direction the side roots go, then trail them out from there. Sometimes it's easier to cut the side root off where it meets the crown to more easily dig it out, but don't lose track of which root is which as there are probably other big roots in the ground— although none as yellow as barberry.

Medicinal uses

Barberry is antibacterial, antiviral, antiparasitic, and antifungal, or as it is said, "It kills things real good." Berberine, the alkaloid responsible for this effect, can also be found in goldenseal, yellowroot, and other

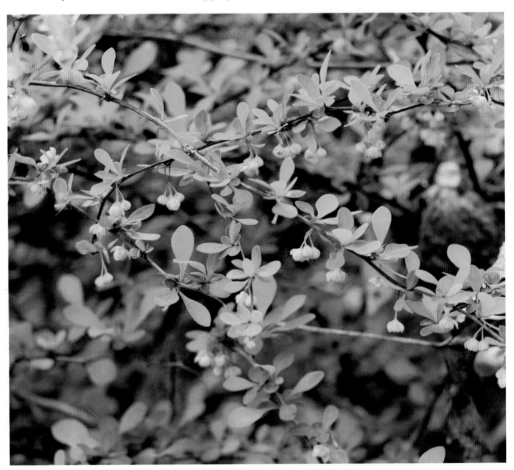

Japanese barberry produces small yellow flowers in early spring that turn into red berries in the fall.

medicinal herbs. It tastes bitter, gives the roots of these plants the yellow color, and is proven to kill many things.

Like other bitters, barberry stimulates the digestive system to produce more enzymes, hydrochloric acid, and other beneficial secretions, while stimulating the liver and gallbladder to produce more bile. Taking bitters before a meal makes the digestive process more efficient and especially improves breakdown of fats and proteins.

This liver stimulation also increases clearance of toxins and helps many kinds of chronic skin conditions like eczema or acne, especially if these are caused or made worse by poor food choices or concurrent allergies, which is often the case with eczema.

When it comes to fighting infections, barberry is an excellent herb for many kinds of sinus infections, respiratory infections, urinary tract infections, or stomach flu. It is one of my favorite herbs for treating any kind of gut infection; it can even help kill parasites, especially when combined with black walnut. It also works well topically as a powder or tincture for skin infections.

It's interesting to note that plants in this genus don't contain enough berberine to have an antimicrobial effect, yet they have a long history of being used for just that. Turns out that there is a chemical in these plants that inhibits the MDR (multidrug resistance) pump in bacteria. The MDR pump flushes out things that could harm the bacteria, such as antibiotics and antimicrobials. By inhibiting this pump, berberine lasts longer and has a stronger action on the bacteria, which is why the whole plant extract works better than isolated berberine. Plants are cool! It can even be taken with antibiotics to help them work better.

And finally, the compound berberine is currently being used in conventional medicine to stabilize blood sugar. Though this isn't one of the traditional uses of the plant, it makes sense to learn from modern medicine as much as modern medicine has learned from herbal medicine.

Future harvests

Japanese barberry is considered a weed, so no worries about overharvesting there. American and European barberry should be harvested only when there is enough, so identifying the right species is important.

HERBAL PREPARATIONS

Works as a tincture or glycerite, fresh 1:2 at 95%, or dried 1:5 at 50%. It could also be used as a decoction, but it is pretty bitter.

bayberry

Morella cerifera (*Myrica cerifera*)
PARTS USED root bark, tree bark

A stimulating and drying herb for sinus congestion and dental issues.

How to identify

Bayberry (wax myrtle, southern bayberry) is a shrub 10–20 feet high with gray bark. The trunks don't grow straight up; instead, there are usually several main trunks that rise up at different angles. The leaves are evergreen and somewhat leathery but not tough, have just a few (if any) teeth in the upper half, and are pleasantly aromatic when crushed. The leaves and usually the twigs also have small yellow resin dots that are visible under a magnifying lens. Plants produce small but abundant gray berries in the late summer and fall; these berries, clustered up and down the branches, used to be used in candle making, as they are waxy and aromatic.

Bayberry could be mistaken for live oaks, but those have thicker leaves, no berries, and the leaves aren't aromatic when crushed. Curiously, it is one of the few plants outside the pea family that can fix nitrogen in the soil because of a symbiotic relationship with soil bacteria.

Where, when, and how to wildcraft

Southern bayberry is one of the most abundant plants of the coastal plain from New Jersey to the tip of Florida, and all the way

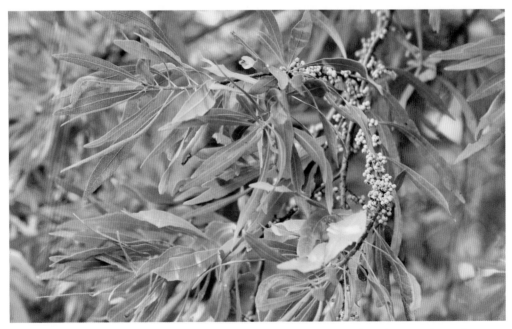

The thin long leaves of southern bayberry, with clusters of the berries that have been used to make scented candle wax.

west to Texas. In Florida, no need to even be near the coast, since the whole state is a coastal plain pretty much. Northern bayberry (*Morella pensylvanica*), which grows mostly from Maryland and Delaware north to Quebec, can be used similarly; it has thinner non-evergreen leaves that are wider than southern bayberry, being an inch wide instead of half an inch.

The roots or branches can be harvested pretty much year-round. Michael Moore held that stressed (partially exposed) roots tend to make better medicine. If digging the root, be prepared to be there for a while since plants can have a huge network of roots. Sometimes I've harvested just one branch of a root and left the rest so I didn't have to take the whole plant. But they are often a dominant shrub where they grow, along with live oak shrubs, so don't feel bad about digging one up.

To process the bark (root or branches), the best way is to put them in a burlap sack, set it on a hard surface, and pound it with a blunt tool. This will loosen the bark, and then it can be removed from the bag and the loosened bark stripped off.

Medicinal uses

Everything bayberry is about can be summed up by saying it is an astringent and circulatory stimulant. This combination of actions is excellent for the kind of mucous membranes that become loose and boggy, allowing fluids to accumulate and cause congestion. It doesn't treat a disease so much as a tissue state.

It's an excellent herb for congestion in the nose and sinuses, but it is also a great herb for gum disease. And many old school herbalists used it for digestive complaints such as chronic diarrhea and mucous colitis, and even vaginal problems that met the same criteria of lax and oversecreting mucous membranes.

It can easily be used as an adjunct for sinus infections—not as an antimicrobial, but to clear the thick mucus that backs up and allows the bacteria to make their home there. Add in an antimicrobial like barberry or goldenseal, stop eating dairy, sugar, and wheat for a week, and you'll be good to go.

Bayberry's also great for gum problems. In gingivitis, the gums pull away from the teeth, which creates a space for bacteria to enter and cause inflammation. Diseased gums are usually white and puffy, lacking in good blood flow. Bayberry is perfect for tightening the gums against the teeth while simultaneously clearing out that excess fluid that's hanging around in the gums. For this purpose, it does well as a mouthrinse.

Consider it for any mucus membranes that are lacking in tone and congested with excess fluids, whether it's the digestive system, the mouth, or even as a douche for excessive vaginal secretions.

Future harvests

This is an abundant plant, and when harvested well, future harvests shouldn't be a problem. Don't harvest from the ocean front dunes, which are a delicate ecosystem.

HERBAL PREPARATIONS

Tincture fresh 1:2 at 95%, or dried 1:5 at 60%. Put the tough roots in a canvas bag and smash the crap out of them with the back of an ax or a wide hammer. After this, the root bark comes off easily. Much less work than trying to whittle it off.

bearsfoot

Smallanthus uvedalia (Polymnia uvedalia)

PARTS USED root

A powerful lymph mover, especially for an inflamed or infected spleen.

How to identify

Bearsfoot (aka hairy leafcup) is a robust plant growing from 4–8 feet tall with large opposite leaves, as wide as they are long, with 3 shallow palmate lobes and big teeth that can be as deep as the lobes at times. Even though it's related to sunflowers, its leaves are more remarkable than the flowers and are what draws the eye. With a little imagination, you could see the similarity to a bear's paw.

The flowers look like many other plants in the aster family (Asteraceae) blooming in late summer with a yellow-orange disk and oval yellow rays. The flowers are always found at the top of the stalk in a bold display. Because they normally form stands, there will usually be several of these plants around.

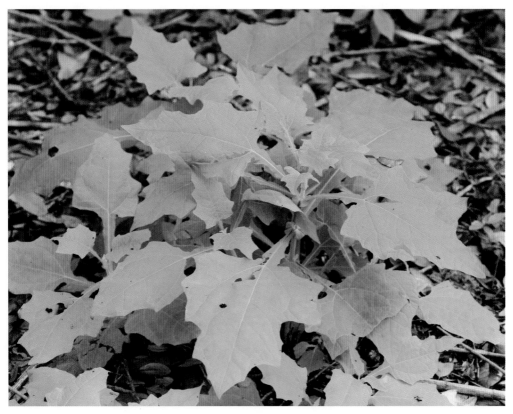

Looking at the leaves, it's easy to understand the common name of this herb, though it is the roots that are used as a deep lymph mover.

Where, when, and how to wildcraft

It is fairly common throughout the Southeast, down to central Florida and west to Arkansas, Louisiana, and to some extent even eastern Texas. There will usually be a cluster of plants coming from one root and then a stand of many clusters. It tends to like moist forests bordering on fields. It flowers in mid to late summer, so harvest either in spring or after the flowers have passed and the plant starts dying back in the fall.

This plant has octopus tentacles for roots. They don't go down so much as extend out, often getting larger as they get further from the plant. If you use a shovel to dig it, you'll lose half your roots from the get-go. The best bet is to use a digging fork (carefully) to loosen the soil in the area, then go in with a soil knife and trail out the individual root tendrils.

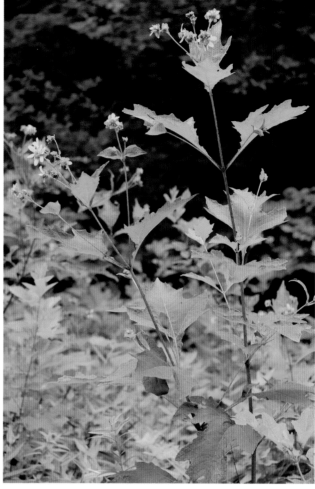

Bearsfoot in flower.

Medicinal uses

This niche herb isn't commonly used anymore, nor is it found in stores. Bearsfoot was highly valued by 19th-century herbalists for spleen problems, which makes it an excellent herb for mononucleosis and other "slow" viruses like Epstein-Barr.

The spleen is a mass of lymph tissue, and what bearsfoot really does is help move lymph fluid deep in the body. This helps the body's immune system as the lymph fluid is the playing field of the acquired immune system. If I didn't have this herb, I would use red root, a better-known lymphatic herb with a broader spectrum of use, which is readily available commercially.

This is almost a specific herb for mononucleosis and could also be used for any kind of viral chronic fatigue syndrome (CFS). Some people never get their energy back after they recover from an infection, which could indicate that the virus is still thriving deep in the body. The most well-known and well studied is Epstein-Barr Virus, a common cause of CFS, and there are other viral suspects as well, including one in the herpes family. Regardless of the particular pathogen, this root could be a useful part of a holistic protocol to address the underlying cause of viral CFS.

Bearsfoot was also used historically for enlarged liver as well as enlarged spleen. Though I've never heard of modern herbalists using it this way, there is some overlap in function between the spleen and the liver, so it could have some direct effect on the liver, or it could help the liver by stimulating the spleen and taking some of the metabolic pressure off.

A curious sidenote—an ointment made from these roots used to be used to treat male pattern baldness. Don't know if it works, as there are a lot of herbs with this reputation, but passing it on if anyone wants to try it!

Future harvests

These roots are best harvested when you find a stand of plants in a field, not isolated individuals. When one does find it, there is often an abundance of plants, but just a couple will give you all the medicine you need for a while. Bearsfoot grows well in disturbed areas near woods, and I have seen poison ivy growing nearby, so be careful those toxic plants are far enough away, or you'll be treating yourself for a skin rash, too.

HERBAL PREPARATIONS

Fresh root tincture 1:2 at 95% alcohol, or dry root decoction.

beggar ticks

Bidens alba, B. pilosa
PARTS USED aerial

*A common plant that is good for many kinds of infections,
and especially for excess mucus in the respiratory tract.*

How to identify

All the approximately 12 *Bidens* species that occur in the Southeast have some medicinal use, and all have the same common name of beggar ticks, but this entry will focus on *Bidens alba* (aka Spanish needles, romerillo, amor seco, picão preto), which is commonly used across the tropics and may or may not be the same plant as *B. pilosa*, which has a widespread history of use. These plants have a yellow disk and 3–8 white rays with opposite, sharply divided pinnate leaves. Botanists might recognize them as separate species, but many folk herbalists see them as the same and use them interchangeably.

All the species have opposite leaves and can be either simple and sharply toothed, sharply lobed, or even pinnately divided. The easiest way to tell a plant in this genus without getting into technical botany is by looking at the seeds, which are long, thin, and flat, and have two hooked prongs at the tip that

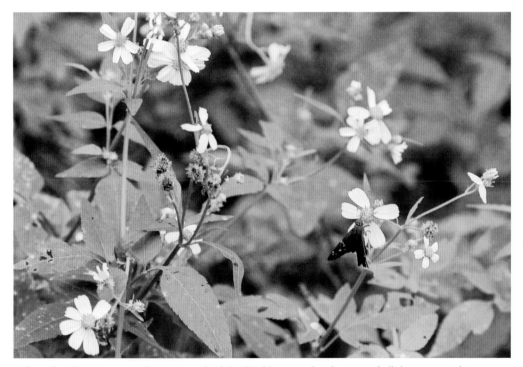

Bidens alba, the species used across much of the Caribbean, is the showiest of all the genus with its yellow disk and white rays.

stick into pants, sweaters, and fur. These two prongs give the genus its name (*bi*, "two"; *den*, "teeth"—think dentist). The way they stick to clothes after walking through the woods lends the plant its common name of beggar ticks.

Where, when, and how to wildcraft

Several species across the Southeast can be used. *Bidens alba* is a common weed along the coastal plain of South Carolina, Georgia, Alabama, and Louisiana, and then all over Florida and throughout the Caribbean, usually covered in orange Gulf fritillary butterflies in the fall.

Harvest the whole plant in late summer and early fall when in full bloom. Usually it can be found in large stands lining roadsides and filling fields. I've seen it from Jekyll Island, Georgia, to St. Petersburg, Florida, to the Yucatán peninsula, Mexico.

Medicinal uses

Whether it's *Bidens alba* and/or *B. pilosa*, the white-flowered bidens is considered a major medicine in the tropics worldwide, and much is written about it, based on the traditional medicine of the Caribbean and tropics. This tropical bidens is used for so many different conditions that it's hard to list them all. But one of its main uses is as an antimicrobial herb for many different kinds of infections, and there has been a lot of medicinal research about this use. Some reports even say it is effective against staph infections. But at the same time, it is also very high in nutrients, and the leaves can be boiled and eaten like kale. Strange that something so powerfully antimicrobial should also be an edible, but plants can do strange things.

All the species can be used to create better tissue tone in the urinary and respiratory tract and to dry up excess mucus. In the United States, bidens is mostly used for two things—helping with urinary tract infections and for respiratory congestion and allergies, much like its fellow weed goldenrod. Like goldenrod, it is a slightly aromatic astringent with antiseptic properties as well as being a decent diuretic. Both qualities strengthen and improve the tissue tone of the mucosa that line the urinary and respiratory tract, making them more resilient to invasion by bacteria, viruses, and allergens. Physical barriers are the first line of defense of our immune system—if something can't get through then it can't start a reaction.

These actions plus its antimicrobial properties make it helpful for urinary tract infections and upper respiratory infections as well, useful in both treating acute infections and for prevention in people with recurring infections. Because it is very drying, it's best for colds with excess mucus and congestion. Stephen Buhner called bidens a "systemic antibiotic" herb, but I never really believed it until Dave Meesters, an herbalist in Marshall, North Carolina, reported using a local species successfully for an infection that other herbs didn't touch. He used large doses (a teaspoon of tincture every 2 hours for 2 days), and it turned the infection around. This gave me new respect for the power of this plant. There are dozens of *Bidens* species, so the one in your area might also have the same actions—experiment and see.

Future harvests

In almost all their range, *Bidens* species are extremely abundant, some would even say weedy. Overharvesting is not an issue.

HERBAL PREPARATIONS

Standard infusion, or tincture fresh 1:2 at 95% or dry at 1:5 at 50% alcohol.

---

blackberry

Rubus pensilvanicus, R. allegheniensis

PARTS USED root

A common and useful astringent, especially for acute diarrhea.

How to identify

All the many species within this genus, which includes blackberries and raspberries, have edible fruit. Most are tall and spreading bushes, but a few species run along the ground. The two species mentioned here are the most commonly used.

It is important to differentiate blackberries from raspberries as they are used very differently for medicine. The easiest way to tell the difference is by the fruit, which are actually an aggregate of many tiny fruits attached to a base called a receptacle. In blackberries the receptacle comes with the fruit, actually inside so that it is one whole oval fruit. In raspberries the receptacle stays on the plant, giving the picked fruit a cap-like appearance. This is why black raspberries are not blackberries.

There are a few other ways to tell the two groups of plants apart: blackberry canes have longer thorns on smooth green canes, where raspberries tend to have shorter prickles, on reddish stems that often have a white coating. Blackberries have 3 or 5 palmate leaflets, fan-like, where raspberries will always be pinnate with a central stem extending beyond the first two leaflets.

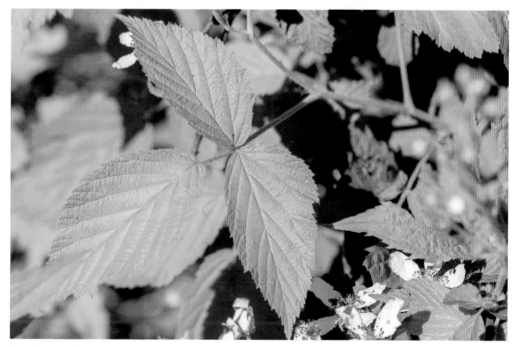

Blackberry in flower.

Where, when, and how to wildcraft

Blackberries are easy enough to find, and often their thorns will find you first! They are a very common plant of fields, meadows, and (if you don't mow often) yards. It's easiest to harvest plants that are on the edge of a stand. The roots are preferable to dig in the fall as the energy starts going back down into the roots then, and also because you can wear thick clothing that will protect you from getting scratched all to hell.

The first thing to do is get out your pruners and cut the canes back close to the ground, leaving just enough so you can still

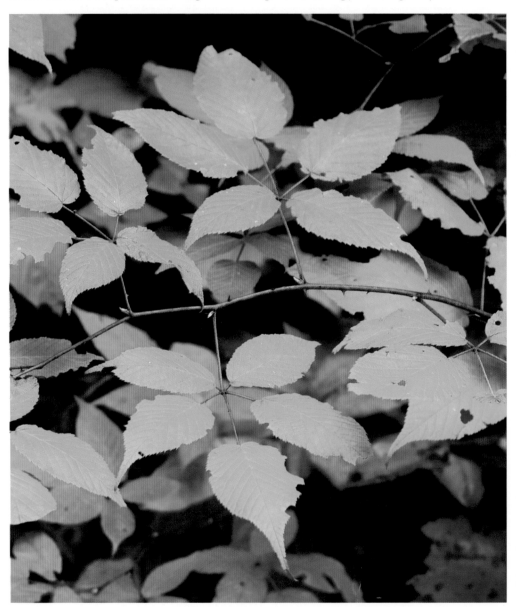

Blackberry leaves can have 3 or 5 palmate leaflets.

find the root crown. Clear these cut vines out, then get out a digging fork and dig around the plant to loosen the soil. Then get your nursery shovel and start going in. These roots are tough and deep, so take your time and have patience.

Medicinal uses

Blackberry is an astringent, plain and simple. Astringents are herbs that are used to dry, tighten, and constrict tissue, and blackberry is specifically used to stop up acute diarrhea. There is a reason why we get diarrhea, and blackberry won't treat the cause, it will just stop the symptom. When the gut finds something irritating (such as food spicier than you're used to) or possibly dangerous (such as an amoeba, paramecium, or a virus), then the best strategy is to get it out of the body as fast as possible instead of trying to spend precious energy attacking it. Just speed up gut motility, produce some protective mucus, and be done with it.

The problem is that this doesn't give the large intestine time to reabsorb all the fluids that have been secreted into the gut, which is why stools are looser. If diarrhea gets bad, it can quickly result in dehydration, which is why diarrhea is a major cause of death in children worldwide. It is also exhausting and inconvenient.

So when you realize you've drunk bad water and you're a two-day hike into the wilderness, or when you have to take that 11-hour bus ride back to New Delhi to catch your flight the next day, or you're just losing more fluids than you can tolerate, then blackberry root is perfect. A really handy thing to keep around in your first aid kit.

Future harvests

This is an abundant and resilient plant, and there is little risk of overharvest. It's also unlikely that you'll need more than one or two plants' worth of root.

⚠ Caution

This can really stop you up so is best for short-term use to get someone through. For chronic diarrhea, there are better remedies. Also, again, be aware that although it stops diarrhea it does not treat the cause of diarrhea.

HERBAL PREPARATIONS

Blackberry root can be prepared as a decoction for maximum effect. The tincture, made from the dried root at a 1:5 ratio with 50% alcohol, is also very effective.

black cohosh

Actaea racemosa (Cimicifuga racemosa)

PARTS USED root

A powerful medicine that relaxes muscles, balances hormones, and helps with joint pain.

How to identify

Black cohosh (aka fairy candles) is a big, conspicuous plant, especially in June and July when it shoots up an 8-foot-high flower stalk. The compound leaves themselves fan out to create a flat light-catching surface, a trick of many woodland plants. What helps differentiate black cohosh is that the individual leaflets are smooth (not hairy) with sharp teeth on the edge. There is also a black dot on the stem at every leaf joint.

In mid-summer, it produces a tall flower stalk topped by a short raceme of white flowers. The flower clusters point straight

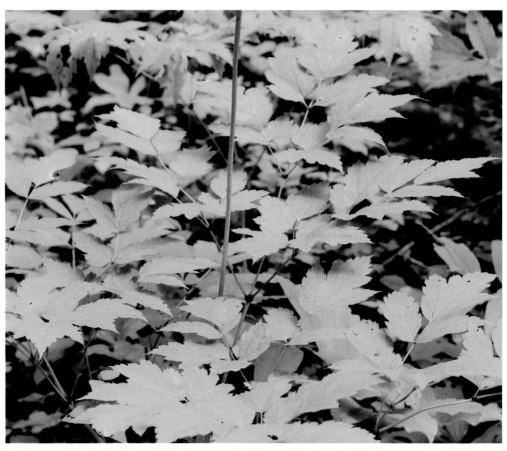

The leaves of black cohosh are divided into many leaflets, and there is a black dot at every leaf joint.

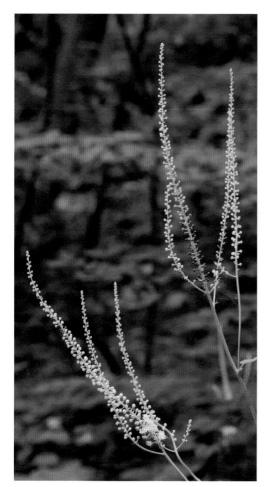

The "fairy candles" of black cohosh make it easy to find during the summer.

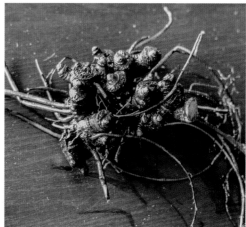

Black cohosh is one of the most useful medicinal roots in the Southeast, but the root is so convoluted that you'll usually find more dirt as you chop it.

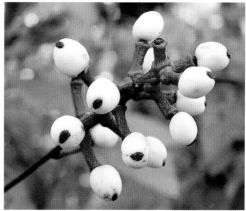

White baneberry looks a lot like a small black cohosh plant but has these distinctive white berries.

up, occasionally branching, but even then they continue to point upward. Two common look-alikes, goatsbeard (*Aruncus dioicus*) and false goatsbeard (*Astilbe biternata*), both have flower stalks that branch out at a 45-degree angle from a central stalk.

Both the goatsbeards, although not related to each other, have fuzzy leaves and stems, compared to the smooth stems and leaves of black cohosh. If all else fails, taste a leaf and spit it out. If it's nasty and acrid like something in the buttercup family should be, you have the right plant.

Harder to tell apart are a few plants in the same genus. Mountain or late black cohosh (*Actaea podocarpa*), which is endemic to the central and southern Appalachians, blooms in August and September and has a deep, broad groove in the petiole of the basal leaves. And throughout the Southeast are white (*A. pachypoda*) and red baneberry (*A. rubra*). These plants, although less common, look almost identical to black cohosh,

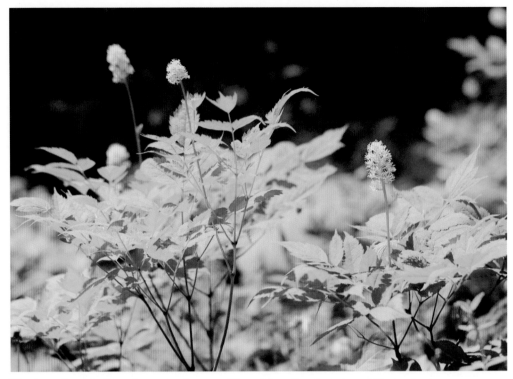
The dense flowers of baneberry are also very different from the airy spires of black cohosh.

but they are generally only a third to half the size, though a large baneberry does looks like a small black cohosh. The baneberries have fleshy berries on racemes 2–3 feet high instead of dry pods 6–8 feet high, so seeing them in fruit makes it easy to tell them apart.

Where, when, and how to wildcraft

This is one of the plants that grows on north-facing wooded slopes in coves and hollers along with bloodroot, stone root, wild yam, and maybe some ginseng if you're lucky and no one has poached it yet.

It's easiest to find the plant in June and July when it's in flower, and that's the best time to do a stand count to see how many plants are in an area. But the roots are best harvested from September through November when the weather starts turning cool and the leaves start dying back. Use

a soil knife to dig up the lateral rhizomes, cutting the thin lateral rootlets as needed or keeping them.

The root is twisty and convoluted, trapping dirt. Wash it well with a vegetable brush, then chop it into small chunks where it curves and wash again to get the dirt pockets. Even then I keep a bowl of water ready on the table because as I chop it into small enough pieces for extract there will still be dirt pockets.

Medicinal uses

Black cohosh, one of the top ten herbs of the early 20th century, remains one of the top ten herbs a century later but for different reasons. In modern times it is mostly popular as a hormone-balancing herb, but it used to be used more for rheumatism and as a muscle relaxant. Both are true though—it has actions on hormones and the musculo-skeletal system.

Black cohosh is an excellent antispasmodic for any kind of cramps or muscle spasms, whether skeletal muscle or smooth muscle (the muscle that's in our internal organs). It can work wonders for menstrual cramps, especially combined with black haw or wild yam. Historically it was also used for whooping cough and spasmodic asthma because of that same muscle-relaxing ability. I've seen it really help an irritated spasmodic cough when remedies like wild cherry and mullein didn't pull through.

Since it relaxes the skeletal muscles, it can be used for sore or tight and overworked muscles; it's also a great herb for whiplash and muscular pain. It can even help treat the symptoms of fibromyalgia, though of course a complete treatment protocol will go much deeper than just this one herb.

Black cohosh is specific for tight and congested tissue states because it relaxes the structure as well as relaxing the blood vessels to allow for greater movement of blood (and therefore oxygen and nutrition) in and out of the tissue. Think about it for a dull and achy kind of pain.

Its relaxant effect also affects the muscles surrounding the blood vessels, allowing them to dilate and lower blood pressure slightly. This also helps relieve some migraine headaches, which are caused by spasms of the blood vessels of the head. Look for dull pain or headaches caused by eyestrain, cold,

or congestion—though if used in excess or in the wrong person, it can also cause a frontal headache or nausea, which can allegedly be cured by green tea.

It also contains some phytoestrogens and has been used to help with menopausal symptoms, especially for hot flashes.

Future harvests

Black cohosh is a bigger plant and is more abundant than ginseng or goldenseal ever were, which can lead one to think it's abundant. I didn't realize how much had been harvested already from our national forests until I started walking around private land and seeing how incredibly abundant it can be in places. Estimates are that 95% of the black cohosh harvested in the wild is exported to Europe, where it is prescribed by doctors.

In other words, harvest sparingly and only when you find an abundance. A good practice is to break off the front few inches of the root, the part containing next year's bud, and replant it, so the plant will keep growing.

⚠ Caution

Not for use during pregnancy due to uterine stimulation.

HERBAL PREPARATIONS

The tincture of the fresh root is best, tinctured fresh 1:2 at 95% alcohol, though it can also be tinctured dry 1:5 at 75% alcohol.

black haw

Viburnum prunifolium
PARTS USED root bark, tree bark

One of nature's best antispasmodics.

How to identify

Black haw is a small tree up to about 15 feet high with simple, oval, toothed leaves that resemble cherry leaves (hence the epithet). Unlike cherry, however, the leaves are opposite and not quite so large. It sends out underground runners and puts up new shoots every 5 feet or so, tending to form tight stands that can be quite abundant in places.

The flowers are in beautiful white umbels (though it is in the Adoxaceae, not the Apiaceae). This is the easiest way to spot the plant as these can line roadsides and field edges when they burst forth. Every spring I am surprised at how much black haw I've been walking and driving by.

Where, when, and how to wildcraft

It is a fairly common plant of the Piedmont and mountains of northern Georgia and South Carolina north through Virginia to southern Pennsylvania and then west

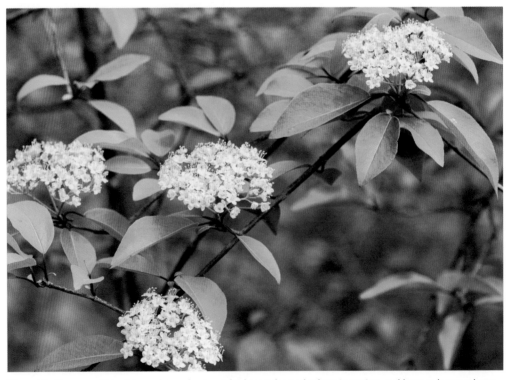

The white flowers of black haw shine along roadsides and wood edges in spring and let you know where you can harvest this wonderful antispasmodic tree.

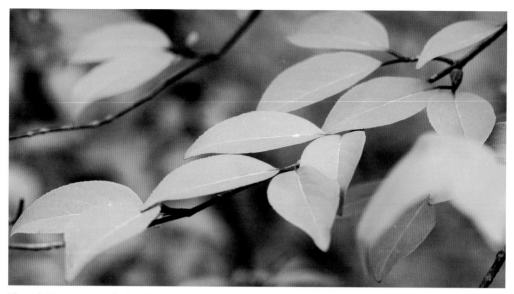
Though it's easiest to find in the spring, I prefer to harvest black haw when it's not in flower.

through Kentucky and some of Tennessee, Arkansas, and Louisiana.

If I'm harvesting the bark then I harvest it in May or June while the new bark is still fresh on the tree, and the roots are best dug in the fall. But harvest it when you can: better to have some than to not have some.

Medicinal uses

This is one of our best antispasmodic herbs, good for almost any kind of muscular cramp or spasm. It is less known than another plant in the same genus, crampbark (*Viburnum opulus*), but is just as powerful and perhaps even more so—it just doesn't have as obvious a common name.

Black haw is mostly used for menstrual cramps, especially combined with wild yam, but can be used for many types of pelvic pain from uterine spasms to painful testes. It also helps with the deeper pain of passing a kidney stone, probably by relaxing the ureters, which can seize up in pain around the stone, making it harder to pass and more painful.

Relaxing these muscular tubes can make for easier passage.

There is a long history of its use to prevent miscarriages. This use comes to us in a sad and unfortunate way. Enslaved Blacks would sometimes use cotton root tea as a way to induce an abortion. If plantation owners learned of such an attempt, they would force the woman to drink black haw tea to prevent the miscarriage.

Future harvests

Harvest this plant when you find it in a large stand. Harvesting limbs and stripping the bark is very sustainable, and even the roots can be dug by thinning trees in a stand that wouldn't make it because they are growing too close together.

HERBAL PREPARATIONS

Fresh root bark is considered the best, fresh tree bark second best, but the dried bark works pretty well too.

black walnut

Juglans nigra
PARTS USED fruit (hulls), leaves

An excellent antifungal and antiparasite, used both topically and internally.

How to identify

This tree can grow straight up to 100 feet tall and have dark bark with prominent vertical ridges. The pinnate leaves have 7–17 sharply toothed leaflets, though they often drop the terminal leaflet.

What is most noticeable about these trees are the tennis ball–sized fruits in late summer through fall that smell like a citrus cleaning product when scratched. They are round and yellow-green, which differentiates them from butternut (*Juglans cinerea*), which has more football-shaped nuts. Butternut used to be the more common tree and was extensively written about in 19th-century herbal books, but a disease has wiped out most of the trees, so now they are difficult to find.

Where, when, and how to wildcraft

Black walnut trees are common throughout most of the eastern United States, though it only grows as far south as the Florida

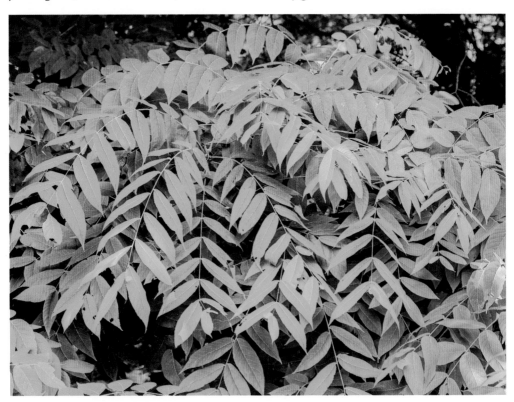

The long compound leaves of black walnut with pointed leaflets.

panhandle. They like sun and are usually found on the edges of yards and fields or along waterways, wherever squirrels forgot they buried them.

The best time to harvest the fruits from the tree is after some have started falling to the ground but there are still some on the tree—usually August through October. It is OK to harvest very recent ground-fall, but if they've been on the ground longer than a couple of days, they often have worms in them and have started degrading. Picking off the tree yields higher-quality medicine. Typically there will be an abundant mast year every 2 or 3 years, and some years in between there will be next to nothing.

Because the juice of the fruit will stain anything it comes in contact with, it is wise to wear dishwashing gloves while processing the hulls (the fleshy part around the nut); otherwise, your hands will be stained brown for 2 weeks. To process, cut the fruit in a circle through both ends, then spin it a quarter turn and cut it in the same direction again so that you have equal quarters.

Peel the hulls off the nut, pop them in a jar, then cover immediately with alcohol. Some add vitamin C powder at this point so the fruit don't oxidize and turn brown. Leave the nut for the squirrels or let it cure in the shell for a couple of months before cracking open for food, perhaps with a sledgehammer or a medium-sized rock.

Medicinal uses

Black walnut is one of the best-known anti-parasite herbs in the United States. Parasites can be single-cell organisms that you'd get from drinking bad water, such as giardia or amoebas, or multi-cell organisms like pinworms or hookworms. Although some herbs work for both types, this one works better for worms.

It can be used when there are signs of acute worm infestation such as excessive hunger (especially carb cravings), eating a lot without gaining weight, fatigue, and other IBS (Itchy Butt Syndrome) symptoms. Parasites are probably more common than Western medicine thinks and less common than alternative medicine thinks.

Black walnut is also an excellent anti-fungal, both internally and topically. It can help tinea infections, including ringworm (a fungus, not actually a worm) and athlete's foot. It works well in a salve with white cedar for this purpose. This is more effective than the standard alternative treatment of tea tree or thuja essential oil.

It is also a mild tonic for the colon, improving tone of the colonic mucosa and helping with diverticula, with the leaves being gentler and a better long-term tonic for that purpose. The fruit is a bit harsh on the digestive tract.

Future harvests

It's difficult to imagine harvesting so much that the future of the tree would be in jeopardy. These trees produce abundantly.

Caution

It does stain the colon brown, so be aware of this if you are about to do a colonoscopy. Taking for too long a time has a negative effect on digestion.

HERBAL PREPARATIONS

Tincture the hulls fresh 1:2 at 95% alcohol, or infuse in extra-virgin olive oil to make a topical infused oil.

Sanguinaria canadensis

PARTS USED root

A potent remedy that can be applied topically to treat fungal infections and burn away growths.

How to identify

This plant is most obvious and easy to identify in early spring when clusters of white flowers dot the woodlands. The flower, with 8–15 white petals, blooms first, while the young leaf stays wrapped around the stem. The petals are delicate, and sometimes a light wind will knock them off.

In time the flower turns into an oval seed capsule, while the leaf grows taller and wider, usually about 6 inches across. The leaf is leathery, round, and has 2–8 notches at the edge, though sometimes it is barely notched at all. There is one leaf and one flower coming off each root or sometimes each end of the root. The root itself oozes blood-red when broken (hence the common name).

Where, when, and how to wildcraft

One of the first signs of spring in March are the beautiful white bloodroot flowers in the woods or small roadsides. They are done flowering before the leaves even come out on the trees, typically growing in small clusters.

Plants can be found in many types of rich woods from New England west to Minnesota, and south to northern Louisiana and sporadically across the Gulf Coast states, but they are more common from the Carolinas, Tennessee, and Arkansas north.

The roots of most plants are dug in the fall, but this plant will be long gone by then,

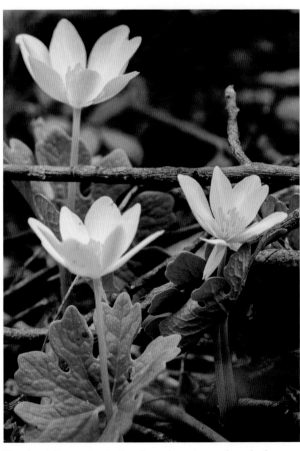

Bloodroot flowers in clusters in early spring and can be harvested at this time.

so it is one of the few plants that is usually harvested in the spring. The roots are small and run parallel to the ground, so it's almost easier to find and dig them with fingers instead of using tools. The only tool you might need is a soil knife to pop up the roots or cut off the tendrils holding them in place.

Medicinal uses

Although it is a famous and recognizable medicinal plant, bloodroot is rarely used in herbal medicine these days. It is mostly used topically as an antifungal and to burn off warts; it is also included in small amounts in some toothpastes for its use for killing the bacteria in the mouth that cause cavities.

Bloodroot is probably most famous (and most controversial) as an anti-cancer agent. It is one of the ingredients in the tradition of "black salves" applied topically to skin cancers. Though I haven't used it this way for clients, I have heard about some positive results as well as other times when it did nothing. So use at your own risk, and even though the cancer might appear on the skin, it comes from within, so systemic remedies should also be used whether those are mainstream medicine or holistic or preferably both.

Mostly I use bloodroot as an infused oil or salve for ringworm and other fungal infections caused by *Tinea corporis*. This same fungus is also responsible for athlete's foot and jock itch, and bloodroot can be used for either of these too, though avoid using it directly on sensitive areas like the genitals.

Although bloodroot does have some history of internal use, it is a very strong herb and should be used only by knowledgeable herbalists. It was traditionally used in doses of 1 or 2 drops in a tincture blend to break up thick stubborn mucus in the sinuses or as a stimulating expectorant for phlegm in the lungs once the active infection is mostly passed. One drop of the tincture on the tongue will cause a burning sensation that can last for a good 20 minutes, so don't use this herb by itself.

Future harvests

Even though this is abundant in some places, it has been harvested heavily in other areas, so don't take too much. You don't need much anyhow. Sometimes you'll find two plants coming out of each end of a root. If you cut the root in half you can take one and leave one to grow back.

Caution

Not for internal use except by skilled practitioners. Though some sources list it as caustic, there are many stories of it being used to paint the skin, so it seems safe enough for short-term use—in "black salves," usually another agent was added for the caustic effect. Definitely not safe internally for pregnancy or for breastfeeding.

HERBAL PREPARATIONS

Despite historical use, this herb is way too intense for internal use. Wash the roots, then let them dry for a day to lose some of the water weight, then chop coarsely and make an infused oil using the heat method. However, it is so antifungal that using the time method and letting it sit for a few weeks would probably be fine too—it just seems to make a stronger product with some heat. You can also use the alcohol intermediary method by adding just enough pure alcohol to the cut roots to moisten them a bit. Let sit for another 4–24 hours, then use the heat method to make the oil. Leave the lid off, and most of the alcohol will evaporate off during the process.

blue cohosh

Caulophyllum thalictroides

PARTS USED root

A powerful pelvic blood mover and a potent herb for menstrual cramps.

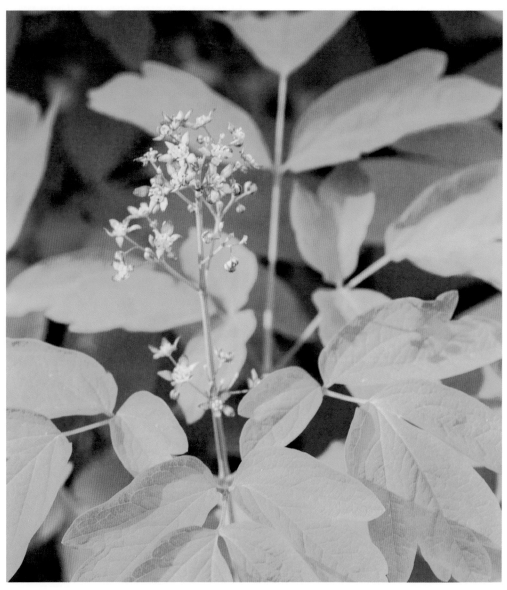

The yellow flowers of blue cohosh come out when the plant first arises in spring and quickly fall, slowly turning to blue berries in late summer.

How to identify

Blue cohosh has a blue-green tint to the leaves, and the leaf edge is smooth with 2 or 3 lobes at the tip of each leaflet, somewhat resembling meadow rue (*Thalictrum*; hence the epithet). When it first arises in early spring, there are small dark yellow flowers that later in the year turn into inedible blue berries.

It is in the barberry family and not related to black cohosh, which is in the buttercup family, and these two woodland plants don't look similar except that they both form a plane of leaflets to catch the sun through the trees. The similarity in names is based on medicinal use, not botany.

Where, when, and how to wildcraft

These are woodland plants, plain and simple; they need shade. They come up in small patches in early spring before the trees leaf out and die back early, so harvest the roots in August and September when they start to yellow. Or harvest during the winter, once you get to know the straw-colored stalks divided into 3 with the clusters of blue berries still attached.

This is a more northern plant; it can be found along the mountains through western Virginia, West Virginia, and Kentucky, down through North Carolina and Tennessee with patches in northern Georgia, northern Alabama, and then sporadically in the Ozarks. The further south you are, the higher the elevation you will need to look; in the southern end of its range, blue cohosh is usually found at over 3,000 feet elevation.

The roots are not large and can easily be dug with a soil knife.

Medicinal uses

This is first and foremost a pelvic stimulant and blood mover. It is a powerful herb for getting things moving in the pelvic area and can be used for feelings of congestion in that area, including uterine fibroids.

Blue cohosh brings more blood to the uterus and really seems to open up circulation, and so it can be helpful for someone whose period is late or slow coming on. It can also help with menstrual cramps when there is a feeling of congestion in the lower belly, or with a heavy or bearing-down sensation, especially in someone whose cycles are 30 days or longer or have already had a baby.

Even though it's often written about as a women's herb, there really is no such thing—plants affect us all. Blue cohosh can be helpful for orchitis, for example, a painful swelling of the testicles. It helps move stuck blood out of the pelvic area and relieve the pressure.

Future harvests

Gather carefully and only when you find an abundance of plants: at some places in the Southeast, these plants are at the very edge of their range.

Caution

This potent herb is definitely not safe for use during pregnancy. Though it has been used to stimulate contractions and bring on labor, even that might be dangerous as there are reports of babies born with heart problems from mothers who have used blue cohosh to induce.

> **HERBAL PREPARATIONS**
>
> Blue cohosh can be tinctured fresh 1:2 at 95%, or dry 1:5 at 60%. It is so intense-tasting that it is seldom used as a tea but could be used as a decoction.

Verbena hastata

PARTS USED aerial

Stimulating for the liver, blue vervain helps relax resistance and anger, moving stuck emotions while relaxing nervous tension.

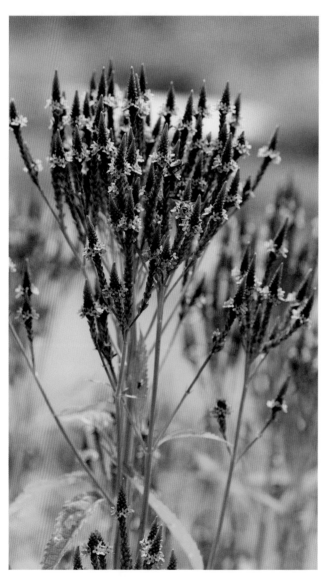

Blue vervain has beautiful spikes of small bluish purple to purple flowers.

How to identify

A native plant of wet areas, blue vervain has long and sharply toothed opposite leaves. The whole plant is very angular, rising straight up in the air with branches shooting out at exactly 45-degree angles.

But what is really noticeable are the gorgeous spikes of small purple flowers that wave like flags on top of the 5-foot-tall plants. Each individual flower in the bunch has 5 equal petals. The plant that most closely resembles it is purple loose-strife (*Lythrum salicaria*), and both grow in clusters in wet places. The best way to tell them apart is the color—loosestrife has reddish purple flowers and blue vervain is more of a bluish purple. The individual flowers of loosestrife are also a little bit larger.

Where, when, and how to wildcraft

Blue vervain is found around pond edges and in wet mead-ows, often alongside other wetland medicinals like boneset and elder, plants that "like to have their feet wet." And your feet will probably be wet too when you go to collect it.

The best time to harvest is mid-summer when the plant is in full bloom. Harvest the entire plant just above the lowest usable leaves and use the leaves and the stem down to where it starts getting tough and woody. Like the unrelated mint plants, it will grow shoots out each side and continue growing.

Though widespread in the Northeast and Midwest, in the Southeast blue vervain is found only in Virginia, West Virginia, and some parts of Kentucky. Some southern herbalists use Brazilian vervain (*Verbena brasiliensis*), a garden escapee, as a direct replacement. I have tinctured white vervain (*V. urticifolia*), which grows more in upland woods than the swampy areas of blue vervain; it has tall wavy bunches of small white flowers instead of the stiff purple bundles of blue vervain. It is a milder remedy but acceptable if that's all you have.

Medicinal uses

Blue vervain is relaxing and opening, having a direct action on the nervous system. It is great for tight and tense muscles in stressed-out people who are holding themselves stiffly. Interestingly, in Europe the native species, *Verbena officinalis*, is used more as a flu herb than as a nervine. But in the same way this species can relax and open up the flow of emotions, it can also relax and open the pores of the skin to help sweat out a fever. In the same sense it is also considered an antispasmodic. In Chinese medicine it would be called a qi mover or regulator.

Its primary use is to relax tension in the nervous system, what in the old days would have been called "liverish energy." In both Chinese and traditional European (Greek) medicine, the liver is the organ related to anger and frustration. Blue vervain is

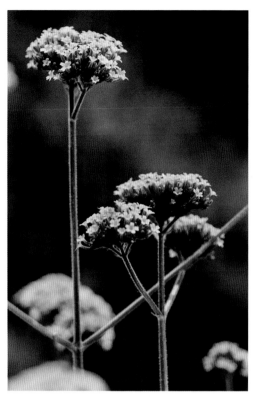

Brazilian vervain, a common garden plant that can escape into nearby lands, is a good substitute for blue vervain.

commonly used to help relax people who tend to hold onto anger and frustration for too long.

It's good to note here that anger has its purpose and its time; it can be a totally appropriate reaction and get us out of negative situations. But there are also times when anger can be misdirected or tucked away for too long only to explode. Vervain is great for those times.

It's also a great herb for migraine headaches, especially combined with mad-dog skullcap (*Scutellaria lateriflora*) and other herbs as appropriate. Though it is specific for those who have a hard time expressing anger, it also just helps release the shoulders and neck.

Many of the vervains have a long history of use for viral infections. The herb itself is not antiviral it seems but rather acts as a diaphoretic to help sweat out a fever. It is also very bitter, which helps bring excess heat down out of the head. On the whole it is used much like boneset to help sweat out a fever, though the latter herb does have more antiviral properties.

And lastly, blue vervain has a traditional use for epilepsy and seizures along with skullcap, passionflower, and other nervines. Though I wouldn't recommend going off antiseizure medication, the combination of skullcap and blue vervain could be helpful at the first sign of a prodromal aura signaling the onset of a seizure. There are some scientific connections between migraines and seizures, which could be why vervain and skullcap can be useful for both.

Future harvests

In the middle of its range, it is easy to harvest sustainably. But as one goes further south and gets closer to the edge of its range, care should be taken not to overharvest. Again, other *Verbena* species, some of which are weedy and abundant, can be used instead.

HERBAL PREPARATIONS

Tincture fresh leaves 1:2 at 95% alcohol, or in half glycerin and half vinegar. Though it can be used as a tea to sweat out a fever, the taste is strongly bitter, so tincture might be preferred.

Ligusticum canadense
PARTS USED root

A lesser-known but potent lung tonic and adaptogen.

How to identify
Though this plant is also known as angelico, it is not in the genus *Angelica*, even though they look similar and are both in the parsley family (Apiaceae). Great care should always be taken when identifying plants in this family since in addition to edible and medicinal plants, it holds some of the deadliest plants in North America. Be 100% sure of your ID before harvesting as even experienced herbalists and botanists have made mistakes, and plant medicine is not worth dying over.

The leaves divide into 3 from a central stem, then each leaf has 5–7 egg-shaped leaflets with toothed edges. It's not a very distinctive plant, so it's a little hard to notice unless you're looking for it. It puts up a tall flower stalk with an umbel of light-colored flowers during the spring.

This plant is in the same genus as oshá, a medicinal in the Rockies that is much more aromatic, but it's more similar in taste to the species used in Chinese medicine, chuan xiong (*Ligusticum wallichii*). Like oshá, there

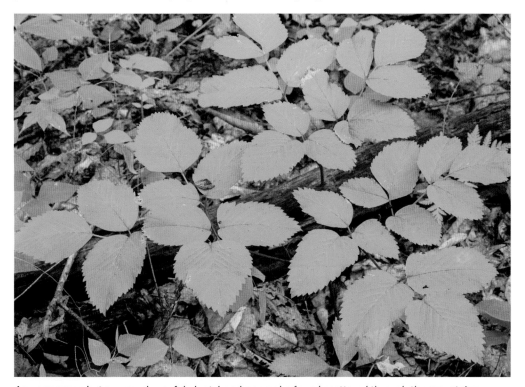

An uncommon but supremely useful plant, boarhog can be found scattered through the mountains.

is a distinctive ring of hairs around the top of the roots, reminiscent of a boar's bristles (hence the common name); these stiff hairs are actually threads from last year's stalks.

Where, when, and how to wildcraft

Though most abundant in the mountains and adjacent Piedmont of the East Coast states, boarhog has some presence in many places in the Southeast, usually on ridges and slopes with rich soil. Mostly one finds a few plants here and there; rarely, I have seen large stands of this plant.

Harvest before the leaves die off completely in late summer and early fall, after which it is impossible to find. The roots are small but can be long, so dig carefully and be patient.

Medicinal uses

Boarhog is a surprisingly useful herb with a long history of folk use, yet very little is written about it. It is a good respiratory herb both as a tonic and for acute infections, and it is also a nourishing adaptogen used somewhat like ginseng in some parts. It's even been used as a sexual tonic.

Much like oshá, its cousin in the Rocky Mountains, boarhog root can be used for colds and respiratory infections. It is not as pungent and hot as osha so it won't be quite as good at breaking up congestion in the lungs and sinuses, but it still does a good job of tackling a head or chest cold by clearing out mucus and stimulating the immune response. And it is also a good respiratory tonic for long-term use, clearing dampness from the lungs and strengthening the ability to transpire oxygen. It's hard to say exactly how it works, but it might be a bronchodilator like oshá.

It is considered an important tonic in southern folk medicine, especially for people feeling run-down and tired. It is more warming and moving than American ginseng for this indication but not quite as warming as spikenard, though any of the three can be used for people who are worn out or tired and have weak lungs prone to infections.

It is also considered an aphrodisiac in the African-American folk tradition. Traditionally it was taken for a few weeks for men feeling run-down and needing a little pep in their step to bring the fire back in their lives. This might be another reason for the common name as in the blues tradition, boars rutting the earth with their phallic tusks is a common metaphor for sexual liveliness. In Chinese medicine it might be considered a kidney yang tonic for this same reason.

Future harvests

In my experience this is not an abundant plant, and the roots aren't that large. Occasionally one can find large stands, but always harvest with great care and take only what you need and what the stand can afford. If you don't find many, there are other more abundant plants out there that do similar things. To put it plainly, don't harvest this plant unless you know what you're doing—both for ID purposes and for the health of this plant in the wild.

HERBAL PREPARATIONS

Traditionally used as a tea or chewed, it also makes a delicious tincture from either the fresh or dried root. Tincture fresh 1:2 at 95%, or dry 1:5 at 60% alcohol.

boneset

Eupatorium perfoliatum
PARTS USED leaves, flowers

A strong antiviral herb that helps with muscle aches.

How to identify
Boneset is pretty unique-looking—the opposite leaves grow together, making it look like one big leaf with the stem poking through. It grows to 5 feet tall in stands in marshy areas and blooms with an abundance of small white florets in mid-summer.

Be aware the upland boneset (*Eupatorium sessilifolium*) is similar-looking but not medicinal and possibly even a little toxic. It can be told apart by the leaves, which although they lack a leaf stalk, aren't sewn together like in boneset.

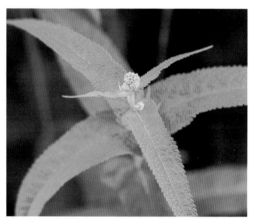

The opposite leaves of boneset join together to look like one large leaf perforated by the stem.

Where, when, and how to wildcraft
Boneset grows in wet areas because it likes to have its feet wet. So, like blue vervain and calamus, it grows in areas where your feet might get wet when you go to harvest it. It is usually found in wet seeps and low meadows, as well as on pond edges.

It is found from the Northeast and upper Midwest south to South Carolina, sporadically in northern Florida, west to Kentucky and Tennessee, then south again to Arkansas, Mississippi, and Louisiana. It is uncommon in Georgia and Alabama.

Medicinal uses
The most classic use of boneset is for a viral infection with accompanying muscle aches, such as happens with the flu. Boneset is a great antiviral with a long tradition of use for colds and viruses; for this purpose it is often combined with echinacea and other immune stimulants. Though it is specific for viral infections with accompanying muscle aches (the result of interferons and other chemical messengers from our own immune system), it can be used for any acute viral infection.

It is also a great diaphoretic—that is, when drunk as a hot tea, it will cause a sweat. Sweating is the body's way of releasing heat and cooling off, so this will help lower a mild to moderate fever. For this purpose boneset is often combined with elder flowers and yarrow flowers. Catnip can be used if there is more agitation, upset stomach, or congestion.

In the 19th century, boneset was taken for breakbone fever (as dengue was then called), hence the common name. Fourth-generation southern folk herbalist Phyllis D. Light (2018) reports it is also used throughout our

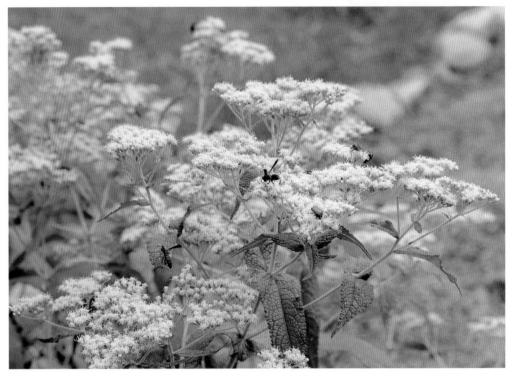

The flowers of boneset can make it easier to find, but make sure to look at the leaves too because many plants in this genus have the same flowers.

region for healing broken bones, and she's seen good success with this use.

Boneset is a simple herb that is remarkably effective for what it does. It is a great herb to have around for a simple cold or even a viral pandemic.

Future harvests

This is a relatively abundant native plant, so the best way to keep it going is to harvest only the top half of the plants before or during flowering time. The plant will sprout back from the cut with more branches and more flowers. It is also a perennial so will continue to grow after being cut. Harvest only from decent-sized stands, and then observe the usual rule of harvesting no more than one out of four plants.

 Caution

There is debate about the long-term safety of using boneset. It does contain some pyrrolizidine alkaloids (PAs) and can, with long-term use, potentially cause liver damage. But it seems to be safe for short-term use.

HERBAL PREPARATIONS

This plant is traditionally used as an infusion, especially for its sweat-inducing properties. But because it is extremely bitter and unpleasant-tasting, it can also be used as a tincture. The tincture can be used as an antiviral and pain reliever, and if the sweating effect is desired, the dose of tincture can be put in hot water and drunk like a tea.

Aesculus flava, A. glabra, A. pavia
PARTS USED inner seed (nut)

A pelvic blood mover helpful for hemorrhoids and varicose veins.

How to identify

In the spring, buckeyes are some of the first plants to leaf out. They are unique in that the leaves are opposite and palmately divided into 5–7 toothed leaflets. Yellow buckeye (*Aesculus flava*) can grow to be a fairly large tree, 50–70 feet high.

In late summer and fall the trees produce round nuts that split open along 3 seams to reveal what looks like a chestnut but is decidedly not edible. The interior flesh of this nut is what is used for medicine, though the leaves can be used as a weaker substitute if needed.

The horse chestnut (*Aesculus hippocastanum*) is native to Europe but can occasionally escape from cultivation. This is the species more commonly used in medicine and the main one found in herb books, but all trees in this genus can be used identically. The easiest way to tell the difference is that horse chestnut has spiny fruits, whereas all the buckeyes have smooth fruits. It also has 7–9 leaflets as opposed to buckeyes which have 5–7.

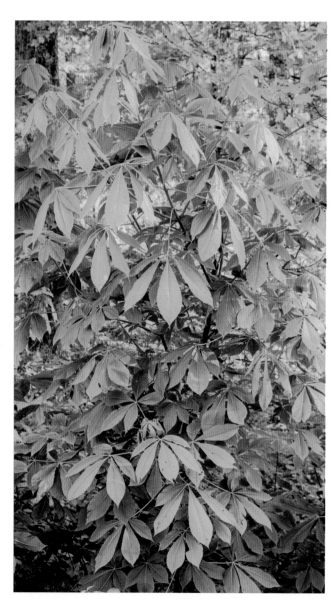

Buckeyes can be large trees with abundant palmately compound leaves, but it is the nuts that are medicinal.

Where, when, and how to wildcraft

Buckeye trees can grow tall in deep woods or can be found at woods' edge in semi-shaded areas. In late summer and early fall its nuts litter the ground in some areas and are easy to pick up and collect. I usually use pruners to split the nut in quarters before throwing into tincture or oil. They also make great worry stones to carry in your pocket and rub when needed.

Medicinal uses

The horse chestnut tree is one of the most popular medicines in Europe for hemorrhoids and varicose veins. Our native buckeyes have been used since the 19th century as a direct substitute for the European nut. Though buckeye can be used for any type of hemorrhoid, it is particularly effective for hypertonic tissue—hemorrhoids in the young and active with little bleeding. The specific indication is a feeling of heaviness or congestion in the rectal area.

It seems to work by helping reabsorption of congested blood and also by clearing congestion in the portal vein, which drains the pelvic area back to the liver.

Future harvests

Gathering nuts from the ground will not endanger the future growth of this abundant tree.

Caution

Be careful with the dosage of this plant, as too much can have a somewhat narcotic effect on the nervous system, causing vertigo or other unpleasant symptoms.

HERBAL PREPARATIONS

The best preparation is the fresh nut tinctured 1:2 at 95% alcohol, and the second best is the dry nut tinctured 1:5 at 50% alcohol. Recommended dosage is 5–15 drops, but don't exceed one dropperful 3 times a day.

The nut can also be infused into olive oil, then made into a salve that can be applied directly on hemorrhoids or varicosities. Because the nuts are particularly tough and dense, I would recommend putting the jar of oil in a hot water bath for 4–8 hours to speed up extraction.

bugleweed

Lycopus virginicus
PARTS USED aerial

Lowers thyroid, relaxes the mind, and helps the heart.

How to identify
Like most plants in the mint family, bugleweed has square stems and opposite toothed leaves, but it is a little different in that the leaves lack a petiole, just narrowing down to the main stem, and it is lacking in any kind of minty smell. The tiny white flowers are clustered in the leaf axils up and down the plant. Though the flowers aren't showy, the ladders of white flower clusters make this species, the most common bugleweed in the Southeast, easier to find. Plants grow closely clustered together in the troughs next to trails and in wet areas.

Where, when, and how to wildcraft
This plant can often be found in small stands, growing along the edges of trails and in

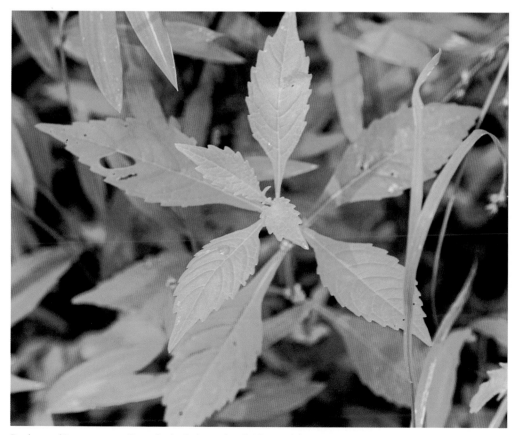

Bugleweed is a common if overlooked plant of trailsides and damp open areas.

wet meadows. Harvest the whole above-ground plant when it is in bloom, mid to late summer.

Medicinal uses

Mostly used as a niche herb for hyperthyroidism, bugleweed actually has a nice range of uses including calming the mind, reducing fast heart rate, and helping heal the lungs.

It is one of the main herbs used for hyperthyroid symptoms—motherwort is another.

Hyperthyroid could manifest in a fast heart rate, fast digestion, racing mind, and insomnia—really just fast everything. Since the thyroid is like the thermostat of the body, controlling the base metabolic rate, when it is overactive then everything goes too fast and when underactive everything goes too slow. This is usually caused by an autoimmune condition, so although none of these herbs stop the causes of hyperthyroid, they can help manage symptoms.

In the 19th century, bugleweed was used like motherwort for fast heart rate and anxiety with palpitations. Though it works best for this when the cause is hyperthyroid, it can also be used for tachycardia and palpitations when not from thyroid issues.

The herb itself tastes peculiarly like skullcap and has a similar use for anxiety and racing mind. Though skullcap is stronger, bugleweed is much easier to find, so use what you've got.

There is a long tradition of using this herb for respiratory issues as well, specifically coughing up blood. Though it doesn't taste particularly astringent, it seems to have some ability to stop bleeding as it was used for coughing up blood, peeing blood, and bleeding in the intestines. It's not the first herb I would use for this and in fact I haven't used it this way, but it's always good to have options. And then go to a qualified health practitioner to find out why there is blood there.

Future harvests

Bugleweed is native but relatively abundant. Just follow the normal rules of not harvesting more than one out of four plants, and it should come back the next year.

HERBAL PREPARATIONS

Tincture the whole fresh aerial plant 1:2 at 95%. It is much more effective fresh.

burdock

Arctium minus

PARTS USED root, seeds

An abundant weed that is both nourishing and cleansing.

How to identify

Common burdock is a relatively common weed of meadows and yard edges. Tiny white hairs give a lighter color to the underside of its leaves, which are wide and easily 2–3 feet long—large enough to be used as a hat in the rain or a dinner plate at a smorgasbord. Dock is an Old English word for any broad-leaved plant. It is not related to yellow dock (or the plant favored by a certain mischievous rabbit, what's-up dock).

Like some other aster family plants, it is a biennial. In the first year, it will just put out basal leaves from the root crown to store up energy in its roots. Then the second year it will use that stored energy to put up a flower stalk 6–7 feet high with scruffy heads of pretty purple flowers, which, by late summer, turn into spherical burs that stick to anything and everything that passes by. Apparently the inventor of Velcro got the idea from looking at burdock seed pods.

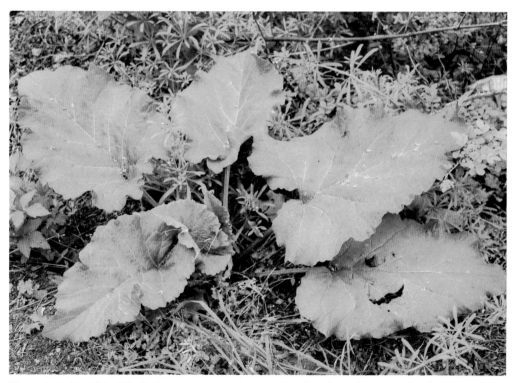

Many plants have "dock" in their common name because they have large leaves, but burdock leaves have "earlobes" at the base and are whiter underneath.

Where, when, and how to wildcraft

Like many common weeds this plant is native to Eurasia but is found in all kinds of disturbed soil like open meadows, yards, and roadsides. It is common from the Northeast through Virginia and West Virginia and south to Tennessee and western North Carolina but is rarely found in the coastal plain.

The root is best dug in the fall of the first year when the plant is still a basal rosette, or in the spring of the second year when the leaves may be large but before it has put up its flower head.

Use a nursery or trenching spade to dig; this root goes deep and straight down, and to make it worse, it is rather fragile and easily breaks off. If planting these roots for later harvest, then plant in loose soil or even in compost.

The seeds are easy to harvest: just walk through an overgrown field in the fall wearing a wool sweater! But as easy as they are to harvest, they are a real pain to process. And I mean really a pain, as the pappus that's mixed in with the seeds will get into your skin like fiberglass and cause you to itch for a day or two.

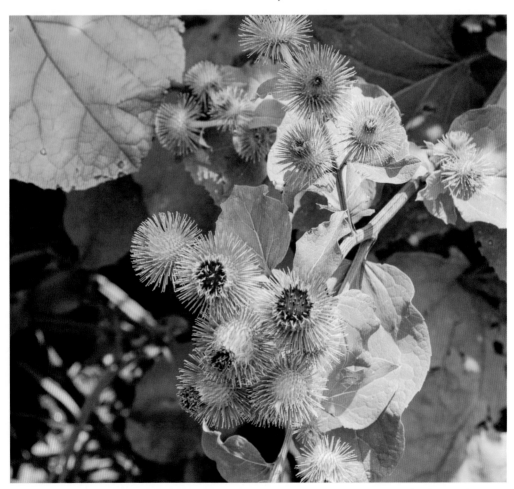

Burdock flowers look like thistle flowers because they are in the same family, but it is hooks, not thorns, that make them stick to things.

I advise you just buy the seeds. But if you still want to wildcraft your own rather than buy, here's how to do it. First put the burs in a canvas shopping bag you're not going to use for groceries anymore or a burlap sack and smash the hell out of it to break up the seedpods. Then open up the pods and lay them out on an old cleaned window screen. Standing outside on a windy day or with a fan blowing over them, bounce them up and down so the white fluff (pappus) all blows away and you're left with just the actual seeds.

Medicinal uses

In Western herbal medicine we mostly use the root, but in Chinese medicine the seed is the main part used. Both plant parts are alterative, cleansing toxins from the liver, kidneys, and lymph specifically. This makes it a great remedy for chronic liver and skin conditions. The root is more soothing and nourishing, and the seeds, though harder to find in commerce, are actually a stronger herb.

Burdock root is somewhat moistening and nourishing to the liver, a bit like peony root is in Chinese medicine. This is a nice change as most liver herbs are bitter, cold, and dry, and this makes it a nice choice for dry skin conditions or people who tend to be dry generally. Even though the seeds are stronger, this unusual characteristic makes the root a better choice at times.

The root also contains inulin, a prebiotic polysaccharide that helps feed the gut flora. Inulin is more water than alcohol soluble, so if using burdock to increase the health of the gut microbiome, be sure to make a tea and not a tincture.

It really is such a sweet and gentle liver tonic that it needs to be taken for long periods of time for best effect. In Asia, gobo (as it is known) is thought of more as a medicinal food than as an herbal medicine and is used in macrobiotic cooking as a healing food that is grounding and helps balance out sugar indulgences. It is also used medicinally for skin diseases and arthritis.

Burdock seeds are a similar medicine that are more active at cleansing the blood and lymph stagnation but not quite as moistening, although it is used in Chinese medicine to moisten the intestines for chronic constipation. All in all, it is actually a stronger medicine for arthritis and for dry and flaky skin conditions.

Interestingly, it is mostly used in Chinese medicine for a totally different use, to help with the initial stages of an infection with a fever to help move the invading pathogen up and out to the surface of the body. This could mean it was used to sweat out a fever, but it could just be a metaphor for pushing an invader out of the body before it penetrates too deeply.

In general, burdock cools off liver heat and so helps with anger and emotional irritability as well as dry and irritated physical conditions, and it does this while also moving liver and lymph stagnation. It's a great medicine to have around, is superabundant in many areas, and it even tastes pretty good.

Future harvests

No worries about damaging these populations. It is an abundant weed in most of the East Coast.

HERBAL PREPARATIONS

Root as a decoction or tincture fresh or dry. It is also delicious cooked up in a stir fry or in soup. The seeds are easiest to use in tincture, but they are traditionally decocted in Chinese medicine.

calamus

Acorus calamus, A. americanus
PARTS USED root

A "lighthouse in the fog" that clears the mind, stimulates digestion, and clears phlegm.

How to identify

Because this plant grows tall, straight, grass-like leaves in marshy fields and pond edges, it can easily be mistaken for cattails (*Typha* spp.) or yellow iris (*Iris pseudacorus*). Cattails have similar-looking leaves, but calamus has a strong vein that runs down the middle of the leaf. Cattails also have a distinctive flower and fruit, starting in May, that looks like a corn dog on a stick; these fruits can often still be seen in the winter.

Yellow iris has similar long flat leaves, but they arise from a flattened base like a paper fan. Calamus is distinctly aromatic where yellow iris is not, so you can break off a piece of leaf to see if it has a distinctive smell. And of course if you find yellow iris when flowering, then there's no mistaking those glorious flowers. The calamus of the Southeast rarely flowers and when it does it is a somewhat phallic greenish protuberance that juts out at 45 degrees from the plant.

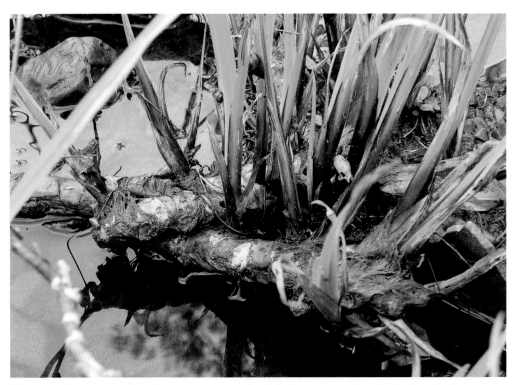

The roots of calamus are found in or near water and send out long leaves in a cluster from their ends.

Two species of calamus occur in North America: the native *Acorus americanus* (American calamus), which is more common up north, and *A. calamus* (sweetflag), native to Eurasia and the more common species in the Southeast. It is challenging to tell the difference without seeing both, but the main thing to look for is how thick the midvein is. Sweetflag has a prominent rib running down the length of the leaf, whereas in American calamus the midrib is still present but is more of a gradual rise that blends into the rest of the leaf.

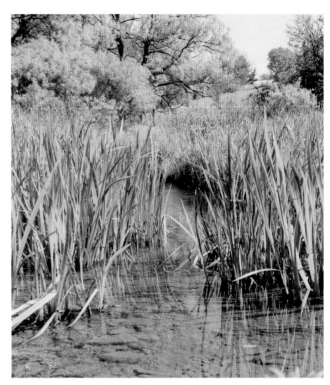

Large stands of calamus can be found mixed in with cattails along the edges of ponds.

Where, when, and how to wildcraft

This is an uncommon plant, and most times I think I've found it what I've actually found is a stand of cattails, so double-check your ID before getting too excited. It is mostly found in Virginia west to Arkansas and south to North Carolina and Louisiana. It's a plant that likes to have its feet wet, so it's found in the muck at the edge of ponds, in wet fields, and sometimes in the Piedmont in slow-running creeks and drainages.

You need only three things to harvest calamus—mud boots, a soil knife, and a lot of patience. To harvest you're going to have to stand in water or a marshy area, and then get in there, get down and dirty, and dig. The roots (actually rhizomes) run laterally and in a good stand form mats that are held in place by tiny rootlets that project out. Cut these strands with your soil knife and often the main rhizome body will come out much easier.

Medicinal uses

The way that this plant juts up tall and straight out of the swampy muck speaks to its medicinal use as a "lighthouse in the fog." It has been used across Europe, Asia, India, and North America as a treasured medicinal, in North America it was often dug up and replanted when a community moved to a new site. There are even records of it being used in Egypt over 3000 years ago.

This root cuts through the dampness in three ways—it helps clear brain fog, it stimulates boggy digestion, and it helps dry up and clear excess mucus from our sinuses and lungs.

In Western herbalism it is primarily used as a brain herb, and it is my favorite herb for brain fog, sometimes combined with ginkgo or gotu kola. Ayurveda uses the herb similarly, to "open the mind and improve concentration, clarity and speech" (Pole 2012). This works better for those who feel like something is clogging up their gears rather than those who feel too tired to put thoughts together. It is great at clearing excess, but those who have cloudy thinking from exhaustion or a lack of nutrients might need more building and nourishing tonics instead.

In Chinese medicine, calamus (shi chang pu) is primarily used to remove obstacles to seeing the world clearly ("clearing phlegm from the Heart orifices"), and as such it is used for manic behavior, schizophrenia, and delirium. It also has an aspect of calming the shen (spirit), so it is sometimes used for insomnia and forgetfulness. It is even used to help restore speech after a stroke.

Calamus is a great digestive herb, similar to angelica. Both are aromatic bitters that warm up digestion. It is especially indicated when there is a feeling of heaviness or bloating after eating, or for those people who don't have sufficient digestive power to digest even simple foods. It is also an excellent appetite stimulant and has been used for anorexia nervosa. Not that you'll gain weight, as it is also used in Ayurveda for reducing obesity. Think of it for rumbling stomach, flatulence, and indigestion. If fennel and peppermint aren't helping enough, calamus might just do the trick.

Finally, it is used to help wet coughs, sore throat, and sinus congestion. Its hot and dry qualities make it useful as a decongestant, whether the mucus is from allergies, a head cold, or the aftereffect of poor digestion. For allergies, combine it with fresh nettle leaf and ragweed leaf. For a head cold, add it in with red root and echinacea.

Future harvests

Calamus is not very abundant in the Southeast, and caution should be used not to overharvest. When it finds a place it likes, however, it can easily spread and take over areas; so when you find a good stand, it is perfectly acceptable to harvest in appropriate quantities. Harvest in places where there is an abundance of plants and dig around the edges of the stands so as to damage as few plants as possible. Native or non-native, calamus is special and deserves respect.

⚠ Caution

Some fiery people might find this herb too mentally stimulating. Because it is heating, those who are already hot-natured might get a headache from consistent use.

Some varieties of calamus contain the chemical beta-asarone, which has some toxicity, but the amount of the chemical varies widely according to the specific plant and where it grows. American plants have far less than the Eurasian plants, but it's worth checking the current research before using any calamus long-term.

HERBAL PREPARATIONS

The root can be made into a tincture either fresh 1:2 or dried 1:5, or can be mixed with gentler herbs as a small part of a tea. This herb works best in small doses, so only 5–10 drops of a tincture are needed at a time, even in a formula. Some like to chew pieces of the fresh root for mental stimulation—more like nibbling, as it is far too spicy to hold in the mouth for long.

catnip

Nepeta cataria
PARTS USED leaves

It might be stimulating to cats, but catnip is calming to humans.
It also helps dry out mucus in the upper respiratory tract.

How to identify

Like many plants in the mint family (Lamiaceae), catnip has square stems, opposite leaves, and irregular flowers. The leaves have pronounced veins and rounded teeth; when crushed, they give off a pleasantly stinky mint-like smell. The stems are upright and fuzzy, growing 2–3 feet high in thick stands. Plants bear tight clusters of small white flowers in mid-summer.

Where, when, and how to wildcraft

A native of Europe, catnip is found in disturbed areas, near old gardens, homesteads, barns, and peculiarly is very common on I-81 through the northern half of Virginia. Not that I would gather it that close to a highway.

Like most plants where the leaves are used, catnip is preferentially harvested just before flowering or in the early stages of bloom. That would be the ideal, but let's

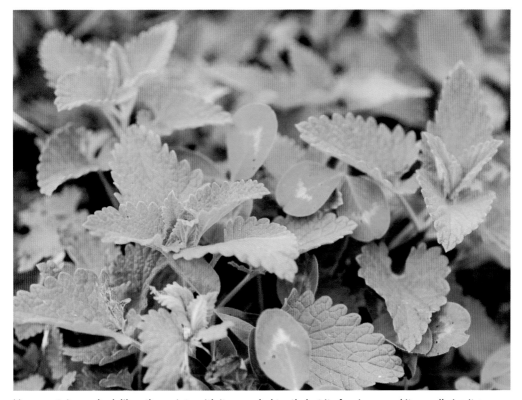

Young catnip can look like other mints with its rounded teeth, but its fuzziness and its smell give it away.

face it—getting harvesting times right can be challenging, and it works to harvest this plant any time before frost.

Like most aromatics, it is best gathered on a sunny day when it hasn't rained the day before but still early in the day. The sun tends to bring the essential oils in aromatic plants to the fore, and rain tends to dilute.

To harvest, use pruners or even scissors to trim the plant just above any less-than-prime leaves. This saves time processing them out later, and the plant, like most mints, will sprout again from the cut.

Medicinal uses

Though it makes most cats freak out adorably, catnip is actually very calming to humans. Like many other aromatic mints, it stimulates digestion but has the added ability to break up and dry out excess mucus in the upper respiratory tract. It is gentle enough for agitated children but strong enough for adults irritated by allergy symptoms.

Because of all this, I think of catnip as being a stronger version of chamomile. Both calm the nervous system while stimulating digestion, and seeing as stress impairs healthy digestion, that's an especially beneficial combination. Catnip is a stronger calming agent and perhaps stronger at stimulating digestion as an after-dinner tea, tincture, or glycerite.

But whereas chamomile is moistening and soothing, catnip is drying. This makes catnip a better choice when there is excess mucus—whether chronic drippy runny nose from poor food choices or acute problems like allergies or even a head cold. The species name is actually a reference to catarrh (a thick mucus), and not (as one might think) to "cat."

Catnip combines with lemon balm for a nice-tasting tea for kids majorly irritated by a minor cold. It can combine with nettle or ragweed for seasonal allergies, or with chamomile, peppermint, and ginger for an after-dinner tea for indigestion or a weak digestive fire.

Future harvests

This non-native plant can be very persistent—there is little worry about overharvesting. Just leave enough for your local feline friends. To be honest, I think that some cats plant this plant themselves. Just a suspicion, though.

HERBAL PREPARATIONS

The dried leaves make a lovely infusion with a bit of honey added. I also tincture the recently dried leaves or make a glycerin extract. This last preparation is probably my favorite for digestive issues because of the soothing nature of glycerin itself.

cleavers

Galium aparine
PARTS USED aerial

A weed that heals the urinary tract, soothes skin conditions, and cleanses and moves the lymph.

How to identify

Cleavers (aka goosegrass, sticky willy) is a common weed that forms small mats of short reclining vines in the springtime. Each stem is square and has many whorls of 6–8 leaves, and both stem and leaves are full of tiny hooked barbs that make the plant stick (or cleave) to things.

There are tiny, white, 4-petaled flowers in the leaf axils. These turn into tiny green balls that stick to clothes and fur as a way of dispersing the seeds far and wide, which seems

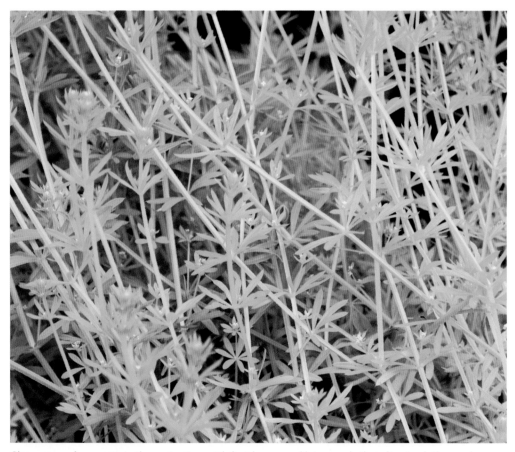

Cleavers can form mats in the springtime with first leaves and later seeds that cling to clothes and fur alike.

to work well for the plant. Confusingly, the same species is considered both native and non-native to North America.

Other plants in this genus, usually called bedstraws, look almost identical but lack the bristles that make cleavers stick to things. None of these other species are medicinal, or at least not in the same way.

Where, when, and how to wildcraft

Harvest the plant in early to mid-spring when the plant is vibrant and green, either before flowering or when the flowers still look fresh. Usually by the time the plant goes to seed, the leaves look wilted but could still be used.

Further north this plant lasts longer, but in the Southeast these plants die off when the weather starts warming up.

Because these plants grow in disturbed areas, it is important to make sure that the environment where you are harvesting is clean. Make sure the area doesn't get sprayed by herbicides, is more than 10 feet from the nearest road, and doesn't get runoff from farm fields or parking lots.

Harvest the plants by grabbing a bundle with one hand, then taking a sharp knife in your other hand and cutting low on the plant, leaving the bottom of the plant that is yellow and full of dirt. Like giving the plant a haircut.

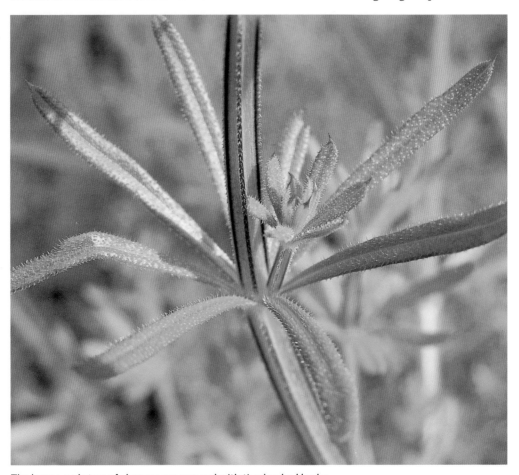

The leaves and stem of cleavers are covered with tiny hooked barbs.

Medicinal uses

This plant works by clearing toxins throughout the body and then eliminating those toxins through the urinary tract. This makes it a great herb for swollen lymph glands, chronic skin conditions, and kidney stones, as well as tonifying the urinary tract.

This herb is primarily used in modern herbal practice as a diuretic and as a powerful herb for the entire urinary tract. It stimulates the kidneys to help clear excess fluids from the body, which makes it great for edema, water retention of PMS, and as part of a protocol for high blood pressure.

More than just moving fluids, it can also help the kidneys excrete more waste such as excess uric acid. I have found it very helpful for gout, combined with shepherd's purse and nettle leaf. It is also an anti-inflammatory used for the irritation and discomfort that accompanies urinary tract infections, prostatitis, and even interstitial cystitis—any kind of inflammation or irritation of the urinary tract or the prostate and accompanying anatomy. It's ability to move things in the UT while reducing inflammation makes it useful for kidney stones, too, though for that purpose I usually prefer using gravel root, stone root, and wild hydrangea.

Cleavers is also an excellent herb for moving and clearing lymph fluids. It is a slower herb than echinacea and red root so it's more for chronic or subacute swollen glands, not for swollen glands accompanying a head cold. It can be used topically as well as internally for this purpose.

Topically cleavers has a long history of use for slow-healing wounds, skin irritations, sunburn, and chronic skin conditions such as psoriasis, eczema, and acne. Because most of these are treated by herbalists with internal cleansing herbs, it can be useful both topically as well as internally.

The infused oil or salve of this herb is great for soothing irritated skin conditions as well as clearing some of the underlying toxicity creating the condition. Some older books indicate it for topical cancers but it's hard to know what the authors mean, as this word could indicate either what we think of as cancer today or a canker, a slow-healing wound.

Overall it is a very useful if slow-acting herb, so it takes some time to have the best effect. Use larger doses of tincture or use the juice for faster action.

Future harvests

This is an abundant plant that spreads easily, so there is little worry you'll harm it long-term. Because it is an annual, always leave some to go to seed so there will be more next year.

 Caution

Do not use if a diuretic is contraindicated.

HERBAL PREPARATIONS

The fresh herb tincture is considered superior, which is odd because most other diuretics are used dry as tea. It can also be used as a succus—plant juice preserved with alcohol. Wheatgrass juicers seem to work best for this purpose, and I have a hand crank juicer I use just for juicing cleavers.

For topical use, the fresh plant can be infused in olive oil, and this can be used as is or made into a salve. There is also a history of using the whole fresh plant mashed up as a poultice (but this seems like it could be prickly) or a wash of the tea (which seems easier).

---

clematis

Clematis virginiana
PARTS USED aerial

A low-dose medicine for migraines.

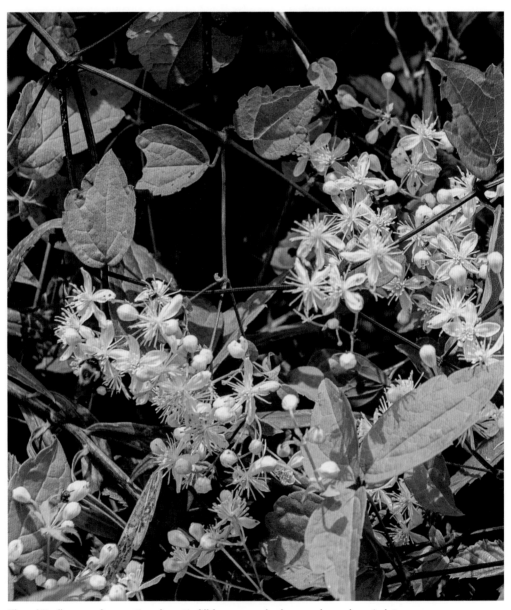

The white flowers of our native clematis fill fencerows, hedges, and meadows in late summer.

How to identify

This clematis (aka virgin's bower) is a weed, plain and simple, even if it is native. It is a long thin vine with opposite pinnate leaves that are sharply toothed. When it blooms in mid to late summer, the 5-petaled white flowers perfume the air with their delicious scent until one is almost sick of it after a while. It has toothed leaflets, whereas Japanese clematis (*Clematis terniflora*), which is even more common, has smooth leaflets

Where, when, and how to wildcraft

It is abundant in roadsides, fields, meadows, and about anywhere else that is left unmowed for too long, climbing up fences and following train tracks. It grows in much of our region except the Piedmont and coastal plain of South Carolina and Georgia.

Harvest the whole upper vine in mid to late summer, and tincture it fresh.

Medicinal uses

This is a great herb for certain types of migraine headaches. It probably works because it is a vasodilator, and if you take too much you'll feel what that means. It is a low-dose botanical; more than 5 drops often causes upset stomach, uncomfortable spaciness, and a cold clammy sweat. Not fun.

But when it is the right herb, it can really help migraine headaches that feel tight and constrictive, like a band across the head. The sufferer might also feel cold, look pale, and want to huddle under blankets. It doesn't work for everyone, and like any migraine medicine it needs to be taken as early as possible because it's hard to turn around a full-blown migraine. But when it works, it works well.

Future harvests

This clematis is an abundant weed—no worries about overharvesting.

 Caution

Use only 5–10 drops at a time, never more. Too much can really upset the stomach and cause vasodilation, leaving someone feeling cold, clammy, and pale, as well as generally uncomfortable. Because it is a vasodilator, it is inappropriate for people who are already feeling hot or those with heat signs.

HERBAL PREPARATIONS

The whole fresh vine, tinctured 1:2 at 95% alcohol.

---

cotton

Gossypium hirsutum

PARTS USED root

A plant that powerfully stimulates the uterus and can be used as a birthing herb and oxytocin synergist.

How to identify

Cotton is in the same family as hollyhocks and marshmallow, and the flower looks it. The plant is an erect herb 3–4 feet high with alternate leaves that have 3 deep palmate lobes. The flowers have 5 even yellow petals that turn into a fruit in the fall; this boll, as it is known, eventually opens up into 5 white poofs, which are the part used for fabrics.

Note that it is actually illegal to grow cotton in your backyard in many southern states; home crops can harbor boll weevils that can then transfer to large farms.

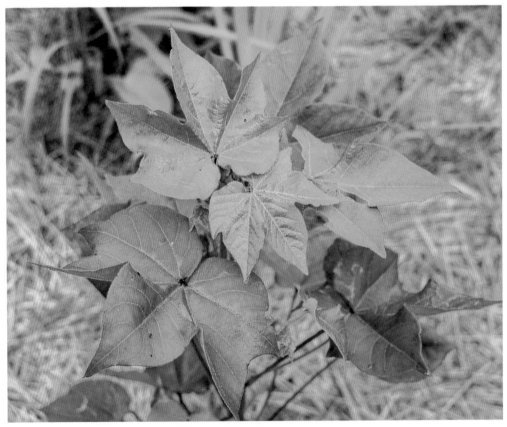

The leaves of cotton aren't nearly as famous as the puffy seeds we make fabric from, but they are a good way to identify the plant in summer.

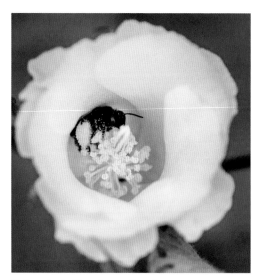
Pollen-dusted bee in a cotton flower.

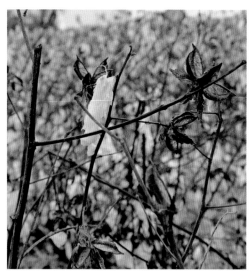
Fields of ripe cotton cover parts of the Southeast.

Where, when, and how to wildcraft

Cotton is actually a perennial that is grown as an annual to prevent pests, so it can sometimes be found growing wild near cultivated fields. If you ask to harvest from someone's fields, make sure they are growing it organically because there are a lot of chemicals dumped on cotton otherwise. Cotton is traditionally grown across the coastal plain and into the Piedmont from Virginia south to Louisiana, then from western Texas to southern California. In all these places, it is still a major cash crop.

The root is the medicinal part, which isn't too hard to dig in the fall. The leaves die back after the first frost, leaving flat white fields stretching for acres. Find a farmer and ask permission; not all cotton plants get used every year.

Medicinal uses

Cotton root is rarely used these days as it is a very strong medicine, but if you know what you're doing it can be a powerful helper when needed. It acts as an oxytocin synergist, a strong uterine stimulant.

It helps bring on a delayed menses, and it is used in midwifery to help bring on a post-term birth. It can also help bring on the afterbirth when the new mother is too exhausted, but it also stops excessive postpartum bleeding. It is an excellent emmenagogue.

Future harvests

Cotton is commonly cultivated, so not a consideration unless you find a wild stand that you can tend.

Caution

Because it is potentially abortifacient, cotton is obviously not safe during pregnancy. Daily use may cause sterility in men.

HERBAL PREPARATIONS

Tincture fresh 1:2 at 85% alcohol and 10% glycerin, recently dried 1:5 at 50% alcohol and 10% glycerin.

Heracleum maximum (H. lanatum)

PARTS USED root, unripe seed

A topical application that both numbs pain and stimulates nerve growth.

How to identify

Cow parsnip is a big plant, even by parsley family standards. The umbel flower head can be a foot across, and the plant easily reaches 8 feet in height. The 2-foot-wide leaves are unusual for this family in that they are not finely divided like a parsley or carrot leaf but only divided into 3 deeply lobed leaflets. The petiole of this plant can form a sheath around the stalk, like the closely related angelica does, but otherwise looks quite different.

It is very important to differentiate this native plant from the closely related giant hogweed, a European species that has recently made its way to the states. Though rarely found in the Southeast at present, it spreads easily and it causes one hell of a rash—putting poison ivy to shame. Giant hogweed can be twice as tall as cow parsnip, growing up to 18 feet high, with leaves up to 5 feet across. Giant hogweed also has purple splotches on the stem, and neither stem nor leaves nor any part of this plant should be touched, ever, because of the risk of caustic burns.

Where, when, and how to wildcraft

Cow parsnip is more common in the Northeast, northern Midwest, and West, but it is found in the Southeast from Maryland south along the Virginia–West Virginia mountains and into the North Carolina and Tennessee mountains as far as northern Georgia.

As this photo shows, cow parsnip is a tall plant that usually grows in large stands, but it's not nearly as tall and robust as giant hogweed, its cousin up north, which can cause a bad skin rash.

The unripe green seeds can be harvested in late spring or early summer and made into a topical application or dried for later use. The roots can be dug in fall.

Medicinal uses

This is a very strong plant that should be used with caution, but it can be really helpful when needed. An extract of the root can be applied topically to a recent injury to help nerves regrow; the green seeds can be chewed for mouth and tooth pain.

Like many, I learned about this plant from Michael Moore, who used a fresh root liniment directly on nerves within a few weeks to a few months after an injury to stimulate nerve regeneration and repair. Unlike St. John's wort, which helps with nerve pain and inflammation, cow parsnip causes some therapeutic irritation for places that are numb or tingling either at the site of an injury or distal to the injury (further from the body's center).

It could also be used for carpal tunnel syndrome, trigeminal nerve pain, and Bell's palsy. He believed it worked like a counterirritant to stimulate nerve growth. It could even be used for recent localized paralysis, again topically only. Keep applying it as long and as often as possible until sensation returns.

The unripe green seeds could be used this way but are not quite as powerful. They are aromatic and stimulating as well as numbing, like a stronger version of angelica seeds. Mostly the seeds are either chewed or a tea swished for almost any kind of dental pain. It's not the best flavor, but it does numb the mouth as well as the upper digestive tract while also stimulating digestion. Like many plants in the parsley family, it is a great carminative.

The main caution in all these uses is the danger of making the skin much more sensitive to sun burn. Brushing up against the plant before sun exposure is the main way that this can happen. Some herbalists have reported it happening from alcohol extracts applied topically as well; others have never seen it cause a problem. It seems the further north the plant grows, the more of these photosensitizing furanocoumarins are produced and the more likely it is to cause a skin reaction. Sometimes these are mild burns and sometimes they leave the skin stained for months afterward (not months of pain, just discoloration).

So use with appropriate caution, but when needed cow parsnip can do what hardly any other plant can do.

Future harvests

The seeds are never a problem, and usually when you find one plant you find a bunch of them, so digging a root or two is rarely a problem either. And a root or two is all you really need.

Caution

Be careful with topical application and sun exposure as blistering can occur in some.

HERBAL PREPARATIONS

The liniment can be made by infusing the fresh roots or fresh green unripe seeds in isopropyl alcohol. It is potent enough to be made somewhat dilute. The seeds can be chewed or made into a tea for a mouth-rinse. The original Latino New Mexican tradition is to make a decoction and put it in a bath.

crossvine

Bignonia capreolata
PARTS USED flowers, leaves

A southern folk remedy used as an energy tonic as well as a blood cleanser.

How to identify

This vine can climb fairly high and is green when young but woody as it gets older, sometimes forming several shoots from a single root that overlap each other. The leaves are opposite with 2 leaflets on each side, creating at each junction an interesting 4-leaf pattern, like a cross when free-hanging. The tendrils that the plant uses to climb are where a third leaflet would usually be.

The flower is large and tubular with 5 lobes at the opening, looking much like trumpet creeper (*Campsis radicans*), which is in the same family, except crossvine's flowers are red on the outside and yellow on the inside (where trumpet creeper is either red or yellow).

Where, when, and how to wildcraft

This plant can be found from southern Virginia south to central Florida and west from

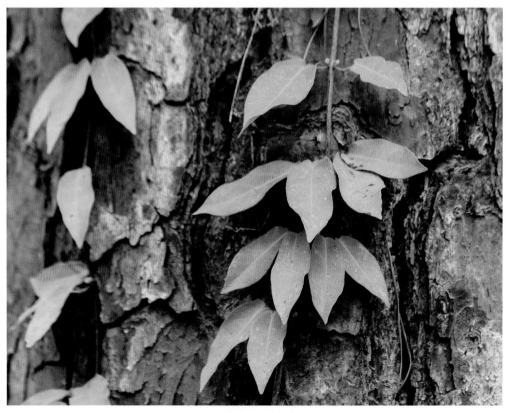

Crossvine is an unusual vine, having 4 leaves coming out from the same place on the stem.

Kentucky to eastern Texas. It is most common in wet woods and bottomlands of the Piedmont and coastal plain, only rarely making it up into the mountains. It sometimes grows in drier forests but remains stunted and doesn't flower or fruit.

Harvest the leaves and flowers during the summer when the plant looks vital.

Medicinal uses

Crossvine deserves more attention and research. I first learned about it from Phyllis D. Light (2018), but it is not much talked or written about. It was used as both a tonic and a cleanser by the indigenous

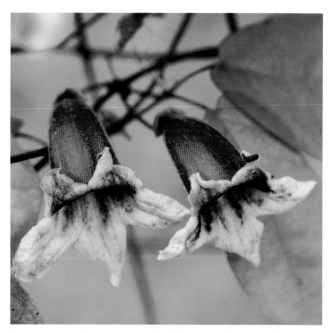

Crossvine also has these beautiful flowers, which resemble those of its close relative, trumpet creeper.

people of the Southeast, and it remains abundant. It is useful enough that it should be re-remembered, though to be honest I'm just learning this little-known plant myself.

It is an interesting plant to get to know, with the possibility of being a true American adaptogen: it was used for cases of exhaustion and debility in people and in animals and had the reputation of being able to give strength back to people who were depleted. For this purpose it was combined with ginseng or other roots.

But then it's also a bit like sarsaparilla or sassafras, in that it has a reputation for cleansing the blood as well as building energy. Maybe part of why it is energizing is because it gets the toxins out of the way.

Another take on it is as a nervine—Thomas Easley and Steven Horne (2016) recommend it as a relaxant to help people who are overly driven to stop and get the rest that their body needs; and yet at the same time once they stop working it also helps restore their energy.

Future harvests

It is fairly abundant where it grows. Just make sure to leave plenty when you harvest.

HERBAL PREPARATIONS

Traditionally an infusion was made of either the leaves or flowers, but the tincture seems to do pretty well too, fresh 1:2 at 95% or dry 1:5 at 50% alcohol.

dandelion

Taraxacum officinale
PARTS USED root, leaves

*A powerful liver herb and blood cleanser
that is also one of our most common weeds.*

How to identify

It seems like dandelion wouldn't need a description since it's such a common weed, but there are several weeds with similar leaves or similar yellow flowers, so be sure to pick the right plant.

All the leaves are basal, meaning they come directly from the root; there are no leaves on the flower stalk. The leaves themselves can be very variable, but the shape is always widest at the tip, and the leaf shape can range from big teeth that angle back toward the root (the original French name was *dents de lion*, "lion's teeth") to barely toothed, often on the same plant. And the leaves are invariably smooth; rarely, a few downy hairs lie along the leaf.

The smooth leaves are quite different from the erect hairs on the underside of hawkweed, chicory, and wild lettuce. Though the latter two are very similar to dandelion, their leaves are also usually bigger.

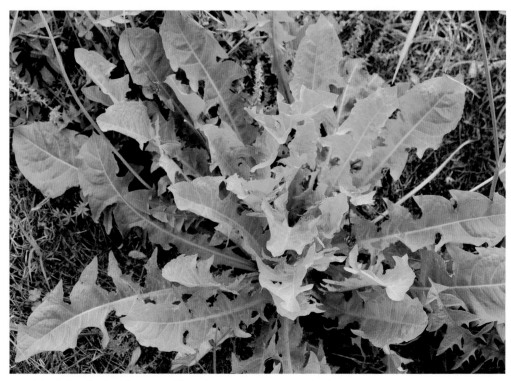

Dandelion's familiar basal rosette of leaves.

Though the distinctive yellow aster family flowers should be a giveaway, there are similar flowers out there in yards and meadows. The way to tell the difference is that unlike sow thistle, salsify, and hawkweed, the flower stalks of dandelion are hollow, leafless, and unbranching.

Where, when, and how to wildcraft

Dandelions can be found anywhere, much to the consternation of gardeners, farmers, and meticulous lawn keepers. They are a European import, originally brought here to beautify lawns, with their yellow flowers and short stature (they never grow up to be tall weeds)—which makes you wonder why nowadays people try to get rid of them. In fact, one of the most important things to be aware of when harvesting is to make sure that the area hasn't been sprayed with herbicides. The next most important thing is to find loose soil to dig in. Sure, you can dig these right out of your front yard if you're at least 10 feet away from a house, but it is so much easier to get the roots out of a garden bed than from compacted turf soil.

Although the plant can be found almost year-round, it is easiest to notice in early spring, when it seems every dandelion blooms at once; I have seen them in flower almost every month of the year in the Southeast.

That said, the roots make slightly better medicine in the fall or early spring. And the leaves seem to be sweetest and best for eating in the spring, but more bitter and best for medicine in the summer.

Most people would describe dandelion as ubiquitous, and it is present in every state but Hawaii. But it is actually far less common in Mississippi, Alabama, Georgia, and Florida. It grows well in disturbed areas, including meadows and lawns.

Medicinal uses

This forgotten and cursed backyard weed is an amazing herb to detoxify the whole body. The roots are more specific for cleansing the liver and the leaves are more specific for cleansing the kidneys, but the whole plant is what's used in Chinese medicine and really both do both. The flowers too are edible and tasty, with a high amount of beta-carotene.

This plant helps clear toxins from the liver, kidneys, and blood, and these days, with so many toxins floating around in the air, in our water, and in our food—who couldn't use some dandelion? I find it ironic that the same herb some spray with chemicals could help clear those very same chemicals from the body.

The root is the part I use most often. It is a gentle but powerful liver herb with a flavor that is both bitter and sweet; the starches in the root help balance out the bitterness. This is a mainstay liver tonic, stimulating bile, stomach acid, and other digestive secretions, clearing toxins, and nourishing and protecting the liver. It has even been used as part of formulas for jaundice and hepatitis.

It is a great digestive bitter, meaning it can be taken before meals to "prime the pump" and get our digestive secretions going so we have better assimilation of food. By stimulating bile flow, fat is broken down more completely and gallstone formation is slowed. It can also help move stones already present, but avoid use if there's a possibility that a stone might be blocking the bile duct.

The root also clears heat from the liver, reducing inflammation and irritation. Look for symptoms such as acne, eczema, chronic dull headaches, brain fog, or nonspecific inflammation such as joint pain. It can even reduce irritability and outbursts of anger. These are some signs that a general detox is needed, and herbs like dandelion, barberry,

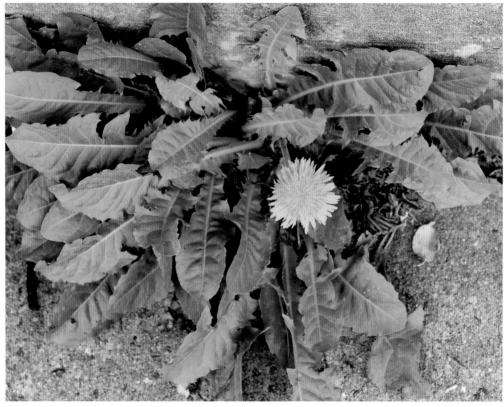

Dandelion can pop up in yards, sidewalks, or even out of concrete like this one.

and other liver herbs can help with that.

Those starches in the root have a somewhat balancing effect on blood sugar. Not enough to treat diabetes, but it can still help with intermittent blood sugar instability. The same starches are also prebiotics, nourishing the gut bacteria.

The leaves work more on the kidneys as a strong diuretic. Diuretics can be useful for those experiencing edema (water retention), including premenstrual edema, and can also help lower blood pressure. Many pharmaceutical diuretics used for this purpose cause depletion of potassium, but dandelion is so loaded with potassium that it creates a net gain. Use dandelion leaf when there is a roundness to the face, a look of "water weight" or puffiness to the body.

The leaves are edible but pretty bitter: most of the dandelion sold in produce sections is actually the sweeter chicory leaves that look so much like dandelion. But true dandelion leaves can be mixed in with other salad greens, or sautéed with garlic in some olive oil—again probably with some other greens in there too.

The best thing you can say about dandelion is that it detoxifies the liver from all the things that humans spray to try and kill it. This is a great example of the giving nature of the plant world.

Future harvests

Not a problem. If dandelions ever become endangered, then we have much more serious problems to deal with. In fact, people might pay you to dig up their dandelions. It's great to use less of the woodland medicinals and more of the common and abundant weeds, like this one.

Caution

Substances that stimulate the liver can cause drugs to be cleared from the body faster. The root should be avoided if there is a gallstone stopping up the bile duct, because of the bile-stimulating effect. The leaf should be avoided when someone is already too dry or before a long-distance car trip.

HERBAL PREPARATIONS

Both the root and leaf can be used fresh or dry, as tea, tincture, or capsules. The leaves as an infusion are going to be a better diuretic than the tincture, though you can cheat by putting the tincture in warm water. The leaves can be dried for a simple infusion of a teaspoon per cup of water steeped for 15 minutes, or can also be tinctured dry 1:5 at 50% alcohol.

The best preparation of the root is a standard decoction—put a tablespoon of the dried root in a pint of water, bring to a boil, then simmer for 20 minutes. This has more of the prebiotic inulin and a stronger bitter action. It also makes a decent tincture, fresh 1:2 at 80% alcohol or dry 1:4 at 50% alcohol.

elder

Sambucus nigra ssp. *canadensis*
PARTS USED flowers, fruit, leaves

*Elder is gentle enough to use to prevent illness but
strong enough to be used for the early stages of a cold or flu.*

How to identify

It is easiest to spot elder when it's showing off its big white umbrella-like clusters of flowers, but it can be found throughout the year as well. Look for a tree 10–15 feet high with leaves that are opposite and compound, perhaps growing as a solitary tree or as a small colony when established. The leaflets are slightly toothed and pointed at the end.

Just make sure you're looking at a flat-topped umbel (like a giant Queen Anne's lace) with black berries, not a pyramidal flower cluster with red berries, which marks a less common species, *Sambucus racemosa*, which has some toxicity.

Where, when, and how to wildcraft

This first-succession shrub grows in disturbed areas near streams and wet areas because it likes to have its feet wet. Harvest flowers in late May through June, berries in August and September. Either way, just clip whole

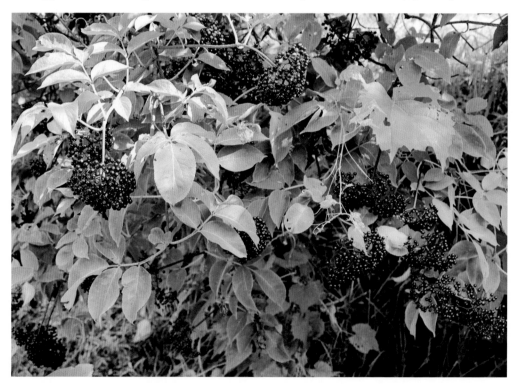

The berries are the most famous part of elder and can easily be made into an antiviral syrup.

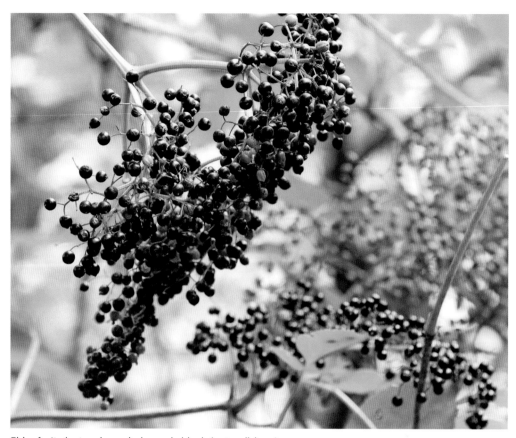

Elder fruit clusters have dark purply black (not red) berries.

umbels into a basket (leaving some for the birds) and sort it out at home. Pick off just the main stems; you don't need to pick off every tiny little floret. Elder is common in every state of the Southeast but occurs only sporadically in Georgia and Alabama.

Medicinal uses

These flowers make you sweat, and that has been one of elder's main uses for a long time: helping sweat out a fever. Recent research has shown the berries to have immune-stimulating and antiviral properties that make elder ideal for the first stage of many acute viral infections such as the common cold or a flu, so now the berries are more popular, but traditionally the flowers

were used more. Some research shows the leaves have some positive benefits as well.

In numerous cultures around the globe, sweating therapy is a primary way to treat colds, fevers, and the flu. From the Nordic sauna to the Japanese sweat bath to Chinese herbs to "release the exterior," sweating has been seen as healing for these acute conditions. In the European tradition, this plant was used as part of a classic sweating tea formula: equal parts elder flower, yarrow flower, and peppermint, then into a hot bath with you.

Raising the heat on a fever may sound strange at first, but there is a reason our bodies respond with a fever: heating the body is the body's natural defense against bacteria

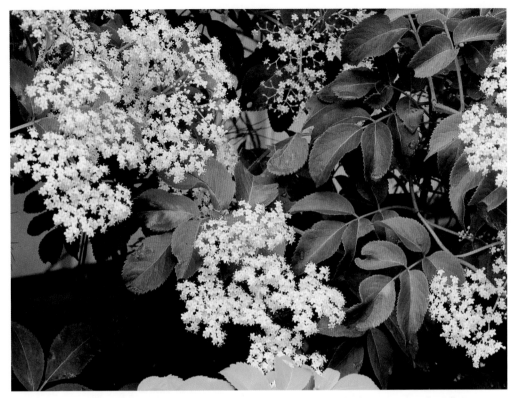

Elder flowers announce the beginning of summer and are often overlooked as an antiviral medicine.

and viruses. Just be careful not to overheat—don't raise fevers of 104 or higher or when someone is already very uncomfortable.

The flowers are also drying to the sinuses and have long been used for congestive (catarrhal) conditions of the nose and sinuses. I've found them helpful in formulas for sinusitis combined with barberry or maybe goldenseal if things get really bad. Less known is their use as an external ointment or oil for burns, bruises, and abrasions.

The berries are high in vitamin C and other flavonoids and have a traditional usage for arthritis and for clearing toxins from the blood. But mostly they are used as a syrup to prevent respiratory infections or to treat them once they've started. They are best for the early stages—they're not strong enough once an infection has set in for a few days.

Future harvests

Even though it is a native plant, it is abundant and easy to harvest sustainably, especially as many of the flowers and berries might be out of reach of most wildcrafters. Just be sure to leave plenty of flowers to create fruits, and plenty of berries to feed the birds who love it. Often that's not a problem: the hard part is getting to the ripe berries before the flocks of birds find them.

HERBAL PREPARATIONS

Flowers (or leaves) primarily used as a hot infusion (for sweating effect). Berries used fresh or dry as a tincture or more commonly as a syrup.

figwort

Scrophularia marilandica
PARTS USED aerial

A deep and slow but powerful blood cleanser and lymphatic.

How to identify

It's one of those plants that's more abundant than you think because it's hard to notice. When it's not flowering, figwort looks like a mint, with opposite toothed leaves on a tall and straight square stem. Then it goes to flower, and the flowers are much smaller than you'd expect from such a large plant—as big

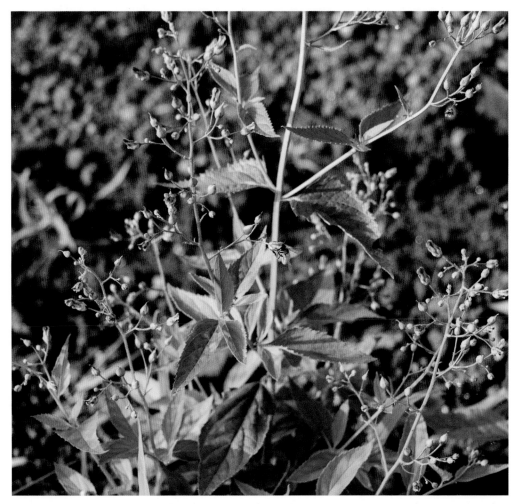

Although figwort flowers are small and brown, the plants often grow in conspicuous clusters on the sides of trails and roads.

as a pinky fingernail and plain brownish; an upper lip juts out further than the lower lip and is redder, the bottom lip greener.

What's more noticeable is that the flowers, although small, are in large branched clusters at the top of the plant with 3–7 flowers coming out of each branch. Those brownish-reddish clusters on top are what can clue you in to stop and look closer, and then you'll see the 2-parted flower.

Where, when, and how to wildcraft

This plant is mostly found in Virginia and West Virginia, and then scattered throughout the rest of the Southeast—south to South Carolina and west to Louisiana and Arkansas, and more common in the mountains. It is said to grow in rich woods, but I see it more often on roadsides, trails, and cleared areas near the woods.

Harvest when the plant is tall and in bloom, which could be all summer long, June through September. Use the whole aboveground plant but especially the leaves. It's OK to harvest before flower if you are sure it is the right plant, but it looks like other plants until then.

Medicinal uses

Figwort is above all a blood cleanser and lymph mover. As such it has a long history of use in chronic skin conditions, lymph swellings, cancer, and even tuberculosis. It is slow to act, but it goes deep in the body to treat obstinate conditions.

Both the common and scientific names of this plant refer to the lymphatic swellings (aka figs, technically scrofula) of cervical tuberculous lymphadenitis, a type of tuberculosis that causes inflamed and irritated lymph nodes in the neck. Though not nearly as common as it once was, it still affects some severely immune-compromised people.

More to the point, this tells us something about what this herb is good for—although not antibacterial itself, it helps to move the lymph tissue, reduce inflammation, and stimulate the immune system in the case of long-term infections. It has even been poulticed topically for wounds and skin ulcerations.

This ability to get things moving also helps with fibrocystic breasts and has long been used as a part of cancer formulas, as most cancers travel through the lymphatic system.

Historically the root was also used as an analgesic specifically for menstrual cramps and labor pains, but I'm not aware that it is still used this way.

Future harvests

This is a common enough plant; but to be safe, harvest only the top half of plants, leaving the rest to regrow.

HERBAL PREPARATIONS

Standard infusion works well, or tincture fresh herb 1:2 at 95% alcohol.

Chionanthus virginicus
PARTS USED root bark, tree bark

A potent herb to cleanse the liver and help chronic skin conditions.

How to identify
Fringe tree is a small tree, growing to about 20 feet high and wide. With its opposite, ovate, simple leaves, it looks a bit like privet or lilac (all are in the olive family), but its leaves are larger, 3–8 inches long. It has a decorative, rounded habit and is often planted in landscapes for that reason.

The easiest time to spot this tree (almost the only time) is when it is in flower in April and May, covered in a profusion of 4-petaled white flowers with impossibly long petals; during the bloom season, the tree has the appearance of something made up for the winter holidays (*Chionanthus* actually means "snow flower"). It produces small blue-black berries in late summer.

Where, when, and how to wildcraft
It ranges from southern Pennsylvania down through central Florida and west across to eastern Texas but is more common at lower elevations on either side of the Appalachian mountains. It likes some moisture and some light and can be found in floodplains, moist ravines, streambanks, and rock outcroppings.

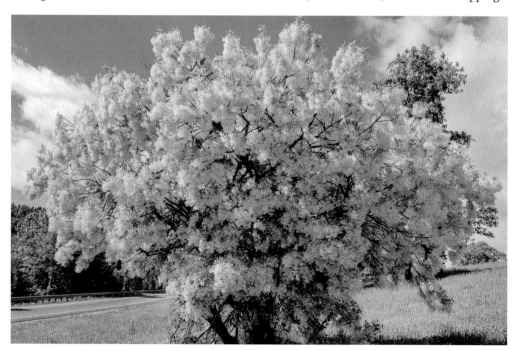

The easiest time to find fringe tree is in the springtime, when the flowers turn the tree into a showy snowball.

Dig it in the fall and either use the whole root or, if the root itself is impressively tough, then just the root bark. The aboveground bark is also decent and can be gathered in the spring. Like some other plants in this book, it is much easier to find this plant when in flower, but it is better to harvest when the tree is not flowering.

Medicinal uses

Fringe tree was one of the favorite liver herbs of 19th- and early 20th-century herbalists, but for some reason it has fallen out of favor. It is an amazing liver herb with a wide variety of uses, including jaundice, gallstones, and chronic skin conditions.

This herb strongly stimulates the liver to cleanse toxins from the body and, like other bitters, also stimulates bile flow and healthy digestion. But it actually tastes better than many bitter herbs—not that it tastes great, it's just that its effect on the liver is stronger than one would expect for how mildly bitter it is, more of a rounded than sharp flavor. It is a great herb to use for jaundice from almost any condition, or any time the skin is yellow, sallow, or has an underlying unhealthy tone to it. It had the reputation of clearing up mild but persistent jaundice that has gone on for years.

It is also an excellent herb for gallstones. It helps stimulate more bile flow to dilute stored bile in the gallbladder as well as stimulating bile release so that it doesn't build up into stones. It can also help pass stones by relaxing the common bile duct, and for this purpose it does well combined with wild yam and black haw to help as antispasmodics and pain relievers.

Herbalists often use liver herbs to treat chronic skin conditions, and fringe tree can work wonders here. Often when working

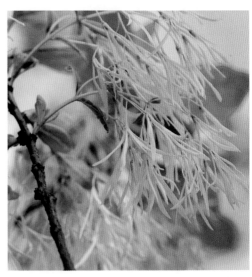

The flowers themselves are small and have 4 thin long petals, which somewhat resemble a fringe.

with a client who has eczema or another type of dermatitis, I find that adding some fringe tree helps amp up a formula and increases its effectiveness.

Fringe tree really is a forgotten but valuable liver herb.

Future harvests

This tree is listed as common to frequent where it grows, but since it is a native tree and the root is used, harvest from places where there is an abundance and be careful not to overharvest.

Caution

Use with caution with active gallstones because this herb can possibly stimulate them to move.

HERBAL PREPARATIONS

Tincture, fresh bark 1:2 at 95%, dry bark 1:5 at 65% alcohol.

---

gentian

Gentiana saponaria, *G. villosa*
PARTS USED root, leaves

Our native version of the most classic digestive bitter.

How to identify

Gentian is an uncommon woodland plant that blooms in late summer and early fall. It has gorgeous deep blue bottle-shaped flowers that are either totally closed or barely open when they are in full bloom. The leaves are opposite, untoothed, smooth, and slightly thick. The whole plant is 1–2 feet tall.

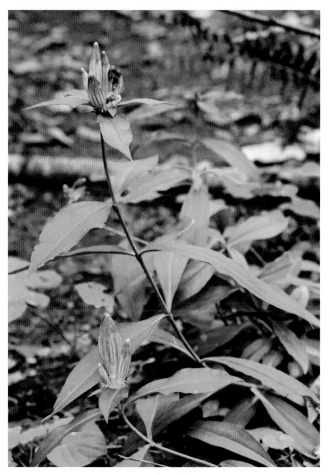

The unmistakable blue of gentian flowers stands out in the fall woodlands, but harvest this plant only when you find it in abundance.

Where, when, and how to wildcraft

Neither of these species is common, but others can be used similarly. Ethical alternatives include European gentian (*Gentiana lutea*), which is commonly cultivated throughout the Southeast, and the bitter-blooms (*Sabatia* spp.), which are more common in the Piedmont and coastal plain.

Gentian can be found blooming from August through October, usually in small stands in rich soil. It likes partial sun, so even though it is a woodland plant it will more typically grow on the edges where some sun can get in.

Though most plants are harvested after flowering, I just dig these roots when in flower because that's when it's easiest to find them.

Medicinal uses

Gentian is the poster child for digestive bitters—it has been used for millennia in Europe, where it is still available as an aperitif at many restaurants and grocery stores. This is probably because the flavor is a pure bitter without any residual yucky flavor and somehow manages to be bitter without being overwhelming.

Digestive bitters are any herbs that taste bitter, as the bitter flavor stimulates digestive secretions by reflex. As such they can be taken 10–15 minutes before a meal to "prime the pump" and get the stomach and liver ready for a meal. They can have a great effect at improving digestion, so are useful for a wide variety of conditions—especially in modern American culture where, except for black coffee, the bitter flavor is almost completely missing.

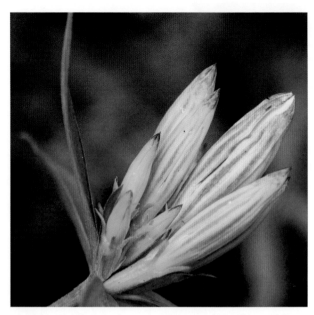

Most gentian flowers don't open any more than this, and if you look closely you may find places where bees have chewed their way through the side of the flower in desperation.

Bitters are great for people who generally have a hard time digesting proteins or fats, those with a poor appetite, or those who feel that no matter how much or how little they eat, the food just sits there: after a regular meal they feel bloated, heavy, and lethargic—the classic "food coma."

Gentian, sometimes combined with other bitters, can also be very useful for lack of appetite caused by pharmaceuticals. This includes the anorexia caused by chemotherapy, where it could be combined with herbs like calamus and prickly ash.

By stimulating bile flow in the liver and gallbladder, gentian also helps the liver function more effectively, as bile is the route the liver uses to excrete toxins into the digestive tract so they can be removed from the body through the feces. Bile also functions as a natural mild laxative and is good for chronic constipation.

By breaking down fats more effectively, gentian can help lower overall cholesterol, especially combined with dandelion and turmeric.

For a simple plant with such a simple action, gentian has a great number of different uses. Typically bitter herbs are considered cooling to the digestive tract so are often mixed with warming herbs like fennel or anise for long-term use.

Future harvests

Gentian is an uncommon plant of deep woods and woodland edges, and as such it should be harvested with great consideration and then only from large patches.

HERBAL PREPARATIONS

Tincture is the easiest way to take this bitter-tasting plant. Tincture 1:2 at 95% fresh, or 1:5 at 50% dry.

ghost pipe

Monotropa uniflora

PARTS USED aerial

An otherworldly plant that helps people disconnect when that's what they need.

How to identify

Ghost pipe (aka Indian pipe, ghost plant, corpse plant) is an unmistakable plant: 8-inch-high clusters of stark white stalks that look like mushrooms. But it does have a pipe bowl of a flower, and the small scales up and down the stem are the reduced leaves. It does not, however, produce chlorophyll and is a myco-heterotroph. That's a long word meaning it gets its sugars from the mycelium of mushrooms that have a relationship with

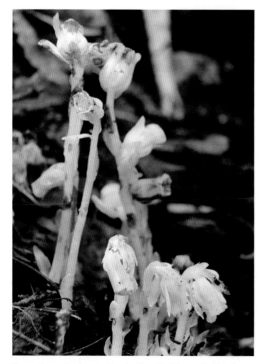

Even though ghost pipe lacks all chlorophyll, it is still a flowering plant, and it does have a symbiotic relationship with mushrooms.

the roots of some conifers—a complex and fascinating relationship with the environment that makes knowing exactly where and when to find it a little unpredictable.

The plants are completely white, sometimes with hints of pink or black, and turning blacker with age or after drying. The single flowers begin pointing down, face sideways when fertile (so they don't collect water but are available to insects to pollinate), and after pollination turn upright, where a dry seed capsule eventually forms. Though they grow in clumps, there is only a single flower per stalk, unlike the related pinesap (*Monotropa hypopitys*), which is thinner, has multiple flowers per stalk, and smells like wintergreen. The latter does not have the medicinal properties of ghost pipe.

Where, when, and how to wildcraft

Though this plant has a huge range, from Maine to Florida and again out west (I've seen it in the forests south of Bellingham, Washington), it is considered uncommon so should be observed and appreciated more than harvested.

It is almost always found near pines or hemlocks, as it is nourished by the mushrooms that have a relationship with those roots. Other than that, where and when it appears is unpredictable, making me wonder if it could be more common than suspected. It can bloom at any time from May through October, after which it disappears back into the soil.

Traditionally the root was the part used, looking more like a tiny bird's nest than anything resembling what one thinks of as a root. But that takes a lot of delicate processing to get clean and takes the whole life of the plant. Most herbalists these days harvest just the aboveground parts of the plant, snapping off a few of the flower stalks here and there. They do the same thing and still turn the tincture a lovely shade of purple.

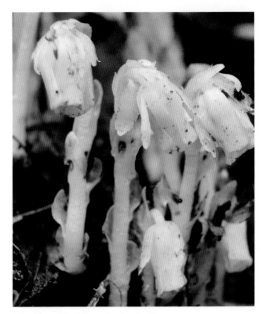

The "bowl" of the pipe is the flower.

Medicinal uses

I like the name ghost pipe because it describes not just what the plant looks like but what it does. It seems to have the strange ability to take one out of one's body a bit, to separate one's self for times when we are too much with the world. Taking enough of it can actually make you feel a bit "ghostly."

Mostly this is used for intense pain. It doesn't so much relieve the pain as make you not care about it, so there's a feeling of looking down on one's body and thinking, "Oh, look at that body in pain." It relieves us of the need to identify with our pain for a while. This effect can be considered somewhat narcotic, though just to be clear I wouldn't call it a "fun" feeling, just a numbness.

This same effect can help when someone is too caught up in their thoughts, in cyclical thinking. Herbalist Chris Marano uses it for PTSD when people get too caught up in their story and need a way to step back. Herbalist 7Song has used it at Rainbow Gatherings for people who are having bad acid trips and are stuck in a loop.

For most people, skullcap would be a much easier and more accessible plant to use for circular thinking and that will do the trick most of the time. Ghost pipe is useful when that plant isn't enough and someone needs a stronger dose of escape.

Future harvests

Sparingly harvest aboveground parts only. It is not a common plant and has become very popular lately, so overharvesting could become an issue. Be gentle with this plant so it can help us in the future.

⚠ Caution

I've had a hard time finding information about the toxicity of ghost pipe, so it is best used short-term. Doses larger than 15 drops can cause people to become spacey and ungrounded, so the traditional "do not operate heavy machinery" warning could be employed here.

HERBAL PREPARATIONS

Fresh extract is best, either a fresh tincture 1:2 at 95% alcohol, or a fresh glycerin extract, 1:2 at 100% glycerin. It doesn't dry well at all. Use doses of 5–15 drops to begin with.

ginkgo

Ginkgo biloba
PARTS USED leaves

An herb that increases microcirculation and
improves brain health, cognition, and memory.

How to identify

Ginkgo is slow-growing, about a foot a year, and is one of the evolutionarily oldest trees extant. It was actually thought to be extinct, but Buddhist monks in China had been growing it and keeping it alive. Now all the ginkgo trees in the world are descendants of that one grove in China.

The trunk is straight with gray bark; the branching habit is pyramidal. The alternate leaves are broad, thick, and flat with strong parallel veins and an indentation at the tip creating two lobes. The leaves turn yellow in the autumn and seem to all fall on (or around) the same day, at the first real frost. It's fun to see a yard covered in yellow as if

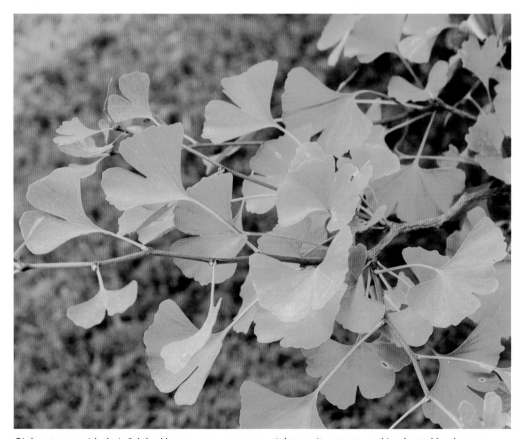

Ginkgo trees, with their 2-lobed leaves, are a common sight on city streets and in planted landscapes.

it's ready for an Andy Goldsworthy project. Often, even in the mountains, the leaves don't fall until November.

There are both male and female trees, and the fruits of the female tree smell like an alluring cross between vomit and dog feces, as one book put it. Let's just say the aroma is strong and far from pleasant, and one never knows whether a tree is male or female until it is old enough to start producing flowers and then it is . . . too late.

Where, when, and how to wildcraft

This popular cultivated tree only rarely escapes to the wild. But it can still be harvested in urban locations, as it is frequently found planted in cities, parks, cemeteries, and such (cemeteries in particular tend to be very quiet). One of the reasons they are planted is because they are incredibly resistant to a number of different environmental factors, including pollution. So be sure to harvest them in a clean area because they could be holding a lot of toxins.

Only the leaves are used, so grab firmly by the petiole and twist off, being careful not to harm the spur where the leaf attaches as that is where next year's leaf comes from. Some flavonoids are highest in the green leaves and some are highest in the yellow leaves, so best practice is to harvest green leaves in June and yellow leaves in October or November, then combine the two for the best medicine. William LeSassier used to pick up the recently fallen yellow leaves for his tinctures.

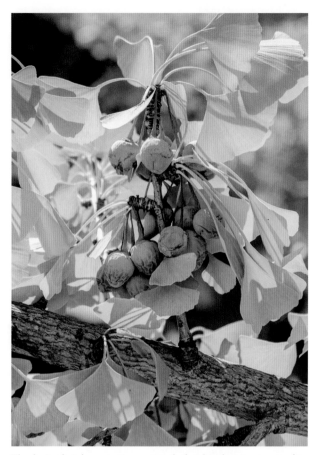

The fruit of ginkgo creates a stench that has been compared to an open sewer and is best avoided if possible.

Medicinal uses

Ginkgo leaves taste a bit like green tea and have similar medicinal properties, though no caffeine—they are powerfully antioxidant and anti-inflammatory, improving the health of the capillaries as well as increasing microcirculation.

Its main effect is as a circulatory stimulant. But somehow it does this without any significant heating, unlike spicy herbs like prickly ash or wild ginger. It seems to gently open up the small blood vessels so that more blood can reach the brain and extremities. It is very useful for poor circulation to the hands and feet, including Raynaud's disease,

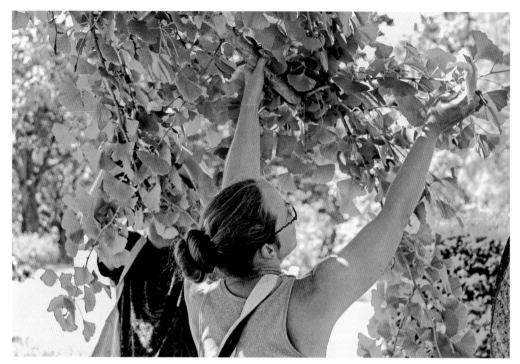
Harvesting ginkgo leaves in a quiet cemetery.

if combined with prickly ash or another heating herb. It can be used for diabetic retinopathy and for erectile dysfunction in men with poor circulation, improving blood flow to the penis, especially if combined with true cinnamon.

This combination of opening up blood flow and its powerful antioxidant and anti-inflammatory effect makes it a great ally for improving cognition and preventing and treating senile dementia. It is sometimes classified as a nootropic, or a cognition-enhancing herb, especially if combined with gotu kola or bacopa.

It has some action on preventing blood clots as well as being anti-inflammatory by inhibiting the action of PAF (platelet-activating factor). It can also help with tinnitus, vertigo, and even intermittent claudication. Its ability to nourish and stabilize blood vessels makes it a helpful preventative for migraine

headaches as well. It needs to be taken for at least a month or two for best effects for these chronic conditions.

Future harvests

This is a cultivated tree, so just be sure not to damage the place where next year's leaves emerge.

Caution

Avoid if also taking anticoagulants (blood thinners) as there is a real risk of interactions. Stop taking 2 weeks before any surgery for the same reason.

HERBAL PREPARATIONS

Mix the dried green and yellow leaves and tincture 1:5 at 60% alcohol. They don't extract well in water, so the best non-tincture method would be to take capsules.

ginseng

Panax quinquefolius
PARTS USED root, leaves

Ginseng is a legendary and powerful adaptogen
that should not be treated as a get-rich-quick scheme.

How to identify

This book is sharing how to identify ginseng (aka American ginseng) so you can observe it, not to harvest it. Because it is getting picked out of the wild so quickly, I strongly advise that you grow it yourself or buy it woods-grown, not wild-harvested. That said, you should know what you're looking at when you're in the woods.

Ginseng has several look-alikes; Virginia creeper is probably the most common and abundant, but that's a vine, not a rooted plant. I once saw someone mistake the berries of Jack in the pulpit for the red berries of ginseng, but besides the fruits they don't look anything alike and taking a bite of that root will make you wish you had never harvested anything at all.

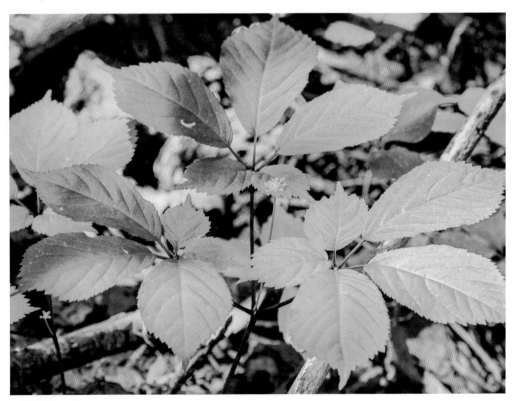

The 5-parted leaf of American ginseng holds a place of magic in southern forests and woodlands but every year is becoming a less common sight.

Look for a plant with palmately compound leaves; typically it will have 3 or 4 prongs, usually with 5 leaflets per prong. If it has more than 4 prongs, it is a very old plant.

The roots of ginseng are tiny compared to the age of the plant, and they are uncommon enough in the wild that it is unusual to find a large enough stand to get any quantity. Another reason not to wildcraft.

Where, when, and how to wildcraft

One word about harvesting ginseng from the wild: don't. It is disappearing at such a rate, even from private land where it is being poached, that we won't have it around to use in 20 years at this rate. There is no wild ginseng in China anymore. Let's not make that mistake.

Many people grow it in their woods. Folks who have been doing it for years often know stands way back in the woods; they have been doing it long enough to recognize that they need to take responsibility for their own actions to protect stands for the future and their grandkids. If you don't get this feeling from the person you are buying from, don't buy it.

Most states where ginseng grows have specific harvest seasons, and you'll need to buy a license to harvest even one plant.

Medicinal uses

Ginseng is a misunderstood and overharvested plant. I am including it because there are specific times when it works really well as a tonic, but too often it is used for the wrong reasons. It is not a stimulant—if someone gets stimulated from taking ginseng, then it is not the right herb for them. It is used for people who are deficient and tired, bringing their energy back to normal.

Now, a lack of energy is one of the most common complaints I hear, but before throwing down 30 bucks on a bottle of ginseng, check out what you're eating and what you're doing in your life. Food has a huge effect on our mood and energy level. And constant stress makes anyone tired, so nervine herbs would help improve sleep and therefore give more energy. Improving digestion is one of the main ways to improve energy in both Ayurveda and Chinese medicine, so either improving diet or digestive ability will always be helpful. These are your raw ingredients.

American ginseng is much more beneficial for us than Chinese or Korean ginseng. Not just because it grows here, but because it is cooler than the other ginsengs. American culture is so full of stimulation that if we take Asian ginseng and are under 40, we run the danger of overstimulating ourselves. American ginseng is less stimulating than Chinese or Korean, though if the wrong person takes it or takes enough for a long enough period of time then it can be overstimulating. This is when it might cause headaches, irritability, and even high blood pressure.

Traditionally, U.S. medicine gave ginseng short shrift because it's not good for any one particular thing. Chinese medicine traditionally loved this herb because it is good for everything. Of course we have to find a middle way.

Ginseng works on the limbic system, which is how the brain talks to the body and the body talks to the brain. The limbic system sets our emotional response to stress, affecting everything from blood pressure to body heat and almost every major hormone in the body, either directly or indirectly. It's at the top of the hormone chain-of-command, the so-called master gland that can affect everything else going on in our body—a powerful place to work, and it's why ginseng can have so many different kinds of action in so many different parts of the body. Many of the herbs called adaptogens also work on the limbic system.

All in all, ginseng doesn't fix anything. It helps our body create more balance and harmony and therefore helps us become more resilient to stress. And that can help a lot.

Future harvests

It is no longer possible to sustainably harvest ginseng from the wild. The exception would be a limited amount of leaves harvested in early fall from a protected stand.

goldenrod

Solidago spp.
PARTS USED leaves, flowers

An abundant plant of autumn that can be used to treat allergies, nasal congestion, and urinary tract issues.

How to identify

All the many species of goldenrod are used fairly interchangeably. This is a general description of goldenrods irrespective of specific species.

Goldenrod is a tall and straight plant, branching occasionally toward the top, with an incredible abundance of small yellow flowers branching off in various kinds of flower heads. Truly a rod of gold if there ever was one. The leaves are long and thin, with a few teeth along the edge. When crushed they have a peculiar smell that is very specifically "goldenrod" but hard to describe exactly.

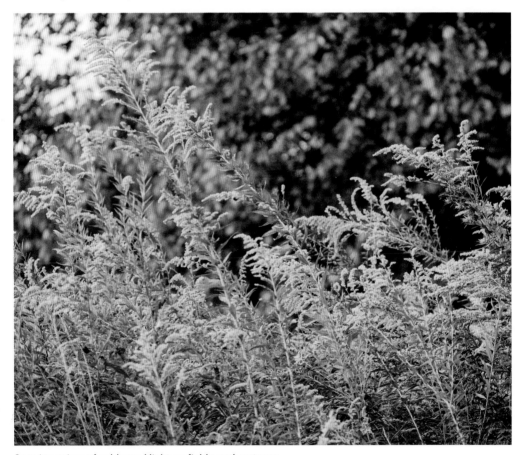

Swaying spires of goldenrod light up fields each autumn.

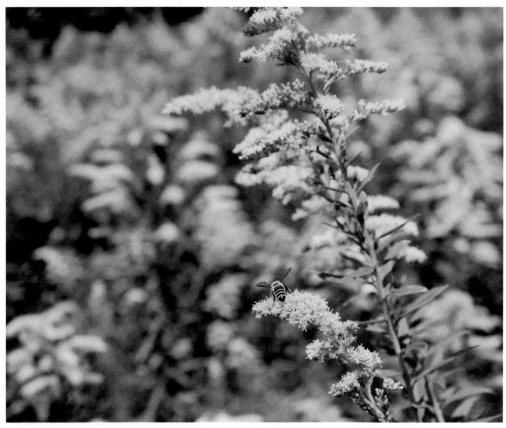

Goldenrods are among the most important late-season pollinator plants, laden with both nectar and pollen for this bee and many others.

Where, when, and how to wildcraft

This is not a hard herb to find, being the most obviously abundant flowering plant of late summer and fall, filling fields with its golden color. You could think of it as one of the colors of autumn. No need to even plant it—just let a corner of your yard go for a year, and goldenrod will be one of the herbs that pops up the next fall.

Goldenrod is abundant throughout the Southeast, and one species or another is found throughout the continent. Just find a meadow or even a roadside in late summer or fall and you'll find some goldenrod.

To harvest, clip above the lowest usable leaves and either strip the leaves fresh or let hang upside down to dry. Put a newspaper down underneath it to catch the flowers as they go to seed or you'll have a mess on your floor, but other than that they dry quickly and easily. Or harvest when they are still in bud and they won't seed out as much.

Medicinal uses

The leaves have a beneficial action on the lining of the respiratory and urinary tracts. As such, goldenrod's been used for allergies, minor colds, and sinus infections in the respiratory system, and for chronic recurrent infections of the urinary tract.

This is not an antiseptic plant; rather, it has a tonic action on the mucosa, the tissue that lines the respiratory, digestive, and urinary tracts. So it's not really killing bacteria or stopping immune reactions so much as it is strengthening the protective membrane in these organs. This is important because it is our first line of defense.

When people think about the immune system, often the first things that come to mind are antibodies, white blood cells, lymph glands, and other players in the immune response to invaders. But our first and most effective lines of defense are our physical barriers—our skin and our mucosa. It's called mucosa because it secretes a layer of mucus that adds an additional layer of protection as well as forming a kind of "fly paper" to trap microorganisms and irritating particles so they can be eliminated from the body before they cause problems.

By strengthening the integrity of these linings, goldenrod helps prevent allergic reactions, urinary tract infections, and other infections. The bugs can't harm us if they can't get through the gate! And because the plant is also astringent and aromatic, it can help dry up and move the excess mucus that is symptomatic of an inflammatory reaction. It helps clear up the debris on the road so traffic can get through again.

It is also a diuretic, helping to get rid of excess water and edema and stimulating the kidneys to excrete more fluid, so it can also be helpful for the urinary tract by flushing the system.

Goldenrod is ridiculously abundant in the fall, easy to harvest, and is a solid preventative/tonic medicine. Go get you some!

Future harvests

Not a problem. There is an abundance of goldenrod in the world.

HERBAL PREPARATIONS

It works best as an infusion—a hot tea usually, but the cool tea is more diuretic and less diaphoretic. Fairly serviceable as a tincture as well, fresh herb 1:2 or dry herb 1:5 at 40% alcohol.

goldenseal

Hydrastis canadensis
PARTS USED root, leaves

This rare plant is a powerful antimicrobial and antiviral for entrenched infections.

How to identify

Goldenseal has a few flat maple-like leaves coming from one root with a raspberry-like fruit coming off one of the leaves. This woodland plant is pretty uncommon and getting more rare; most of the time when I think I've found goldenseal, I've actually found waterleaf (*Hydrophyllum* spp.).

Where, when, and how to wildcraft

This plant is uncommon to rare in most of the Southeast. It is found mostly west of the Appalachian mountains—West Virginia, Kentucky, and Tennessee west to the Ozarks in Missouri and Arkansas. It grows in relatively flat woods, and unlike ginseng it can form large colonies. This makes it easy to

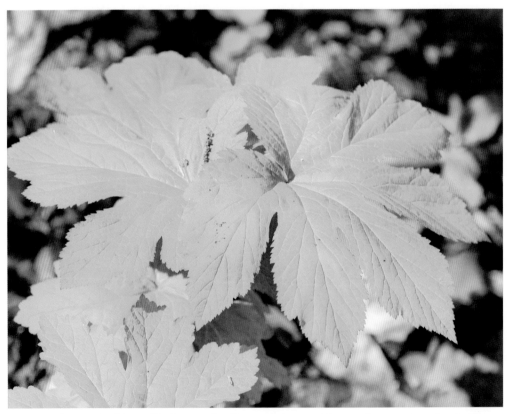

The paired leaves of goldenseal look somewhat like maple leaves with a raspberry on top when fruiting, but the roots have been vastly overharvested from the wild.

overharvest, and people have been harvesting this plant too heavily for hundreds of years, so I encourage you not to harvest it but to plant it in the woods and let it spread. If you find it growing abundantly, remember that this is just an undiscovered remnant of what was once a common plant.

Medicinal uses

Goldenseal is one of several plants (e.g., barberry, yellowroot) that contain the alkaloid berberine, and all these plants are bitter, stimulate the liver, and most importantly are antimicrobial, antiviral, and antifungal. But with this plant becoming rare in the wild and the price reflecting that, what makes goldenseal so special? With all these other antimicrobial herbs out there, when would you choose to use goldenseal instead of another antimicrobial?

Think of this herb specifically when there is a lot of mucus and the tissues are generally more relaxed and lacking in tone. When the mucous membranes are overly relaxed but are also irritated and inflamed, goldenseal helps clear not just the infection but also the associated toxins, creating healthier mucosa. This stage usually happens after the initial infection has progressed deeper into the body and the mucous membranes are semi-exhausted. I rarely think about it for the initial stage of infections but only after an infection has gotten worse.

With this in mind, it is an excellent herb for sinus infections, as well as many kinds of digestive tract infections such as a stomach bug or getting the runs from drinking bad water. It can help lingering urinary tract infections, vaginitis, and cervical dysplasia, the latter two as a pessary. It can also help skin infections such as staph. Goldenseal is a potent herb, good for strong or entrenched infections when the illness has penetrated deeper into the body or is just generally more serious.

It also has some action on lowering blood sugar and is a good stimulant for the liver, increasing bile production and secretion. It was historically used for peptic ulcers long before science understood the role of the bacterium *H. pylori* in causing these.

Future harvests

This is not an appropriate plant to harvest in the wild, as it is being picked much faster than it is growing. The exception would be the leaf harvested in the early fall, which can be used the same way as the root.

 Caution

Contraindicated during pregnancy and probably during breastfeeding, as berberine passes through the milk.

> **HERBAL PREPARATIONS**
>
> Dry root, tinctured 1:5 at 60% alcohol or glycerin.

gotu kola

Centella asiatica, C. erecta
PARTS USED whole plant

A nourishing and calming herb for the mind
that helps promote better memory and focus.

How to identify

There is some debate about what *Centella* species actually grows in the Southeast. Some call it *Centella erecta*; others call it *C. asiatica* (Weakley 2019). How we got an Asian species in the Southeast, who knows, but it's either the same species, a variety of that species, or a closely related species, depending on who you ask—but definitely native.

Whatever scientific name you want to call it, the plant that grows here can be used just like the one in Asia, but it is different from

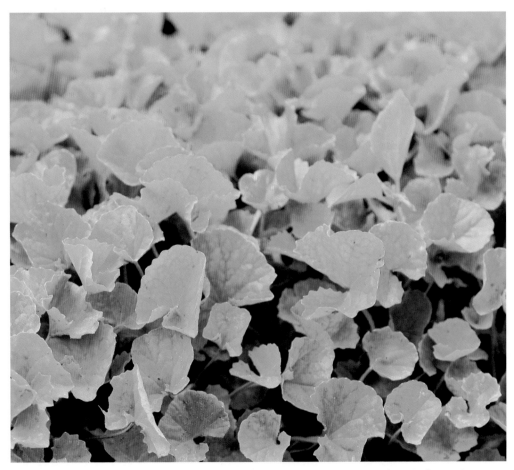

Spreading by runners, gotu kola can form large patches in wet areas next to creeks or in depressions.

its close cousins the pennyworts (*Hydrocotyle* spp.), which may be edible but are not medicinal. In *Centella*, the leaf attaches to the stem at its base, while in *Hydrocotyle*, the leaf stalk is attached right in the middle, shield-like. Half the photos of gotu kola on a recent Google search were actually *Hydrocotyle*, not *Centella*, so this is a quick way to tell the difference. Gotu kola is also a little softer than the leathery pennyworts.

Gotu kola itself runs along the ground, putting shallow roots down and a few leaves up at each node. In places without a frost, it can persist and grow easily. It won't survive outside in places with a frost, so if you think you found it up in the mountains you probably have ground ivy (*Glechoma hederacea*) instead.

The leaves themselves are round to slightly elongated and have scalloped edges. The flowers are in tiny white umbels close to the ground, as the whole plant is close to the ground to begin with.

Where, when, and how to wildcraft

Gotu kola can be found all along the coast, from southern Delaware to the southern tip of Florida, and west through the panhandle and well into Texas. It is usually found in wetter areas than the Hydrocotyle species, next to creeks and ponds where the soil is wet and squishy.

Harvest the plant year-round by simply trailing along and pulling up the runners, then use the whole plant for medicine. If there isn't much but enough to think about harvesting, one could also pluck just the leaves.

Medicinal uses

This is a great herb for calming the mind while enhancing cognition and memory. It grows in similar habitats and has similar uses to bacopa; both are known as brahmi in Ayurveda even though they look different and are not related. Gotu kola is also a good connective tissue tonic.

But mostly it is used as a brain tonic, often combined with ginkgo leaves for help with memory and to improve focus. It's a great herb to take while studying for a test or before meditation. It can even help ADHD, though bacopa has been used more often for that.

The other main use is to help heal connective tissue. It can be used with Solomon's seal to help mend damaged tendons and ligaments, for instance after a sprain or a fracture. Bones actually heal faster than the connective tissue around them, so starting a couple of months after a break, one could add both these herbs to help heal the tissue around the broken bone.

Gotu kola is also used as a skin tonic in Ayurveda, much like horsetail.

Future harvests

Take care when harvesting this plant. It is fairly abundant, but wetlands are fragile ecosystems.

HERBAL PREPARATIONS

Gotu kola can be dried and made into an infusion, or tinctured fresh or dry. A few leaves can also be added to a salad.

Eutrochium purpureum (Eupatorium purpureum)

PARTS USED root

*A great anti-inflammatory for the whole urinary tract;
it also helps move out kidney stones.*

How to identify

Of the five species collectively known as Joe Pye weed (including spotted Joe Pye weed, *Eutrochium maculatum*), only one, *E. purpureum*, is the official gravel root. All are fairly tall plants in the aster family with large clusters of flowers and whorled leaves. Many herbalists use them all the same, but since 19th-century herbalists preferred *E. purpureum*, I will focus on that one species.

Unlike the other Joe Pye weeds that grow abundantly in meadows and wet pastures, gravel root grows in the woods. Since there's less light in the woods, it tends to be a shorter plant, only 3–5 feet high instead of the massive stance of 6–10 feet that many of the others get. And finally, whereas the flowers of most of the others are a beautiful purple, gravel root is barely purple at all—more of a pale lavender. There is usually a purple dot at the leaf node, and if the leaf is crushed it should have a hay-like smell after a couple of minutes.

Where, when, and how to wildcraft

Gravel root blooms from August to September in dry to mesic woods, often on trailsides or in small clearings where it can catch more light. The other Joe Pye weeds bloom July to September, attracting clusters of amazing butterflies and other pollinators.

I usually wait for the plants to go to seed then dig up the roots with a digging fork, if

The real gravel root is shorter than other Joe Pye weeds, grows in the woods, and has flowers that are only slightly purple.

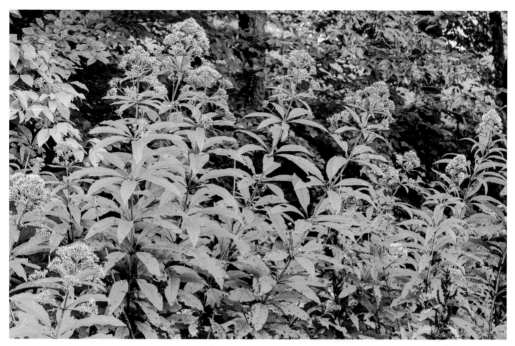

Most American herbalists use all the Joe Pye weeds, such as this spotted Joe Pye weed, interchangeably.

necessary, and a soil knife. The roots are smaller than one would think and tend to grow in dense soil.

Medicinal uses

As its name implies, gravel root is traditionally used for kidney stones or gravel in the urinary tract. Though it does a great job moving stones, it is also a great anti-inflammatory for any irritation or inflammation in the genitourinary tract and is also a pelvic blood mover.

For kidney stones, I combine gravel root with wild hydrangea and stone root and make it as a decoction. Be aware that besides helping to break up stones it can also help get stones moving very quickly, so be prepared. Meaning, be near a hospital in case pain medicines are needed, though black haw will get you through until you get there.

It can also help with prostatitis, a sometimes painful inflammation of the prostate.

Here it works to decrease the irritation and therefore helps with some of the pain. It also works generally for painful urination, though it won't help treat an infection; if that's what's causing the pain, an antiseptic herb like yarrow or pipsissewa should be added.

Gravel root also has some traditional use for pelvic pain with a feeling of heaviness in the loins.

Future harvests

Gravel root is not an uncommon plant, but always harvest with care so as not to disturb its woodland habitat. The field varieties of Joe Pye weed are usually so abundant that less caution is needed.

HERBAL PREPARATIONS

Fresh root tincture preferred, 1:2 at 95%, or dry root 1:5 at 60%.

hawthorn

Crataegus spp.
PARTS USED flowers, fruit, leaves

The best nourishing tonic for the heart, both physically and emotionally.

How to identify

The many species of hawthorn are challenging to tell apart, even for botanists. Not to mention that they often interbreed, making it even more confusing. Luckily, as a group, they are pretty easy to identify.

Hawthorns are small trees that grow on the edges of woods and back in a bit, though they tend to have more flowers and berries where they get more sun. They have long acupuncture-needle-sized thorns that don't branch, unlike those of the related crab apple,

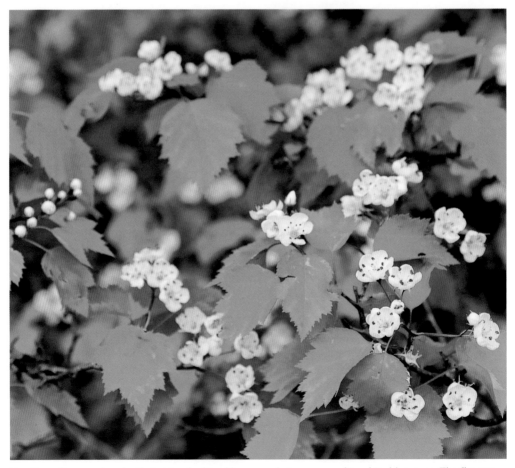

Hawthorn flowers abundantly in May, looking like an apple tree covered in white blossoms. The flowers are just as medicinal, if not moreso, than the berries, which are more commonly used for medicine.

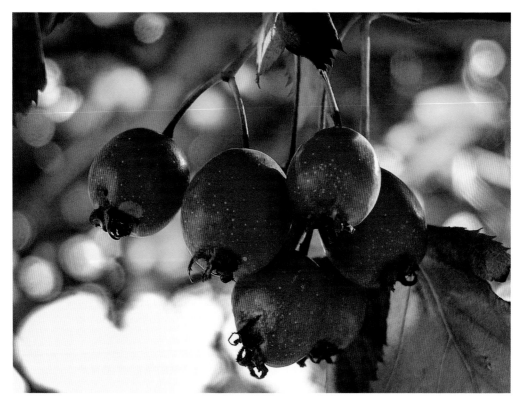
In the fall, the berries can be picked after they turn red; they are a great food for the heart.

which sometimes do. The leaves are variously shaped, but the most common shapes I see are either triangular with sharp teeth or thick, oval, and barely toothed.

The 5-petaled white flowers bloom in clusters in spring; they eventually turn into red berries with yellow flesh. The flowers have a unusual stink about them, typical of many white-flowered plants that are pollinated by flies in spring.

Where, when, and how to wildcraft
Find the flowers in mid-May depending on weather, elevation, and species, and the berries in fall (September–October). When I harvest flowers, I pick a whole branch with a few leaves in there too. Look for fresh new flowers with good-looking stamens at their center. The buds just before opening are

actually higher in flavonoids than the flowers once opened, so be sure to include some buds.

In the fall, I harvest the red berries off of trees after they are ripe but before the bugs get to them. If possible, look for darker-colored berries with more orangey-red flesh because they are more likely to have a high content of flavonoids.

Herbalist Alanna Whitney puts one thorn in her hawthorn tincture and I love that idea, so I've been doing that now too. We need to protect our heart.

Medicinal uses
Hawthorn is almost the definition of a tonic herb: it is literally food for the heart. I can't think of a heart problem it wouldn't help, and yet it's such a gentle herb there is virtually no overdose potential. When I gather

the berries, I often pop a few in my mouth to snack on.

Hawthorn is the queen of heart tonics, at least partially because so many herbs that work on the heart are strong stuff. It is so gentle it can be taken in larger doses over a period of time. These days, several companies make concentrated solid extracts, or for home medicine you can just make jam and put it on whole grain toast every morning.

With time it strengthens and protects the capillaries through its flavonoid content, so it's good for the blood vessels. It also dilates the coronary artery, opening it up to bring more blood to the heart muscle so the heart can function more efficiently.

These are the main modern uses of hawthorn—to protect the blood vessels from damage and from attachment of cholesterol (like blueberries), to nourish the heart to prevent heart attacks, to help with congestive heart failure, and to normalize blood pressure.

But hawthorn is also excellent at stabilizing collagen and healing connective tissue. Tendons and ligaments are connective tissue, and hawthorn can be very helpful in recovery from injury. It is not anti-inflammatory like turmeric or willow but can be used to clean up after the inflammation, so that a short-term injury doesn't become a long-term one. For this, it combines well with gotu kola, some vitamin C, and maybe some plantain and horsetail.

Note that Chinese hawthorn, which tastes much more sour, is used very differently, for food stagnation and indigestion primarily. One of those "I ate too much" kind of herbs, especially if it is too much meat. Our species of hawthorn don't seem to have the same effect.

Future harvests

Not a problem. But still, leave some behind, for the birds and animals who like to eat the berries.

HERBAL PREPARATIONS

Fresh tincture of flowers, fresh or dry tincture of berries and leaves. So many possibilities! Hawthorn syrup, hawthorn fluid extract, hawthorn vinegar, honey, and more.

honeysuckle

Lonicera japonica

PARTS USED flowers, green vines

A common weed that is a powerful antiviral for flu and colds.

How to identify

This tough green vine has opposite, entire, oval leaves that will often survive the winter. The very young leaves can have an oak-leaf shape when they first emerge in spring before becoming the classic honeysuckle leaf shape.

The flowers are paired, long, tubular, and either white or yellow, with a tuft of stamens messily sticking out the tip; these, by summer, have turned into 2 pairs of red berries that turn black when fully ripe. The scent of the flowers is the very smell of spring-time.

Most other honeysuckles, some native and some not, are shrubs in the genera *Lonicera* or *Diervilla*, so although Japanese honeysuckle is the most common of these plants, make sure that the plant is a vine, not a shrub, and that the flowers are in pairs coming from the tip of the plant and from the leaf junctions along the vine. Other species can be emetic or purgative, so make sure to harvest the right one.

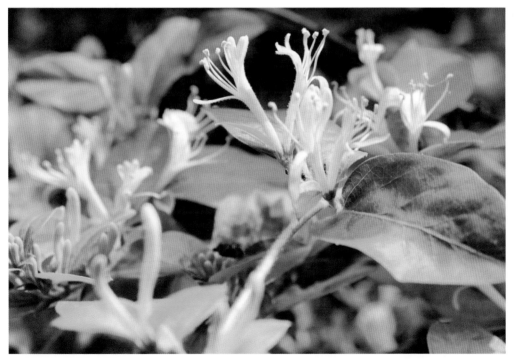

The yellow and white flowers of the honeysuckle vine that perfume the spring air are both a tasty treat and a powerful antiviral.

Where, when, and how to wildcraft

This is a common weed vining up hedges and fences throughout eastern North America, from Ontario and Maine south to Florida and west to Kansas and middle Texas. Harvest the flowers when they are club-shaped buds just about to open. Though it flowers through the summer, the easiest time to harvest is in early spring when there is a lush abundance of these juicy flowers. It takes a long time to gather a pint's worth because they are so light, so bring some friends to help or plan a day around it.

The other option is to use the green stem, the vine itself, harvested in summer after most of the flowers have finished. Though easier to harvest, it is considered less effective but is still official in the Chinese materia medica.

Medicinal uses

Our knowledge of this plant comes from traditional Chinese medicine, where both the flowers and vines are used to "clear heat," which in this case means it helps fight infections. Modern research has shown it to be an effective antiviral and antibacterial as well as being somewhat anti-inflammatory.

The flower buds are considered the strongest medicine and are in some ways the echinacea of Chinese medicine. They are a primary herb used in formulas to treat the onset of head colds and influenza, especially when there is a fever, and can also be used for sinus infections, ear infections, and sore throats. They are antimicrobial but also help reduce the inflammation caused by these bugs. The vines do the same thing, just not as strong.

Japanese honeysuckle can treat diarrhea and dysentery by killing the microbes that are causing the digestive upset. Interestingly it is also considered a mild laxative; maybe it helps flush out the bad stuff. It is not an antiparasite; it doesn't kill worms and other multi-cell critters, but it does seem to be effective against single-cell organisms, such as the kind one gets from drinking bad water.

The plant can also be used topically for sores, abscesses, ulcerations, warts, and other acute skin conditions.

Future harvests

No worries about overharvesting this abundant and invasive weed.

HERBAL PREPARATIONS

Traditionally prepared as a dry flower tea, but the fresh flower tincture or glycerite is great and drying flowers can be challenging.

horsetail

Equisetum arvense, E. hyemale
PARTS USED whole plant

A diuretic and astringent that helps heal connective tissue,
horsetail can also be used as a tonic for healthy skin and hair.

How to identify

The two common species of horsetail in the Southeast are found throughout the northern hemisphere, and both have identical medicinal uses. All horsetails look somewhat like a telescoping radio antenna, hollow with nodes along its length.

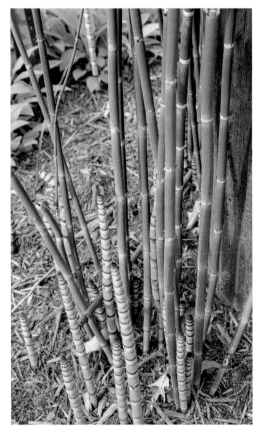

The entire horsetail plant can be harvested for medicinal use.

Horsetails predate ferns in evolution, dating back almost 400 million years, making them some of the earliest vascular plants. The field or common horsetail (*Equisetum arvense*), like some ferns, has two different forms—a fertile form for a short time in spring for reproducing and then a sterile form that photosynthesizes. First there is the pinkish white hollow stalk with a strobile on the top that produces the spores. Then when that dies back, a vegetative stalk grows that looks similar but has whorls of needle-like leaves, which makes it look like a baby pine tree.

The scouring rush horsetail (*Equisetum hyemale*) has dark green stalks shooting straight up without side stems. Instead of alternating two different forms, it has just one form that both photosynthesizes and produces a spore-producing strobile.

Where, when, and how to wildcraft

Horsetails, like ferns, need water nearby for the spores to reproduce, so they are most commonly found on streambanks, wet meadows, and railroad embankments. Common horsetail is found from Canada south to northern Georgia, but mostly in Virginia, West Virginia, Kentucky, and Tennessee, then west into the Ozarks. Scouring rush horsetail is found from Canada south to South Carolina, with a similar range but going further south into Alabama and all along the Mississippi River Basin down to Arkansas and Louisiana.

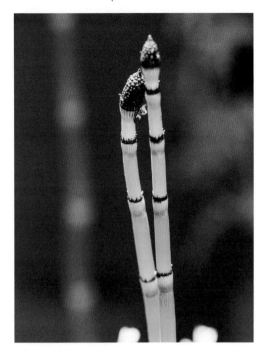

The stems of horsetail are hollow and jointed like an old radio antenna.

Harvest the leafier sterile stems in spring or summer, or even into the fall, but harvesting earlier in the year is considered better by some. Just be very careful about where you harvest because this plant does an excellent job of taking up not just minerals but heavy metals, too. If growing in a polluted area or near commercial agriculture, it can contain a compound that blocks the uptake of thiamine, one of the B vitamins.

Medicinal uses

Horsetail is a diuretic and astringent, making it a great herb for urinary tract conditions. Containing a good amount of silica, it is also a great tonic for hair, skin, and nails as well as connective tissue. And finally, it can somewhat alleviate internal bleeding.

The silica content of this unusual plant is reported to be as high as 25% of dry weight, making it a wonderful nutritive for all kinds of connective tissue. Silica is a necessary cofactor with calcium to build healthy bones, so horsetail can be used to treat osteoporosis and support recovery from bone fractures. It also improves collagen strength, improving the tone and elasticity of hair, skin, and nails, used both internally as well as topically.

As a mild diuretic, it increases fluids more than solid excretion, so it is considered more of a volume diuretic than a cleansing diuretic like nettle, though the two plants go very well together. It has been used to treat urinary tract infections, but what it really excels at is reducing inflammation, pain, and bleeding of the urinary tract, not elimination of any particular bacteria. It has a mild action to reduce internal bleeding in general but is even more specific for blood in the urine. It can be added to any formula for a UTI with pain and discomfort, whether there's blood or not.

Future harvests

Horsetail is abundant where it grows and in some places is considered a noxious weed, even though it is native. There is little danger of overharvesting.

Caution

If harvested near commercial agriculture, plants may contain nicotine and aconitic acids from uptake of nitrates. Also contains thiaminase, which breaks down thiamine. So, not for long-term use, and not for use by pregnant women.

HERBAL PREPARATIONS

Standard infusion, internally or topically. Would probably make a decent vinegar infusion as well.

Japanese knotweed

Reynoutria japonica (Polygonum cuspidatum)

PARTS USED root

An invasive weed that offers great medicine as an anti-inflammatory, antimicrobial, and deep cleanser.

How to identify

Because it can grow up to 10 feet high, Japanese knotweed can easily be mistaken for a shrub, but it is actually a perennial herb. Like bamboo, its hollow stems are jointed and plants grow in dense clusters, but the leaves are quite different. The distinctive zig-zag stalks hold the oval leaves; each leaf is about 6 inches long and 4 inches wide, with a flat base and coming to a sharp point at the tip.

At some point during the summer plants put out elongated clusters of small white flowers. The plant spreads by underground rhizomes, and even a small piece of the root can grow more plants. Outside of Japan almost all plants are female, which is why they don't produce seeds.

Where, when, and how to wildcraft

This common noxious weed from east Asia has spread across the mountains and Piedmont as far south as northern Georgia and scattered further south. By the time you read this, it will have spread even more. It is rated as one of the top 100 most invasive plants and animals by the IUCN (International Union for Conservation of Nature).

It often grows next to waterways, and when flooding washes away some roots, it replants itself downstream. But it's not picky and can also be seen around old barns, in fields, and on roadsides. It can pop up from underneath asphalt and through building foundations and is extremely hard to get rid of.

Japanese knotweed was originally introduced as an ornamental; the wands of its flowers are now seen growing on roadsides and along streams in late summer.

The roots are not easy to dig. They're not deep so much as convoluted and all through the soil, one plant lapping on top of the next. And they break easily so it's hard to get a whole root. It takes some patience and dedication to dig it, but it's well worth it—both for the medicine it provides and to save a place from invasion.

Medicinal uses

Hated as a noxious weed, this plant has so many medicinal uses that it's hard to find a way to sum them all up. It is anti-inflammatory, antimicrobial, anticancer, and antioxidant. It is also protective to the cardiovascular system, and recent research shows it has neuroprotective effects as well. It is used in Chinese medicine for many kinds of pain and inflammation, including acute injuries.

This recent addition to the American materia medica has been used medicinally in Asia (where it's native) for millennia. It is probably best known as an anti-inflammatory due in some part to its extremely high content of resveratrol, the highest concentration in nature. Resveratrol, the famous antioxidant in red grapes, is behind the "French paradox": the people of France have a low incidence of heart disease even though their diet is high in saturated fats. Turns out there's a lot more to this than just red wine, and saturated fats aren't as dangerous for our heart as was originally thought. But this is what made resveratrol famous and led to a lot of the research showing it is a powerful antioxidant that can help prevent and possibly treat cancer, it inhibits COX-2 (a pro-inflammatory chemical in our body), and it restores glutathione levels (an important part of our liver's detoxification pathways).

All this makes Japanese knotweed an amazing anti-inflammatory and antioxidant.

These powerful effects are what make it so useful for everything from joint injuries and pain (acute inflammation) to cancer, cardiovascular disease, and prevention of senile dementia (all made worse by chronic inflammation). It is one of the main ingredients in Zheng Gu Shui, a Chinese remedy for acute injuries and broken bones.

It is also antimicrobial against both bacteria and virus but is more of a slow and deep antimicrobial. In other words, it's not used for colds and flu so much as infections that have gone deep in the body and are hard to get rid of. It is one of the main herbs used in many Lyme disease protocols. Japanese knotweed seems to go deep into the tissues and help clear these entrenched infections, even crossing the blood-brain barrier to help with Lyme-induced effects on the nervous system.

This ability to cross the blood-brain barrier combined with its powerful antioxidant effect make it excellent for preventing Alzheimer's as well as supporting recovery from stroke and brain injury. It has been shown to be very protective to neurons as well as helping in neuronal regrowth.

There's probably even more to this amazing plant, and it is insanely weedy. The more that we harvest and make medicine with it, the better chance our native plants have of surviving.

Future harvests

Please dig it. Dig as much as you can. Please.

HERBAL PREPARATIONS

Fresh root tincture 1:2 at 95% alcohol, dry root tincture 1:5 at 60% alcohol. To make root tea, use a standard decoction. It can also be made into a liniment for topical use on injuries by infusing the fresh or dry root into isopropyl alcohol.

juniper

Juniperus virginiana
PARTS USED fruit, leaves

A powerful urinary tract antiseptic.

How to identify

Junipers are evergreen conifers up to 30–40 feet tall. Instead of having long needles like pines or spruces, they have some tiny needles and some scales, and the needles are usually paired or in a whorl of 3 on younger branches. As they get older, the trees get more scale-like leaves, but there are usually some short needles on younger branches and those lower down.

But the easiest way to tell a juniper is by its fruit, a berry-like cone (which is still technically a cone even though it's commonly called juniper "berry"). There are both male (pollen-producing) and female (berry-producing) trees, so not every juniper will have berries on it. In this species (aka eastern red cedar), the cone matures each year, whereas in some other junipers it takes two years to mature. The fragrant

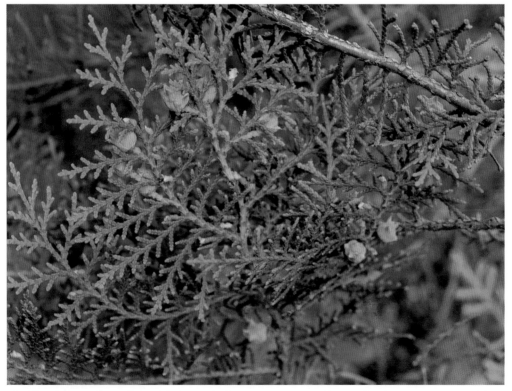

The blue "berries" (actually modified cones) of juniper are a great cleanser for the urinary tract, and the leaves aren't bad either.

heartwood is a beautiful reddish color that makes wonderful incense; it is often worked into cedar chests.

Similar plants include southern juniper (*Juniperus virginiana* var. *silicicola*), white cedar (*Thuja occidentalis*), which has only overlapping scales and no needles, and common juniper (*J. communis*), a low-growing shrub that is found worldwide. Common juniper is actually the species most commonly used in medicine, but it is rare in the Southeast, being more common in Europe, New England, and the western states.

Where, when, and how to wildcraft

This juniper is abundant from Canada to southern Florida and west to the middle of Texas. It grows in fields, along roads, and on wood edges. The fleshy cones/berries mature in the fall, so that is the best time to harvest them. You can harvest leaves any time of the year by trimming some lower branch tips, and they can be used similarly.

Medicinal uses

Juniper is first and foremost one of the best remedies for urinary tract infections, even when they are intense deep infections. But it is also a great blood cleanser and circulatory stimulant, which makes it very useful for chronic joint pain.

This is such a powerful herb for urinary tract infections that it has traditionally been used even for bad infections that have gone deep. It is so powerful as a diuretic, astringent, and antiseptic that it is helpful to add a demulcent herb like plantain in there as well.

It stimulates the kidneys to clear not just fluids but to remove waste products. This makes it helpful as a general body cleanse, especially when there is joint inflammation.

The circulatory-stimulant effect combines nicely with this. It has a long history of use for chronic rheumatism, both used internally and applied externally on painful joints.

It is also an aromatic bitter that stimulates digestion and promotes healthy assimilation. It should be used in moderation though, as using it by itself or in too high a dose can cause too much stimulation and associated discomfort, or griping as it is sometimes called. The leaves make a good addition to a bitters blend, which would work better than just the berries by themselves.

This is a potent heating and drying remedy that can kick a UTI by itself, but it is often best used in combination to avoid overstimulation.

Future harvests

This is an abundant plant and usually produces an abundance of "berries," so observe regular precautions about not overharvesting and it will be fine.

Caution

Juniper is contraindicated during pregnancy because of its blood-moving effects. Although some authors say the berries irritate the kidneys, naturopath and herbalist Eric Yarnell reports that the berries are not toxic to the kidneys. He believes this mistake might have been made for various reasons, including confusion with the volatile oil of *Juniperus sabina*, but the short version is that juniper is safer than generally reported.

> **HERBAL PREPARATIONS**
>
> Dried berry tincture, 1:5 at 65% alcohol, or dried leaf or berry infusion.

Pueraria montana var. *lobata* (*P. lobata*)
PARTS USED root, flowers

Stops alcohol cravings and helps muscular pain.

How to identify

If you don't know what kudzu looks like, then you probably haven't spent long in the Southeast. The tough vine is spreading, climbing, and forms dense mats over acres of land and up trees. Kudzu is a hairy vine with 3 lobed leaflets on each leaf; a hard frost kills back the leaves, but the vine persists and will regrow the following spring. In late summer and early fall there are clusters of wisteria-like purple flowers that smell for all the world like grape jelly.

Where, when, and how to wildcraft

Known as "the vine that ate the South," kudzu was brought to this country to control erosion. It has taken over huge areas and is now growing in our region from southern Pennsylvania south to Florida and west to southern Missouri and eastern Texas.

Because it takes over fields and climbs trees, it can be hard to figure out where the roots are until the frost kills the plant back and the vines can be traced back to the roots. It is said to grow a foot a day, so folks will warn you not to leave your window open at night! At least it's in the pea family, so it fixes nitrogen and improves tough clay soil—if you can ever get rid of it to plant other things.

Once you find the root, your work has just begun. The roots go straight down and they go deep, so you'll need a sturdy shovel, though a

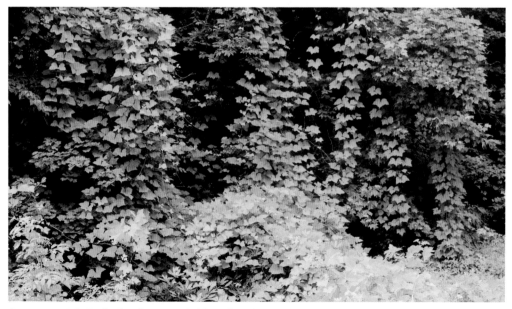

A common sight in the Southeast are fields and yards completely taken over by kudzu vines.

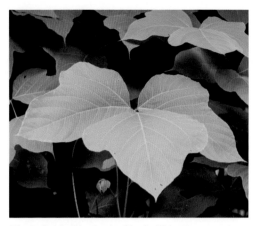

The individual kudzu leaf looks like other members of the pea family with 3 leaflets.

tractor or a backhoe are other options. Dig as deep as you're willing to go (it's highly unlikely you'll get to the bottom), use a soil knife to cut the root, and then just pray it doesn't come back from the part that's left.

Medicinal uses

Kudzu is another Asian herb with a long history of medicinal use in its native continent that has become weedy in North America—much like burdock, mimosa, or Japanese knotweed. Learning to use these herbs helps us appreciate these abundant plants as abundant sources of medicine.

Kudzu root is mostly used in Western herbal medicine to reduce alcohol cravings and help with hangovers, but in traditional Chinese medicine it is used for viral infections and for relaxing tight muscles. For centuries, it has been used in formulas for upper respiratory infections. Although it's not particularly antiviral, this abundant weed helps to open things up and move the pathogen out, and it's specifically used when there's shoulder and upper back tension that comes along with an infection. It is cooling

and moistening and can be used to help clear fevers while nourishing the fluids of both the lungs and the stomach. It has been used for both chronic diarrhea from digestive deficiency and acute diarrhea with fever.

Although I first learned it as relieving muscles aches specifically from an illness, it can be used more generally as a mild antispasmodic for tight and tense muscles, and is starting to be used more broadly for acute neck and shoulder pain and injuries. It can also help sinus headaches.

The flowers and the roots have long been used as an antidote for excessive indulgence in alcohol, both to relieve hangover symptoms and to decrease desire for further indulgence. This is not Antabuse, but it does support someone who wants to quit by decreasing cravings for alcohol; for this purpose, it is usually taken as capsules, tea, or a glycerin extract.

There is a lot of promising research on kudzu for other actions as well, including treating high blood pressure, lowering blood sugar, stopping internal blood clots, and treating coronary artery disease. It is also high in phytoestrogens. That's a lot of claims for one herb, but it does seem worthy of further investigation.

Future harvests

Oh please harvest it! The world needs more medicine and less wild kudzu.

HERBAL PREPARATIONS

The roots fresh or dried can be prepared as a tincture or a glycerite, fresh 1:2 at 95% or dry 1:5 at 50%. It's a nice one to have as an alcohol-free extract for those quitting alcohol.

Packera aurea (Senecio aureus)
PARTS USED leaves, flowers

A useful plant for short-term use for menstrual problems.

How to identify

Liferoot (aka golden ragwort, birthwort, yellow groundsel, female regulator) is the most medicinal of the dozen or so *Packera* species in the Southeast; the others may be toxic. All have small aster family flowers of both yellow disks and rays in abundant open clusters. Liferoot is a stand-forming plant, so sometimes there will be many yards of these plants where found.

This species in particular has two different kinds of leaves—vaguely heart-shaped basal leaves somewhat resembling violets, and stem leaves that are linear and deeply lobed. The basal leaves are more toothed than violets with a rounded, not pointed, apex, and are usually purple on the underside—a type of antifreeze produced by the plant because it comes up so early.

Where, when, and how to wildcraft

This species can be found from Pennsylvania south to northern Georgia and northern South Carolina, and west through Tennessee

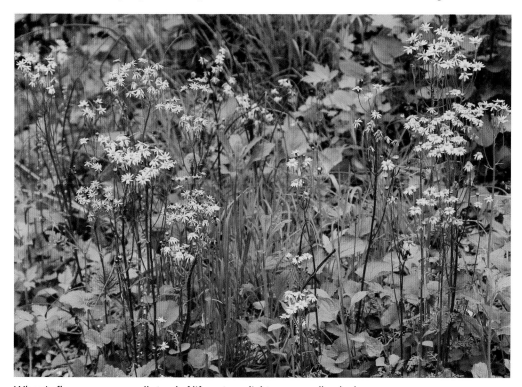

When in flower, even a small stand of liferoot can light up a woodland edge.

to Arkansas, and is incredibly abundant in the middle and southern Appalachians. It is so prevalent, large stands are as easily spotted driving down an interstate highway as on a forest service road.

Plants like moist woods but aren't very particular about where they grow, including roadsides, yards, woods, and wooded streambanks. When not in flower, their round basal leaves mix with violet leaves throughout the growing season.

Harvest the basal leaves and flower heads in April and May when they are in flower. Some herbalists and midwives use just the flowers, not the leaves.

Medicinal uses

Liferoot is a powerful herb for moving pelvic blood flow. Because of this, it can be a helpful herb for menstrual cramps, bringing on birth, and for prostate issues.

It is important to note up front that although this used to be used both acutely and as a tonic, it is now only used short-term: it contains pyrrolizidine alkaloids.

What this herb does really well is stimulate pelvic circulation, which makes it excellent for delayed menses and congestive (as opposed to spasmodic) dysmenorrhea. The latter shows up as menstrual cramps

with a heavy feeling in the pelvis and dull, achy pain. It can also be used for men when there is difficulty urinating or a dragging feeling in the testes.

One of the common names, birthwort, probably refers to its ability to bring on labor. An abundant plant with some good uses, it is rarely used these days because of the toxic potential. Blue cohosh might be a good substitute to stimulate pelvic blood circulation.

Future harvests

It is a native plant but grows abundantly in many places.

Caution

Not for long-term use (longer than 2 weeks). Not safe during pregnancy. The pyrrolizidine alkaloids can have negative effects on the liver, so contraindicated for anyone with a history of liver issues or who has used or been exposed to substances that might be hard on the liver.

HERBAL PREPARATIONS

Tincture of fresh flowers and leaves, 1:2 at 95% alcohol.

Tilia ×*europaea*
PARTS USED flowers

A sweet and gentle remedy for relaxing the nerves and calming the heart.

How to identify

Although several *Tilia* species, all known as basswood, are native to North America, the cultivated European linden, or lime, is the focus here. It is a moderately tall straight-trunked tree with grayish bark. The leaves are heart-shaped, uneven at the base, sharply toothed along the edges, dull green above, lighter green below, and come to an abrupt point at the tip. The main veins branch out straight from the base. The leaves are 2–4 inches wide, much smaller than those of the native basswood trees. Those native basswoods might also have medicinal flowers, but they produce fewer flowers that are borne much higher up in the tree.

The flowers come in a bundle off a long and angled yellowish bract and have 5 even off-white petals that are almost obscured by the abundance of stamens.

Where, when, and how to wildcraft

Like ginkgo, lindens are commonly planted in cities because they are tolerant of a wide

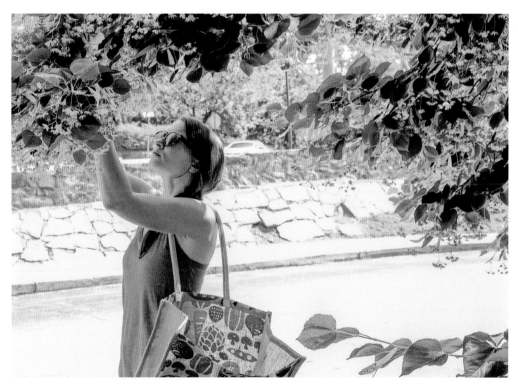

Anna Claire Lotti harvesting linden flowers in a grove planted around a little-used parking lot.

variety of conditions, including pollution. So be sure to always harvest from a clean area. It is rare that they go wild, so it is best to find a planting of linden that is in a seldom-used parking lot or side street.

Harvest the flower with the bract in mid-June when in full flower and the citrusy scent hangs in the air. Harvesting early on a sunny day is best for both the flowers and the most aromatics. Make sure the stamens still look young and fresh; if they are starting to brown, then skip that flower—often different trees right next to each other will ripen flowers a few days apart. Because a lot of pollinators are also attracted to these flowers, be careful not to get stung when harvesting.

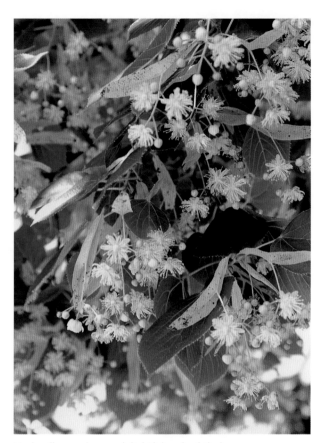

Linden flowers have a delightful and subtle fragrance.

Medicinal uses

Linden is a special sweet plant that is beloved by many, even though it is more of a social tea than a strong medicinal. Taken over time and with intention, even the gentlest remedies can have powerful effects.

Linden flowers, or flores de tilo, is a favorite after-dinner tea in many parts of the world, right up there with chamomile. It is a sweet relaxing herb that has a gentle action on the heart, both the physical and emotional heart. It uplifts the spirit but also gently lowers blood pressure and relaxes the heart muscle, preventing hypertension and arteriosclerosis.

It can be used for palpitations from stress, anger, and nervous agitation. It also has a positive effect on digestion.

Future harvests

No worries about overharvesting; we use only the flowers of this cultivated ornamental tree.

HERBAL PREPARATIONS

Though linden flowers are most commonly made as a simple and tasty infusion, they can also be tinctured fresh 1:2 at 75% alcohol.

Hericium erinaceus
PARTS USED whole mushroom

A tasty mushroom that is good for the immune system and promotes nerve growth.

How to identify

It has been wisely said that you should never harvest a mushroom unless you are 100% sure of its ID, and I completely agree. Great care should be taken with any mushroom, but this is a fairly distinctive mushroom with no poisonous look-alikes (for those who are used to looking at mushrooms). It does have some look-alikes, but they are related and also edible, though they may or may not be medicinal themselves. All the same, please be careful: there are many more poisonous mushrooms than poisonous plants.

That said, lion's mane grows, shelf-like, out of wounds in hardwood trees, primarily oak and beech in eastern North America. It is a tooth mushroom: instead of gills or pores, it has long spines or teeth growing down, which with some imagination resemble a beard or perhaps even the mane of a lion.

The mushroom should be all white. If it is starting to brown or has a bad smell, then it is too old to use. When cooked it tastes like seafood.

Where, when, and how to wildcraft

Typically fruiting in late summer and fall, it can also have a window of fruiting in a late cool spring. The visible mushroom is actually the "fruit," meaning it contains the reproductive or spore-producing parts. The actual vegetative part of the mushroom is the mycelium—the thin white threads that are embedded in the tree.

To ethically harvest, use a sharp knife to cut the

Lion's mane is a type of tooth fungus that grows on damaged trees; this one is growing on an oak in coastal South Carolina.

mushroom from the tree so that the mycelium aren't harmed and they can keep growing and perhaps produce another year. This is true of most mushrooms: harvesting is like picking an apple off of a tree and won't damage the actual organism itself—though it is also important to leave enough around to produce spores.

Once harvested, the soft mushroom can be sliced and either cooked fresh or dried for later use, or it can be made into a double extraction tincture either fresh or dried.

Medicinal uses

Like reishi and many other medicinal mushrooms, lion's mane has immunomodulating polysaccharides that are nourishing and balancing for the immune system. This alone would make it a great medicine, but it also has the unique ability to stimulate nerve growth and repair, making this a supremely useful medicine for many things, such as stroke recovery, healing nerve damage, and prevention of senile dementia.

The immune properties of lion's mane are pretty good, though not as strong as those of reishi and some of the other heavy hitters. There is some research based on traditional use for treating several different types of cancer. It's unclear whether it actually kills cancer cells or more likely stimulates the body's own ability to clear the cancer.

Lion's mane's effect on the nervous system is particularly unique and noteworthy. It has been called one of the most potent inducers of nerve growth factor synthesis, that is, it stimulates neurons to regenerate and grow after damage (Rogers 2011). This property has led to further research on its use for everything from stroke and concussion recovery to prevention of Alzheimer's and other forms of senile dementia. Though some of this research is speculative and is different from most of its traditional use, I have

seen it subjectively help people with recent concussions, especially when combined with other neuro-tropho-restoratives like milky oat seed and skullcap. And this is how it is currently best known in Western medicine.

In traditional Chinese medicine, hou tou gu (as it is known) is used to nourish all the major organs of the body for many types of deficiency, but specifically for weak digestion with fatigue and for gastric ulcers.

This medicinal mushroom is incredibly powerful and also pretty tasty, and deserves much more research and use.

Future harvests

This is a fairly abundant mushroom, but still—leave plenty behind to make spores for future generations of lion's mane. Also, be sure to use a knife to separate the fruiting body from the tree it is growing on so as not to damage the mycelium.

This increasingly popular mushroom is also readily cultivated, and many companies sell kits to grow it at home, which is easier than finding it in the wild and also more sustainable.

HERBAL PREPARATIONS

Like most medicinal mushrooms, it contains polysaccharides, which are more water soluble, and other constituents like saponins that are more alcohol soluble. So, to make a preserved extract, I prefer to use a double extraction method.

First simmer the dried mushroom for several hours, then cool, and add alcohol to the mushroom and tea to both preserve and extract the alcohol-soluble portions. Make sure the final product is at least 25% alcohol by volume in order to remain shelf stable. For complete directions, see page 30.

lobelia

Lobelia inflata
PARTS USED aerial

A potent plant for opening up the lungs and breaking up mucus.

How to identify

Lobelia (aka Indian tobacco, pukeweed) is more common than you would think; it's just hard to notice. In fact, if you see a big showy lobelia plant, then it's not the right species. The species used in medicine is small and thin, 1–2 feet high (occasionally up to 3 feet) and has quarter-inch-long white or bluish white flowers. The flowers, like all lobelias, are distinctively 2-lipped with 2 lobes pointing up and 3 lobes pointing down.

The leaves are alternate and have wavy, slightly toothed edges; the stem is slightly hairy and often branched. Lobelia is slightly more noticeable when it goes to seed, as the seedpods become inflated like tiny Chinese lanterns (hence the epithet).

If the lobelia you find doesn't branch, has more blue flowers, and the seeds aren't inflated, it could be *Lobelia spicata*. If the flowers are large, blue, and showy then it is probably *L. siphilitica*, and if it has large red flowers and grows near water then it is *L. cardinalis*. There is some historical use for some of these plants, but they are not *L. inflata*.

Where, when, and how to wildcraft

You can find lobelia in many overgrown meadows as far south as Tennessee and northern Alabama. It seems to like dry, acidic meadows near the

The most medicinal species of lobelia has small vaguely blue flowers.

woods, maybe with some pine and sassafras nearby. It also seems to like edges—sides of trails, where the meadow meets the woods, and places like that. It is an annual and has an interesting habit of showing up abundantly one year then just about disappearing the next.

The small flowers bloom in mid-summer, but the medicine is a bit stronger if you wait until August or September, when there are both flowers and seedpods on the plant. Seedpods are actually considered the strongest part of the plant, but since the whole plant is pretty strong to begin with, don't worry too much about that.

To harvest, clip the plant just above the lowest good leaf and use the whole thing—stem, leaf, flower, and seed. Plants usually grow back from the cut and make more seeds later in the year. Plan some extra time for the harvest; it takes a while to find enough to make a pint of tincture.

Medicinal uses

Lobelia might be best known as an emetic (hence pukeweed), but it is one of the strongest herbs to open up the lungs. It is commonly used for asthma and bronchitis as both a stimulating and relaxing expectorant. It is also a great antispasmodic and muscle relaxant.

It can work wonders for acute asthma attacks, quelling an imminent attack quickly, though it is no replacement for an inhaler. It works by both opening up the bronchioles and relaxing the smooth muscle. This is a very potent herb and should always be started with a low dose of 3–5 drops, and then slowly increased if needed. When it is needed for acute attacks, it seems that larger doses can be used without encountering the nausea and negative effects, but it is still wise to start small and work up.

The seedpods of this lobelia inflate like Chinese lanterns.

It is also a powerful expectorant for bronchitis, dilating the bronchioles, allowing for easier coughing up of gunk (relaxing expectorant) while simultaneously causing a mild irritation to the lining of the lungs which helps to break up thick stuck mucus (stimulating expectorant).

Because of its ability to stimulate the vagus nerve, taking too much can cause vomiting, and even taking a strong therapeutic dose can trigger the vomiting up of mucus, although sometimes that's needed.

The plant also contains the alkaloid lobeline, which is chemically similar to nicotine (though not addictive) and fits nicotine receptors. This makes it helpful for those quitting tobacco, especially when combined with nervines like milky oat seed and skullcap, and maybe some calamus too.

This lobeline also has a strong antispasmodic effect on the muscles. So this could be used for a spasmodic cough like whooping cough, or it could be used to loosen tight and tense muscles. As a muscle relaxant it is usually used topically, either as an infused oil or an infused vinegar. It is very potent and can lead to generalized floppiness—so imagine some kind of "do not operate heavy machinery after use" warning here.

Future harvests

To harvest ethically, make sure you have a large stand before you start picking. Though I always do a stand count before I harvest any plant, it's even more important with lobelia because sometimes it's not abundant, and even where it is abundant, it is scattered. And it is an annual, so always make sure to leave some plants to make seeds.

 Caution

This is a potentially toxic plant and should be used with great respect and caution. Again, too high a dose will cause vomiting; and for some people, any amount will cause vomiting. But the vomiting will help prevent any further toxic effects.

If for some reason someone takes a large amount and doesn't vomit, it could cause muscular weakness, stupor, sweating, rapid heart rate, prostration, and even coma or death in very large amounts. Note that some reviews of cases where lobelia was blamed for death indicate that the plant was not the cause of death.

Not for use during pregnancy, as one might guess.

HERBAL PREPARATIONS

Fresh is best with this plant, as the dried herb is less complex and has more of the emetic effect. It is so lightweight and so strong that the whole aboveground plant can be tinctured fresh 1:4 in straight alcohol, adding 10% vinegar to help bring out more of the alkaloids. To make an alcohol-free medicine, simply extract it in straight vinegar for best results.

This is a low-dose botanical! Start with 3–5 drops of the extract before giving any more, then if more is needed add 5 drops at a time until it either works or causes too much nausea.

For topical use, infuse the whole plant in a good fixed oil (raw sesame oil, extra-virgin olive oil, almond oil) and let sit for a few weeks before straining. You can also use the heat method. The vinegar extract can also be used topically.

Albizia julibrissin
PARTS USED bark, flowers

An incredibly uplifting plant.

How to identify

Mimosa (aka silktree, tree of collective happiness) is usually a short tree, though it can reach 30–40 feet. The leaves are doubly pinnate, divided into many fine leaflets, with branching leaflets coming off a main axis.

It is easiest to find in bloom, when it is covered in hundreds of pinkish sunset-colored flowers that are easily spotted even while driving down the highway. Each individual flower looks like a fairy paintbrush with numerous stamens protruding in a flat fan.

This species should not be confused with plants and trees of the genus *Mimosa*, also in the pea family (Fabaceae), which have similar leaves but more spherical flowers, and whose leaves curl up when touched. The trees in *Mimosa* have different uses and grow further south.

Where, when, and how to wildcraft

This native of Asia is a common plant of disturbed areas throughout the Southeast and Midwest, often considered a weed tree

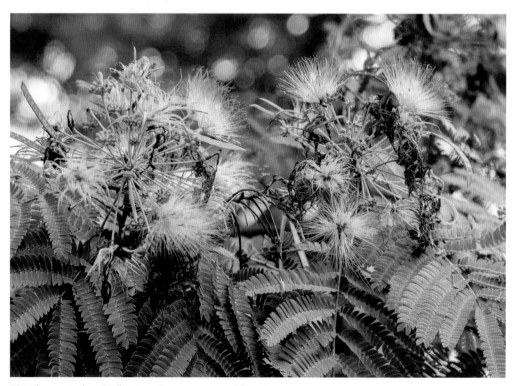

The "fairy paintbrush" flowers of mimosa are uplifting just to see.

because it grows fast and fragile. It is conspicuous along many roads and interstates when in flower.

Blooming from June through August, it is easy to find. The harder part is finding it in a place that is safe to harvest from. So look for it on country backroads, where it might be 10 feet or more off the road, wide trails, and other open disturbed areas. I recommend not gathering it off the side of I-40.

The bark is best in April and May but can be harvested throughout the growing year. Most barks peel off more easily in spring, when the new bark is forming, and mimosa is no exception. Use loppers or a folding saw to trim limbs that are crossing or shading each other out, then strip the bark off—never strip bark off a living tree!

To strip the bark, use a sharp knife to cut a circle around, then a foot away or so cut another circle. Then cut a line between the circles and use the edge of the knife to pry it up a bit. Often the bark will peel off easily from the heartwood this way, giving nice clean quills.

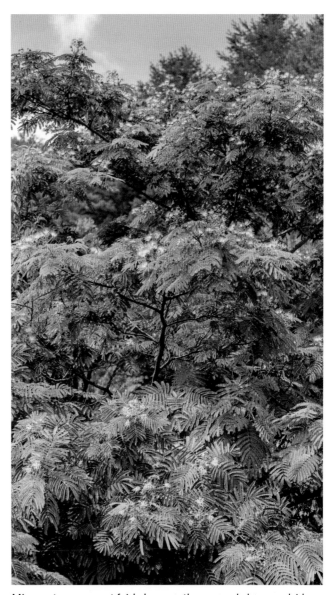

Mimosa trees can get fairly large as they spread along roadsides.

To pick flowers, plan on spending a few hours harvesting. Pick bundles of flowers that have a nice color to them and haven't browned or have too many old flowers in the bundle. This is easier and faster than picking the flowers one by one. Harvest by the flower stalk so that you don't bruise the tender filaments.

Medicinal uses

Mimosa is incredibly uplifting and helps calm a disturbed mind. It is beginning to get popular in Western herbalism, but our knowledge of this plant's uses comes from Chinese medicine. As you might guess from its Chinese name, he huan pi ("collective happiness bark"), it is an excellent remedy for depression, insomnia, trauma, and grief. Really, any shock to the system.

Taking the flowers internally imparts the same feeling as looking at the flowers does—joyous wonder. They are uplifting, a pleasant escape from everyday troubles, and help relieve a troubled heart. They are often discussed as an antidepressant, but they are more like a pause button on worry, like coming home from work and having a drink. They lighten the heart and gladden the spirit for a while.

The bark seems to work more deeply and subtly. It also helps uplift the spirit and treat depression but penetrates more deeply into the body and mind, helping to move stuck trauma and emotions and shift perspectives. Though not as immediately uplifting as the flowers, its effects are more profound; it is useful for working with PTSD, emotional insomnia, and stuck kinds of depression, like a melancholy feeling. It opens things up and allows things to move with more ease.

Because of this ability to get things moving, both bark and flower have a traditional use for physical trauma as well—a remedy for bruises and bangs.

Future harvests

No worries about overharvesting this exotic invasive in our region.

 Caution

There are some reports that the uplifting quality can aggravate mania in people with bipolar disorder. Do not use the bark during pregnancy: there's a possibility of it causing uterine contractions. Although no drug interactions are noted, I would still advise using caution when taking it at the same time as psychoactive drugs.

HERBAL PREPARATIONS

Fresh bark or flower, 1:2 at 95% alcohol. Dried bark 1:5 at 50% alcohol.

---

motherwort

Leonurus cardiaca
PARTS USED leaves

A relaxing herb that helps the heart, calms the mind, and balances hormones.

How to identify

Like most plants in the mint family, motherwort has a square stem and opposite leaves, but unlike most mint plants it is lacking in any kind of aroma beyond just green plant smell. The leaves have two different shapes, both being simple and deeply lobed. The basal leaves and those low on the stalk are palmately and sharply lobed, somewhat like a Canadian maple leaf, but most of the leaves on the flowering stalk are elongated with just 3 teeth at the end.

The flowers are small and purple, in clusters on the top third of the plant. After they finish flowering, the calyx that is left behind becomes sharp and pointy.

Where, when, and how to wildcraft

Motherwort is abundant in Virginia, West Virginia, and northern Kentucky, and is scattered through the mountains of North Carolina, across Tennessee, and into Arkansas. It is so obnoxiously weedy in the Northeast and upper Midwest that plant people from there

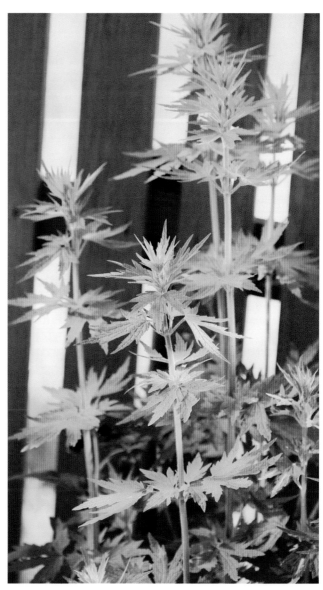

Motherwort can be a weed in some places; plant it along a fence to keep it contained.

laugh at herbalists who plant it in their gardens in the Southeast. Harvest in late spring and early summer when the plants are in flower, though they can be harvested earlier or later as well. The challenge with harvesting them in the middle of summer are those calyxes where the flowers used to be—they're small but incredibly sharp and poky. As long as the leaves are green and looking good, they can be used for medicine.

Medicinal uses

Motherwort is another one of those plants that does so many things it is hard to characterize. It is a nervine herb for anxiety, insomnia, and pain; it is a hormonal herb for PMS and hyperthyroid; it is a heart remedy; and finally, it's a liver herb that also works on the digestion.

First and foremost though, it is an herb for the nervous system. It is a great herb for anxiety and nervous tension, especially if the person gets a fluttery feeling in their chest when they get anxious. It can even help with insomnia where people feel really irritated. It is a great remedy for stressed-out overworked at-their-wits'-end parents—taking some just makes you feel that maybe it's not such a big deal that your kid just dumped ketchup on the table.

It's also a good remedy for nerve pain, especially combined with skullcap and St. John's wort. It can help prevent or shorten a herpes outbreak, and it is one of the best herbs I've seen to help with the intense pain of shingles, used both topically and internally.

The scientific binomial translates to "lion-hearted," and this herb is great for heart palpitations due to nervous tension. It can also be used for mild atrial fibrillations and

tachycardia. It settles a stressed-out heart. It also helps lower high blood pressure due to stress.

For hyperthyroid, it has some action to block TSH action on the thyroid, so it helps to lower circulating thyroid hormone. This can be especially helpful when combined with bugleweed.

A close relative used in Chinese medicine, *Leonurus sibiricus* (yi mu cao, "herb to benefit the mother"), is considered a blood mover. Even if it's not exactly the same as motherwort, it helps explain some of what motherwort does. Specifically it gets things moving, helps with menstrual cramps (especially in a slow-onset menses), and can improve PMS.

And finally, motherwort stimulates the liver and can act as a digestive bitter, though its nervine action is stronger; it would be best used when someone needs a relaxant *and* a digestive bitter.

It's not an easy herb to encapsulate, but it's a great one to have around because it just has so many uses.

Future harvests

It is fine to harvest this invasive European plant in abundance. It will probably come back whether you want it to or not.

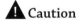 Caution

Be careful using in hypothyroidism. Not for use during pregnancy.

HERBAL PREPARATIONS

Fresh plant 1:2 at 95%, or dry plant 1:5 at 60% alcohol. Standard infusion, a half cup per dose.

---

mountain mint

Pycnanthemum incanum

PARTS USED leaves

An aromatic herb to open the lungs and clear phlegm.

How to identify

The mountain mints are tall and thin mints that prefer wood edges to the typical fields and meadows preferred by most plants in that family. They have opposite, barely toothed egg-shaped leaves that come to a point. The stem is square and branches only in the upper third of the plant. The small purplish flowers are in tight heads at the end of the branches; leaves are directly underneath the flower head.

What's most distinctive about this species is the white dusting on many of the upper leaves, which explains its other common name, hoary mountain mint: it looks like it's been hit by a hoar frost. All the leaves, even the young ones, have fuzzy white undersides.

Where, when, and how to wildcraft

This species is common from southern New York down to South Carolina, west to Kentucky and scattered across the Deep South.

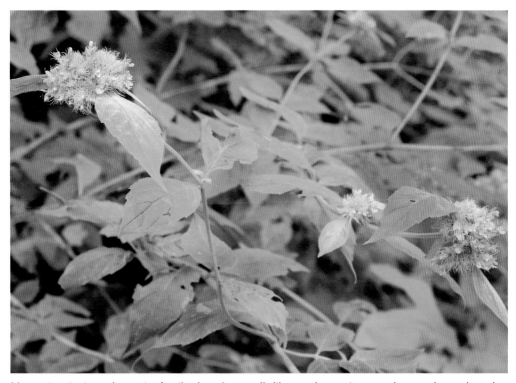

Mountain mint is a robust mint family plant that smells like eucalyptus; its upper leaves, always dusted with white, look as if they've been frosted.

It prefers wood margins and trailsides with mostly shade and some sun but can sometimes be found in fields.

Harvest the whole plant when in bloom in the summer, cutting just above any bad leaves, and bundle and hang to dry.

Medicinal uses

This is not a commonly used medicinal, but it grows abundantly in many parts of the Southeast, so it's a great herb to know about. Most of what it does can be explained by the flavor, which is stronger than most mints—it's like a cross between peppermint and eucalyptus. So like many mints, it helps relieve congestion and improve digestion.

It is a good decongestant and a mild expectorant for colds, helping to clear up mucus and reduce the inflammation. It also helps to sweat out fevers even more strongly than peppermint. It would be a good herb to use as a steam inhalation for sticky phlegm that's stuck in the lungs.

Like all minty-tasting plants, it stimulates digestion. It is specific for flatulent colic, as they put it in the older books, meaning it's good for indigestion that feels crampy and makes one fart.

Finally, it could be a useful plant for soft tissue injuries—sprained ankles and strained muscles. Apply topically, either as a poultice or as a liniment.

Future harvests

This plant isn't uncommon, but still—gather from places where there is a fair amount. As with many other mints, leaving the lower half of the plant will help it spring back.

Caution

Because of the strong volatile oils in this plant, it is not advised for long-term use.

HERBAL PREPARATIONS

Mountain mint can be made into a strong-tasting tea that is tasty if you really like mint, but Patricia Howell (2006) says she prefers the cold infusion because it's not quite so intense. It can also be put into just-boiled water and the vapors inhaled as a steam inhalation by creating a tent over the pot with a towel. The strong aromatics in the plant also make it a useful poultice, mashed up and put on a joint injury.

Verbascum thapsus
PARTS USED leaves, root, flowers

A soothing herb and mild expectorant for lung infections and inflammation.

How to identify
Mullein is a fuzzy plant, perhaps the fuzziest, the vegetable version of flannel jammies. It is green and thickly hairy with long leaves that form a basal rosette the first year; in the second year, the plant puts up a flower stalk with alternate leaves and a spike of yellow 5-petaled flowers. The leaves are fuzzy and soft, and attach onto the stalk so that it looks like they continue down the stem.

Plants are much larger than lamb's ear (*Stachys byzantina*) and have taller flower stalks. Lamb's ear, being in the mint family, has opposite leaves and square stems, and is generally whiter than mullein, though just as fuzzy.

Where, when, and how to wildcraft
Mullein grows across the East Coast as far south as northern Florida. It is common in any disturbed area, such as roadsides and

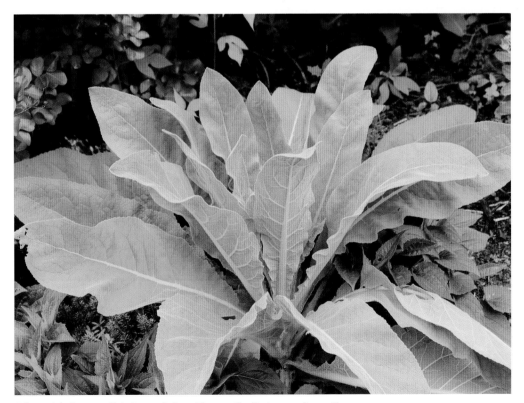

A biennial plant, mullein has only basal leaves the first year of growth.

edges of parking lots and yards. The hardest part is not finding the plant, it's finding it in a place that is safe to harvest from. It just loves to grow in nasty polluted areas.

Harvest the leaves in mid-summer, choosing ones that are not too young and tender but aren't so old as to be bug-eaten.

Medicinal uses

Mullein is probably the most commonly used herb for all kinds of lung problems. It is soothing and moistening yet stimulating enough to expel phlegm. It can be used for everything from bronchitis to asthma. The root is an excellent astringent and diuretic for the urinary tract and has recently been rediscovered as an herb for back pain, and the flowers are a classic for ear infections. An infused oil of the fresh flower can be combined with infused garlic oil and dropped in the infected ear. The garlic is more antimicrobial, and the flowers are cooling, soothing, and anti-inflammatory.

Mostly it is the leaf that's used for healing lung issues. It has the unusual property of being both moistening and drying, and honestly this herb is so broadly useful that it's hard to describe exactly the best time to use it. Although it's listed as a soothing demulcent, it's more soothing because it reduces inflammation and stimulates more fluids to flow to the underlying tissue.

Being a lymphatic herb also helps its properties for the lungs. In the deep part of the lungs where the bronchioles are too narrow for cilia, extra fluid is removed via the lymph system instead of through expectoration—I think of this as "sideways removal" as opposed to the upward removal of expectorants. This in part is how mullein helps in bronchitis and even pneumonia, though it is not a strong expectorant like angelica.

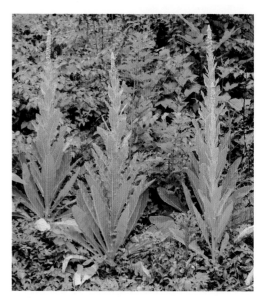

In the second year, mullein shoots up a flower stalk with medicinal flowers before dying completely in the fall.

I have used the root of mullein with agrimony for urinary incontinence, either from age or after pelvic surgery. But I also learned from herbalist jim mcdonald that it is a great remedy for back pain and spinal pain.

Future harvests

This is an invasive weed. Harvest all that you need.

HERBAL PREPARATIONS

Leaves can be prepared as a simple infusion, but be sure to strain the tea well as the fine hairs can get caught in the throat and cause some irritation. They can also be tinctured at 1:6 or 1:7 (it is absolutely impossible to get it to be 1:5, they are so lightweight) at 50% alcohol.

The root can be used as a decoction or tinctured fresh 1:2 at 95% or dry 1:5 at 50% alcohol.

Urtica dioica, U. gracilis, U. chamaedryoides
PARTS USED leaves, seeds, root

*One of the most important herbal medicines with
a host of uses, nettle is both building and cleansing.*

How to identify
This plant looks almost mint-like with opposite serrated leaves and a squarish stem, but
look closer and you'll see lots of little hairs
poking straight out on the stem and on the
leaves. If you brush up against the plant,
you'll notice that these hairs sting like hell,
causing an itchy sensation that can last for
a day.

The hairs are actually trichomes, hollow
tubes that can poke under the skin and inject
a dose of formic acid, the same ingredient
that's in red ant bites, and acetylcholine, a
neurotransmitter. Curiously enough, if you
grasp a nettle leaf firmly, the trichomes crush
instead of poking in and there's less likeli-
hood of getting stung. Word of caution—on
the lower stem these trichomes can get quite
hard; they will never quite crush and do
still sting.

Strings of inconsequential male and
female flowers form at the leaf axils on different plants, both being green-brown at first,
ripening to grayish.

Where, when, and how to wildcraft
Nettles are most common in disturbed areas
around waterways but can also take over old

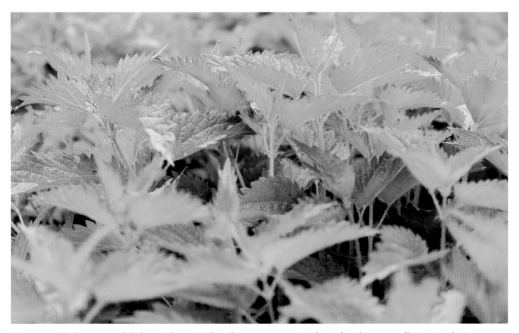

Young nettle leaves could almost be mistaken for a peppermint if not for those small stinging hairs.

fields, meadows, and barn yards; in some places (such as up and down the French Broad River in western North Carolina), they've spread along rivers and creeks into less-disturbed areas.

American stinging nettle (*Urtica gracilis*) is more upright and less branching than European nettle (*U. dioica*) but with hardly any stinging hairs on the stem and only some on the underside of the leaves. European nettle, an exotic invasive, is found from North Carolina and Tennessee north; American stinging nettle can grow as far south as Florida.

In the Deep South one is more likely to find dwarf stinging nettle (*Urtica chamaedryoides*), a native annual plant with shorter leaves and a strong sting. Be aware that when people talk about nettles in Florida, they are often referring to bull nettle, the unrelated *Cnidoscolus urens* var. *stimulosus*, which is not medicinal; besides Florida, it can also be found in mid-Tennessee, Arkansas, and Louisiana.

All these plants are usually found in clusters—if you find one you're likely to find a hundred.

Nettle leaves are best harvested before they go to flower and seed, which means March through late May or June depending on how far south you are, the elevation, and how much sun the plants are getting—plants in the sun tend to flower earlier. Wear gloves and long sleeves while harvesting. You'll get stung anyway, but enjoy it as a way that the plant is helping you be more present and pay attention. Dry them by bundling the bottoms of the stems with rubber bands and hanging the small bundles upside down. Once dry they won't sting, but the stiff

trichomes are still present and can still cause some skin irritation when handled, especially the larger stalks.

Seeds are harvested in mid-summer. There are male and female plants; the male flowers point upward, and the female flowers droop down and eventually produce the brownish seeds. Harvest when they are green-brown and slightly unripe, then dry on a screen with newspaper underneath; thresh or strip them once dry.

The roots are dug in the autumn; they are actually stolons, meaning instead of going deep down they run along just beneath the surface, acting as underground lateral stems, much like many plants in the unrelated mint family.

Medicinal uses

Nettle is one of the most important plants in Western herbalism. In the words of David Hoffmann: when in doubt, use nettles. Mostly the leaves are used for herbal medicine, but the roots have their own specific uses and the seeds are starting to come into clinical practice as well.

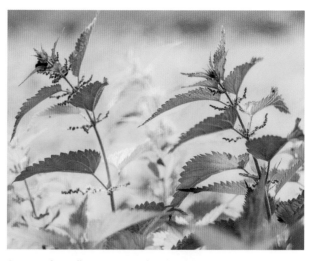

Strings of tiny flowers, several inches long, emerge from the leaf axils in both male and female plants.

Nettle has a long tradition of being used for anemia and nutrient deficiency, especially combined with oatstraw to help balance out its drying aspect. What's amazing about nettle leaves is that they are both nourishing and cleansing at the same time. They are high in many vitamins and minerals, including iron, calcium, magnesium, vitamin C, and vitamin K. Since vitamins and minerals don't extract well in alcohol, they need to be infused in hot water for several hours for best effect, whether in a long infused tea or used in soup or broth. They also do well extracted in apple cider vinegar, which can then be taken by the teaspoonful or used in the kitchen.

The leaves help eliminate toxins from the blood and then stimulate the kidneys to clear those toxins by acting as a diuretic. This ability to both build and to cleanse makes this a very special plant indeed, and it can be used for chronic skin conditions, mild arthritis, and gout. For gout it works well combined with shepherd's purse and cleavers to help clear uric acid from the kidneys.

It's also a great herb for allergies. The dried herb as a tea seems to strengthen the mucosal lining of the upper respiratory system, increasing resilience to allergens. After all, if the allergen can't get through the physical barrier, then it can't cause an allergic reaction. For the same reason it also strengthens the lining of the urinary tract, making it less prone to future infections. For these purposes, drinking a daily tea for a couple of weeks will help prevent allergies and UTIs.

Fresh leaves work quite differently and are a great remedy for acute histamine reactions like hay fever and dust or pet allergies. Take the fresh plant as a tincture, glycerite, or fresh freeze-dried capsule; all produce a more immediate effect than the tea. A combination of nettles and ragweed works best for this use.

The root has a long tradition of use for prostate issues, especially for an enlarged prostate such as in BPH. It seems to function as an aromatase inhibitor, slowing down the breakdown of testosterone into DHT, a hormone that's been implicated in prostate disease. For this purpose it combines well with saw palmetto.

Use of the seed is a more recent introduction to Western herbalism. The first of its two main uses, which I learned about from Jonathan Treasure and David Winston (2013), is as a kidney restorative and nephroprotective. It helps protect the kidneys from damage and helps with recovery after damage has occurred. It could even be used for early stage kidney failure.

The other use is as a gentle adaptogen for people who are so worn out that even mild adaptogens are too stimulating for them. It nourishes the adrenals without causing undue stimulation. It is also physically nourishing; besides having a mineral profile that is similar to that of the leaves, it is high in omega-3 fatty acids, like many nourishing seeds.

Future harvests

Where plants occur, nettle grows abundantly. Overharvesting is rarely a problem, particularly with European nettle.

HERBAL PREPARATIONS

Leaves as a long infusion or vinegar for nutritive properties, and tinctured fresh 1:2 at 95% for antihistamine properties. Seeds tinctured 1:5 dry at 50% or used as an infusion. Roots tinctured 1:2 fresh or 1:5 dry at 50% alcohol. The leaves can also be used as food—in pesto, soup, broth, and about any way you would use spinach besides a raw salad.

Avena sativa

PARTS USED leaves, seeds

*Nourishing and comforting, oats are food for
the nervous system and caretake the caretaker.*

How to identify

Oats are in the grass family (Poaceae) and
they look it. They have stalks that are 3–5 feet
high, long thin leaf blades with parallel veins,
and little green-yellow flowers that hardly
resemble the popular definition of flowers.
What differentiates oats from other grasses is
the way the flowers and seeds have 2 prongs
jutting out, and how each flower is on a lateral stem, giving it the look of a mobile.

Where, when, and how to wildcraft

This is a common cover crop, so it is often
found near cultivated fields or near places
where it was planted for erosion control.
When and where it escapes into the wild is
unpredictable, but it's usually found in areas
with more human influence.

To harvest the leaves for tea, harvest
when the plant looks lush and green, either
before seeding or at least before the seeds get

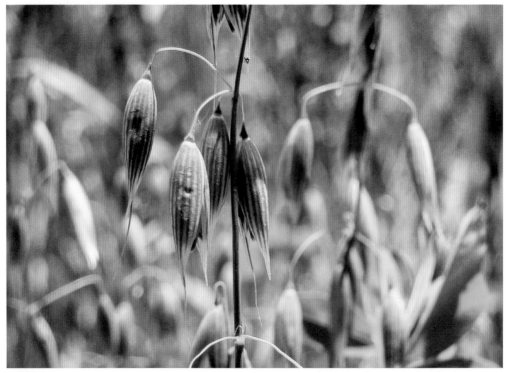

Oat seeds, dangling like mobiles from the stalk, are best gathered for medicine when they are green- and
yellow-striped.

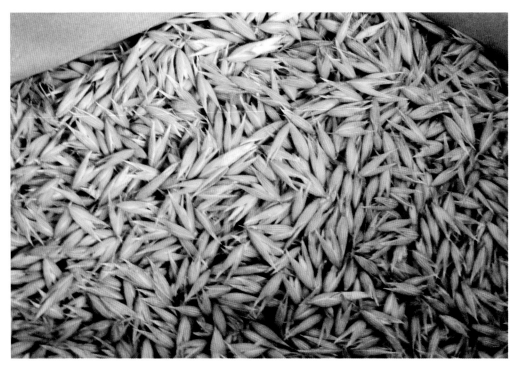
Oat seeds harvested in the unripe "milky" stage.

too ripe. To harvest the seeds for medicine, pick when the plant is starting to yellow but isn't totally straw-colored yet, and the seeds have green and yellow stripes.

Oat seeds are harvested in the unripe "milky" stage. Choose an average-aged stalk in the patch and squeeze a seed. If it is as hard as a sunflower seed, then you might have oatmeal, but it's too late to use the seed for medicine. If you are able to pinch all the way through, then it is too young. But if you squeeze it and it pops to release a milky latex, then it is absolutely perfect. Lean the stalk over your harvesting basket and with fingers on either side of the stalk, run your hands up the stalk to pop off all the seed heads.

If you find a field of these in different stages of growth, test a few seed heads to get a feel for the right ones and then just look for that specific color. They are at the perfect harvesting stage for 1–2 weeks in the spring and again in the fall. This milky oat seed window is shorter in hot weather, longer in cool weather.

Medicinal uses

The leaves are a nourishing tonic for the whole body; the seeds are one of the best tonics for the nervous system, a nervine that's almost an adaptogen.

The leaves (aka oatstraw in commerce) make an excellent blood-building tea, especially when combined with nettle leaves and alfalfa then steeped for at least 4–8 hours in a canning jar with the lid on. This tea is great for blood deficiency and anemia, as well as being an excellent tonic during pregnancy when the body is building up a lot of extra blood. But it is also just great as a general multivitamin, multimineral supplement.

The seeds on the other hand are a very different medicine, a restorative to the nervous system specifically. They are great medicine for those with adrenal exhaustion, burn-out, or folks just feeling depleted—people who are "wired and tired," so worn out that they are anxious, irritable, and maybe even having a hard time sleeping. It's not overstimulation but an exhausted and overreactive "punch drunk" nervous system.

Think of someone who gets stressed out very easily, jumps when someone slams a door on the other side of the house, and is just generally high strung. Though it seems like excess energy, it is actually more of a deficiency condition—the hair-trigger nervous system is firing too easily. Imagine an electric wire with bad insulation—the sparks leaping out are from not enough protection, not from too much electricity. In Chinese medicine, this might be thought of as a type of yin deficiency.

Oat gets overlooked on store shelves because it is not so much for a disease state as a condition of the person. And even then, it can be used by almost anyone as a daily tonic during stressful times when our nerves and adrenals could use more resilience.

In Chinese medicine it could be said that the leaves are a blood tonic, whereas the seed is more of a yin tonic. But in the end both are a great tonic for almost anyone.

Future harvests

This is a commonly cultivated plant, easy to harvest in abundance without threat. Some farmers will appreciate your harvesting their seeds so that they don't grow back where another crop is supposed to go.

HERBAL PREPARATIONS

Oat leaves, or oatstraw, is best made as a long infusion. Pour a quart of boiling water over a tablespoon of leaves and let sit for a minimum of 20 minutes; let it infuse 4–8 hours for the best extraction.

Milky oat seed is prepared as a fresh tincture or glycerite, about 1:6 at 75% alcohol or the same blend of glycerin. This is the only fresh plant that I blend before tincturing. Fill a good blender a third to halfway full with the fresh seeds and mix it right into the menstruum. If the container is too full then the seeds on top won't circulate down, though you can occasionally stop the blender, unplug it for safety, and push the sides down with a spatula. Pour it off into a canning jar and repeat the process, though you may need to pour some of the greened menstruum back in to the new batch.

Repeat the blending until all the seeds are fairly broken up but not necessarily a fine powder. Pour everything into canning jars, cap tightly, and let it all sit for a few weeks to a month; then strain out through a cheesecloth.

partridgeberry

Mitchella repens

PARTS USED aerial

A gentle uterine tonic found in the deep woods.

How to identify

Partridgeberry is usually found with pines and hemlocks, perhaps rhododendrons and sourwood, and probably some pipsissewa and moss around. It runs along the ground on thin vines that can travel many feet but don't climb much. The small leaves are opposite, deep green, and thick, with a conspicuous white vein running down the middle. The white flowers appear in late spring in pairs from which, in a strange exhibit, they form a single red berry with 2 tiny circles on top. The fruit is edible but devoid of flavor, so maybe good enough for small woodland birds.

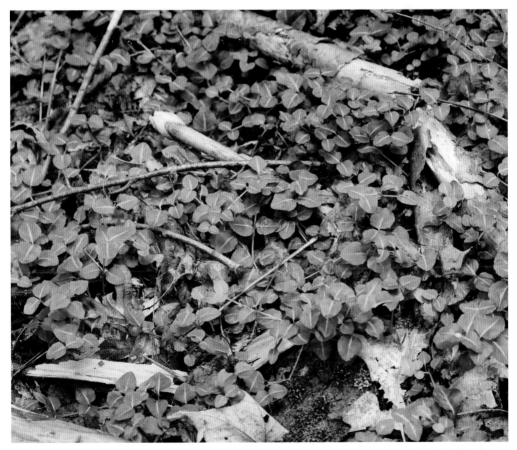

Partridgeberry is a woodland ground cover, often growing in association with pines and hemlocks. The red berries are edible but devoid of flavor.

Where, when, and how to wildcraft

Partridgeberry is pretty widespread across the entire East Coast. Plants are evergreen and can be harvested year-round. Basically, crop back the edges of a large patch, trailing out a few long strands and leaving a good amount in the middle. If the strands are picked when they're going over stones or logs, there will be fewer rootlets to trim off.

Medicinal uses

This is a tonic herb for the pelvic organs, specifically the uterus and prostate. And I mean literally a tonic—it improves and strengthens the physical tone of those organs, which is why one of its main historical uses is to prepare for childbirth.

Herbs that affect the uterus tend to either work on the hormones, which then affect the uterus, or they work directly on the physical structure. This herb is one of the latter. It doesn't seem to have any hormonal action; it just directly helps tighten and tone uterine tissue that is a little slack. Though this is particularly useful in the last trimester before giving birth, it can also be useful for anyone whose uterine issues are due to lack of tone or chronic congestion.

Just as it helps an atonic uterus, it can also help tighten and tone the prostate. This makes it useful for atonic prostate conditions like BPH with dull achy pain in the groin and perineum, again with lack of tone or congestion being key.

Future harvests

This is a native plant, used as a tonic for long periods of time, so look for large stands before harvesting.

HERBAL PREPARATIONS

Typically prepared as a simple infusion. It can also be tinctured dry 1:5 at 50% alcohol or made into a glycerite at the same proportions.

passionflower

Passiflora incarnata

PARTS USED leaves, flowers

A relaxing herb for insomnia and anxiety, despite its misleading name.

How to identify

Passionflower (aka purple passionflower) is a vine that crawls along the ground for a while before clambering up goldenrods, raspberries, and fences to display those unmistakable otherworldly flowers. If it wasn't such a prolific (almost invasive) plant where it grew, people would cultivate it for its beauty. But alas, we always take what is common for granted.

Once you see this flower, you will never forget it. It looks like an alien spaceship, a crown chakra, or an art piece by Antoni Gaudí. The 5 sepals and 5 petals are long but plain and look the same from the top, although the sepals (which enclose the flower in bud) have a small "horn" on the back. Above this, a whorl of beautiful purple-ringed filaments gives the flower its color. Sprouting

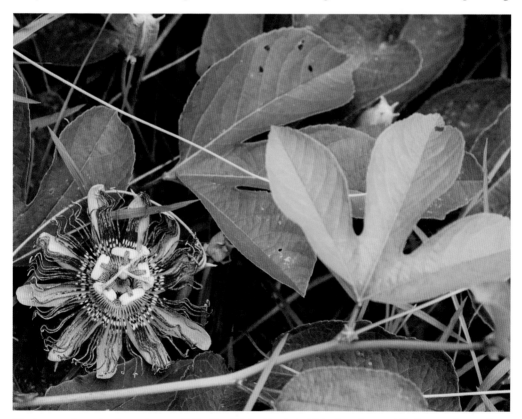

The leaves of passionflower have a distinctive 3-lobed look, but it is the otherworldly flowers that really stand out.

from the middle of this ring is a pedestal with the reproductive parts—5 anthers pointing down to dust the bees with pollen when they come to collect the nectar, sometimes falling asleep in the process, and 3 or 4 pistils crowning the top.

To find it before flowering, look for a tough vine with 3-lobed leaves, climbing by tendrils coming out of the leaf junctions. The large yellow fruit, sometimes called a maypop, has an unusual, pleasant taste, but isn't quite as yummy as its close relative, passionfruit (*Passiflora edulis*).

The smaller yellow passionflower (*Passiflora lutea*), which grows through much of the Southeast, could also be used for medicine. The flowers are a beautiful miniature and monochrome version of the common passionflower, so small that one can fit onto a fingertip. But small flowers make this less-common plant harder to spot; and overall, it is way too small to harvest any kind of quantity, so the more common passionflower is the recommended species.

Where, when, and how to wildcraft

Passionflower is a common vine of fields, meadows, and fencerows through most of the Southeast, though less common in the mountains. I often find it in horse pastures. Like other passionflower species, it can escape from cultivation, so be sure of what species you're harvesting. The vine seems to be strongest in the first flush of flowers from June into July but can be harvested up to September, or as long as the leaves look healthy and there are a few flowers left.

Harvest the top third to half of the vine, wherever it is still soft and pliable, not tough and woody. Keep the healthy leaves and flowers; discard the fruits, or save for making jam or chutney. If a large stand is found, or if you're feeling fancy, one can high-grade and tincture just the flowers for an interesting variation on the medicine.

Medicinal uses

Contrary to what you might think from the name, passionflower has nothing to do with sexual passion. It is a relaxing herb, calming anxiety when taken in smaller doses during the day and inducing sleep when taken in larger doses at bedtime.

It is a nervine, in the same class as skullcap and blue vervain; all three were thought of as nerve antispasmodics and have been used for nerve pain, migraines, and even epilepsy. Think of passionflower specifically when someone is irritable and cranky because they're overtired, that kind of late-night "second wind"—overstimulated and not able to come down.

This is one of my favorite herbs for insomnia. It has none of the heavy or drugged feeling people sometimes get from valerian, an herb that is very popular for insomnia yet has the odd effect of stimulating, not sedating, 10% of the people who take it.

Passionflower has an affinity with the heart, both on a physical and on a spiritual level. On a physical level, it reduces high blood pressure by relaxing the arterial muscles and combines nicely with motherwort for that. On a more energetic level, it opens the heart while cooling the overactive spirit.

There is something special about this plant, an opportunity for spiritual connection. The idea of passion does enter in here, but it's more about divine passion. As a flower essence, it helps us find our passion for life and connects our own individual hearts to the Divine Heart. In terms of the three kinds of love that the Greeks talked about, this is agape, not eros or philos. But then, just looking at it is a heart-opening experience. Tommie Bass said it brings people together because you don't get as bothered by the little things other people do.

Future harvests

This is an abundant plant throughout the Southeast, considered a weed in some places even though it is native. Harvest respectfully, of course, but there's not much worry about overharvesting. It can get mowed and bounce back.

Prunus persica

PARTS USED leaves

A cooling remedy for heat problems, calming the nerves, and reducing irritation and inflammation.

How to identify

Though this is a common tree of yards and orchards, it still bears description as those distinctive fleshy fruits aren't always about. The tree can get to be 30 feet high though when cultivated is often kept shorter to keep the fruits within reach. The leaves are 3–6 inches long and much longer than wide, with a slight curve to them, making them vaguely sickle-shaped. Flowers are pink and 5-petaled and bloom in the spring before the tree leafs out.

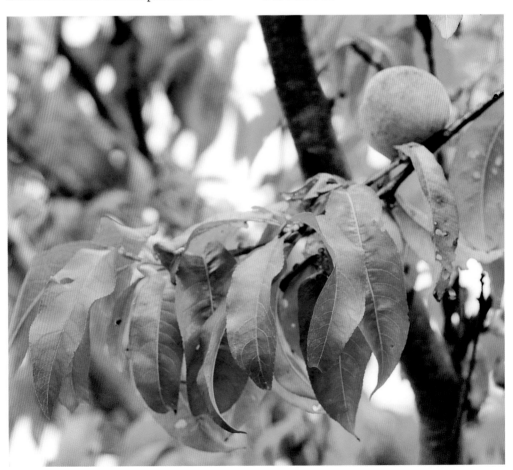

Peaches are usually grown for the tasty fruit, but the long leaves make an excellent medicinal tea.

Where, when, and how to wildcraft

Peaches are native to China, but Europeans thought they came from Persia, which already seemed far away, and that's how the species got named. They were first brought to the Americas by the Spanish and were immediately adopted by the indigenous people; by the time English settlers encountered them, the Cherokee already had peach orchards going strong.

Harvest mid-summer; just pick the leaves off of any unsprayed peach tree. They really could be harvested any time they're around, fresh or dry, but by the end of the summer they do get a bit rough-looking.

Medicinal uses

Peach leaf is just beginning to get recognized in Western herbalism, but it has been used as a folk remedy in the Southeast for generations. I first learned about its medicinal use from Phyllis D. Light (2018).

Peach leaf is easy to describe energetically: it's a cooling herb that clears heat—and that can mean both physical heat and agitated emotions. It can even be used for heat exhaustion; I used it once myself when I had been out in the sun too long and couldn't get cooled off, even after a cold shower and lots of rehydration. It has also been used to help reduce fevers when they get too high, though I prefer to use diaphoretics to sweat out a fever most of the time.

And then it also helps with those hot irritated emotions—helping with agitation, anxiety, and hotheadedness to cool and calm the mind. It's also good for insomnia with agitation and a racing mind.

It can be used topically as a wash of the tea or tincture to help with hot and irritated skin conditions. It works great for poison ivy, insect bites, and allergic skin reactions. I don't know that it affects histamine directly, but it does seem to cool off the body's over-reaction and calm down the irritation. Peach works well for just about any kind of heat!

Future harvests

It occasionally escapes from cultivation, so harvesting isn't a problem as long as you don't take more than the tree can tolerate.

Caution

To avoid any cyanide toxicity, either use the plant fresh or dry it completely, just like its close cousin wild cherry.

HERBAL PREPARATIONS

Infusion of either very fresh or completely dry leaves: if the leaves wilt, they can produce a version of cyanide and be somewhat toxic. Tincture leaves fresh 1:2 at 75% alcohol or in some brandy. I like to throw one peach fruit in a jar of the leaves to give it a nice flavor.

Chimaphila maculata
PARTS USED aerial

A blood cleanser and a great herb for urinary tract infections.

How to identify

Technically this is striped pipsissewa (aka spotted wintergreen, rat vein, prince's pine), but it is more common in our region (growing throughout the Southeast almost as far west as the Mississippi) than its sibling pipsissewa, *Chimaphila umbellata*, which grows in Virginia, north through Delaware into the Northeast, as well as the upper Midwest, the Rockies, and the Pacific Northwest. Luckily, they are medicinally interchangeable. Both species of pipsissewa are small, growing no taller than about 10 inches, and have toothed leaves in whorls that persist

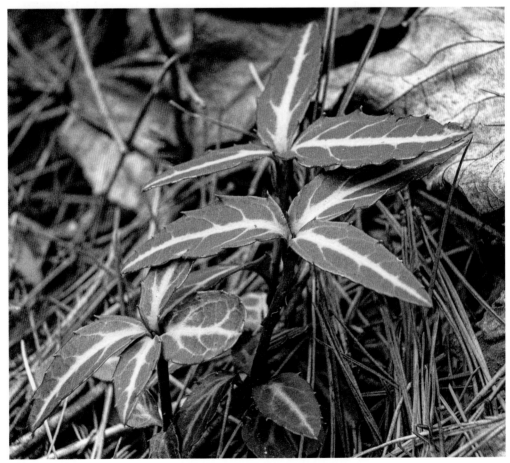

Striped pipsissewa is usually found growing in association with pines and hemlocks.

through winter. Both produce a whorl of leaves each year, so if you find one that has 3 levels of leaves, it is a 3-year-old plant. The leaf of *C. umbellata* is obovate (widest toward the tip), lacks the white stripe, and is slightly softer, where a striped pipsissewa leaf is widest closer to the stem and feels a little tougher.

Where, when, and how to wildcraft

Pipsissewa is usually found in groves of pine and hemlock, but it has some flexibility in terms of habitat: I've found it in mixed hardwood and conifers, and it can also tolerate the acid soil of hemlocks and rhododendrons. This tends to be more of a lower-elevation plant, more common in the Piedmont and coastal plain; but it can also be found somewhat up in the mountains.

The whole aboveground plant can be harvested year-round by clipping the plant at its base. Do use a pruner or scissors to avoid damaging the communal underground root structure. Use the whole plant for medicine.

Medicinal uses

Both pipsissewa species are excellent herbs for helping urinary tract infections. Pipsissewa also has a long use as an alterative for arthritis and skin conditions.

But above all, pipsissewa is a urinary tract herb. It contains arbutin, a constituent excreted through the kidneys that acts as an antiseptic on the tubes of the urinary tract. This makes it great for many kinds of urinary tract infections. It is not astringent, so it won't negatively impact digestion if taken for a longer period of time. But then it also won't help tighten and tone the mucous membranes.

It is said to help kidney stones and that the name comes from the Creek, meaning "it breaks up stones." However, I would tend to use wild hydrangea, stone root, and gravel root more often than this plant. But generally it is good for both acute inflammation and infection as well as many kinds of chronic conditions of the urinary tract, whether with scanty or frequent urination.

It is also a blood cleanser and can be used for dry scaly skin along with barberry. Some sources say it is better for UTIs with alkaline urine. But overall a very useful and pleasant-tasting little plant that I would probably use more often if it grew more abundantly.

Future harvests

This is a slow-growing plant that is not superabundant, so great care should be taken when harvesting. Gather when you find it abundantly and harvest it sparingly. It is hard to find in commerce, but the related uva ursi is easy to find and does many of the same things.

HERBAL PREPARATIONS

Tincture fresh 1:2 at 80% alcohol, or dry 1:5 at 50%. It can also be made into an infusion, but the dried herb will turn brown within a year of harvest.

Plantago rugelii, P. major
PARTS USED leaves

*A common weed that acts as a first aid
remedy, wound healer, and lung healer.*

How to identify

The two species listed here are the most
common broad-leaved plantains, along with
Plantago virginica. Though *P. major* is the
more-cited species in books, it is much less
common in the Southeast, and it is quite
likely herbalists have been using other species without even noticing.

All these plantain species are perennials
with oval basal leaves (other plantains with
more linear leaves might also be useful) and
strong parallel veins. *Plantago major* has
smooth to very hairy leaves with green petioles and is the least common, even though
it is considered an exotic invasive. *Plantago
rugelii* is much more common in the Southeast and has smooth leaves with a reddish
petiole that are easily the largest of this
group. *Plantago virginica* is decidedly hairy
and has smaller leaves that are not as round
as the other two species.

All these plantains put up an unassuming
flower stalk of greenish white flowers that
are barely taller than grass and usually get

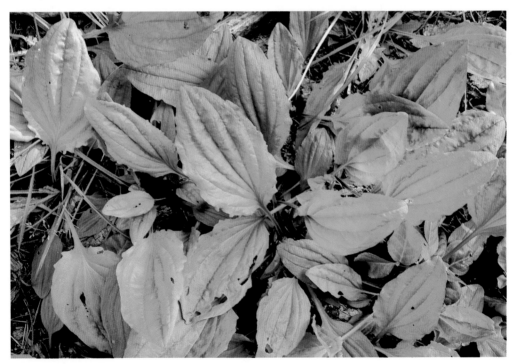

Plantain leaves with their strong veins can be found almost anywhere you would find grass.

mistaken for it. One of the keys to telling it apart from similar broad-leaved plants is to slowly tear the leaf-stalk; the veins that show so strongly in the leaf will jut out like broken threads from one end of the tear.

Sidenote—it is not at all related to the plantain that looks like a banana.

Where, when, and how to wildcraft

The broad-leaved plantains are found so commonly in yards and meadows that they are usually just considered grasses (which they are not). But any place that grass is growing there will probably be some plantain too.

The leaves are up and about spring through fall, even year-round in warmer climates, and they can be harvested anytime, though the fresh young spring leaves are often recommended. Pluck or cut the individual leaves. An easy way to chop them for oil or tincture is to stack a few up, roll them like a cigar, and then cut them into half-inch strips with pruners or even scissors.

Medicinal uses

In the United States, plantain is thought of as the number one first aid remedy, but in the United Kingdom and elsewhere, it is used internally for dry coughs and healing the digestive system. It is a powerful remedy for wounds and is both moistening and astringing.

One of its main uses in first aid is as a drawing poultice, meaning that applying it topically helps draws things up to the surface. I've seen it help many bee and wasp stings; used as an impromptu spit poultice, it stopped the pain almost immediately. It's the first herbal medicine to teach your kids. The drawing effect even works for splinters and other embedded objects—I once had a student who used it on their chin and drew

out a piece of glass from a car crash two years previous within 20 minutes.

The leaves contain allantoin. It is a great herb to stimulate tissue growth and wound healing. It can be used as a poultice for a fresh wound that's not too deep, or after the wound has closed up, it can be applied as an oil or salve to promote faster tissue healing and prevent scar tissue. Curiously, it is both astringent (drying) and emollient/demulcent (moistening), which is a good combination for wound healing.

Though Americans mostly use it externally, it is commonly used internally in the rest of the world. In England it is called ribwort and used for a dry, irritated cough. In Central and South America it is used for peptic ulcers and even stomach cancer. Which makes sense, as anything that heals the skin outside our body can also be used to heal the "skin" that lines the digestive tract.

Plantain is taken for granted because it is so common as to be ubiquitous. But because it is so common, we should be using it even more.

Future harvests

All the plantains are abundant and will even bounce back after a good mowing.

HERBAL PREPARATIONS

The leaves can be made into a fresh infused oil by using a heat method, as letting them sit for a month in oil goes funky half the time. They can also be dried for tea or tinctured fresh 1:2 at 75% alcohol. The most common preparation is the inelegantly named "spit poultice," made by chewing a piece of leaf and slapping it on a bee sting or other acute injury.

pleurisy root

Asclepias tuberosa

PARTS USED root

*A unique and useful lung tonic that redistributes fluid
in the lungs and skin to help rid the lungs of stuck phlegm.*

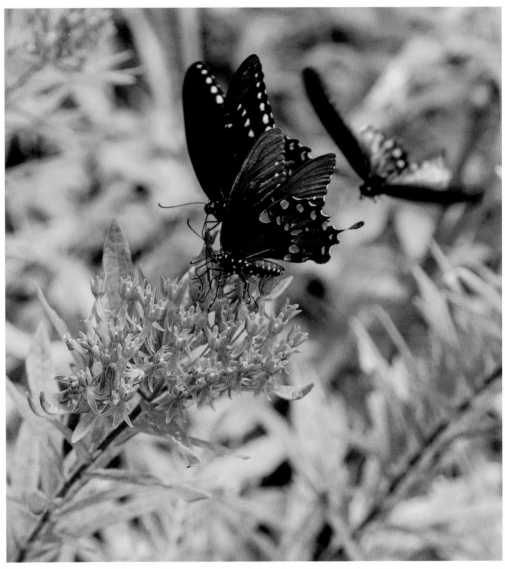

It's not hard to grow pleurisy root in your garden, and it makes a beautiful attractant for an abundance of butterflies and other pollinators.

How to identify

Pleurisy root (aka butterfly weed) is unique among milkweeds in that it has alternate leaves (all others have opposite leaves) and actually has no "milk"—break a leaf in two, and no milky or even clear sap will leak out. This plant is relatively common but almost impossible to spot if it's not in flower. You can tell it is a milkweed because the flowers have the classic hourglass shape, with petals pointing down and a corona of horns and hoods pointing up with the pollinia in between. The flowers are a magnificent bright orange, occasionally heading toward scarlet. Make sure to gather the correct species because some other milkweed species are poisonous, though some are medicinal and some edible.

Where, when, and how to wildcraft

This is a plant of meadows and fields. I associate it with the great plains and Midwest, but it is actually abundant from Pennsylvania and southern New England south through all Florida, and west to Kansas, Oklahoma, and eastern Texas, where it is abundant enough in places to line roadsides.

You'll find pleurisy root in places that get mowed only once a year, and it seems to love horse and cow pastures. I see it more in the Piedmont than up in the mountains, but that could be because it loves compact clay soil that's a bit acidic, with pines and oaks growing nearby.

The roots grow deep down into compacted soil and are surprisingly fragile. I first bought a mattock specifically to harvest these roots. Dig in around the area of the roots, combining a mattock with a digging fork to loosen up the compacted soil, then jump in with a soil knife, digging parallel to the root direction to get the main roots loosened. Don't yank too hard or too early or it will break off.

The flowers bloom June through August, and that's the best (perhaps the only) time to find it. Usually we wait until a plant has finished flowering to dig roots, but this is an exception unless you are positive you are going to be able to find it later. It can be harvested in August or early September if you're lucky—by then the roots have stored up more juice and the flowers have nourished pollinators.

Medicinal uses

Pleurisy root is an herb that is almost impossible to replace in the apothecary because nothing else does quite what it does. It has a unique ability to move fluids in the lungs and the skin (sometimes called the third lung). This makes it extremely useful as part of a formula in bronchitis, pleurisy, pneumonia, and asthma. Pleurisy is really just an inflammation of the pleura, the lining of the lungs.

But for all those uses, pleurisy root is not an antiviral or antibacterial. It treats the ground of the disease by reducing inflammation and changing the fluid balance. As such, it is usually combined with other herbs that are specific for the current condition such as angelica, boarhog, or mullein, for example.

It is not used for one specific disease but for a tissue state that is common to many diseases and problems. This is probably why it isn't more popular, because it doesn't fit well into the herb-for-disease model. But pleurisy root can be incredibly helpful in treating the "soil" in which the disease is growing.

It works by bringing fluids up to the cells that line the surface of both the lungs and the skin (epithelial cells). In the lungs this can really help with thick stuck phlegm by diluting it down so it can be coughed up more easily. It's an herb I use when there is too much fluid in someone's lungs, working deeper in the lungs than other expectorants.

But the interesting and somewhat contradictory use is that it can also help when the mucous membranes of the lungs get dry and irritated, as is the case in pleurisy. Though simple demulcents like slippery elm or plantain can also help by soothing surfaces, pleurisy root works more deeply in the lungs.

The other time I love using it is as after-care for lung infections. Sometimes after bronchitis, pneumonia, or even a chest cold, there can be a lot of thick phlegm deep in the lungs that lingers even after the virus or bacteria is gone—what's called residual phlegm in Chinese medicine. Sometimes there is a rattling cough that lasts for days or weeks after the infection has passed, and this can weaken the lungs and make another infection more likely, so it is important to clear this excess fluid out. Pleurisy root and spikenard are the two herbs that I most commonly use at this clean-up stage.

It can also bring more fluids to the skin and induce a sweat without raising body temperature like other herbs. Sweating is an important way of cooling off and bringing down a fever. More than just sweat, it also helps the skin excrete serous fluids and waste products.

Future harvests

Pleurisy root is beloved of many pollinators and is one of the major host plants for monarch butterflies, so harvest only when there's an abundance of plants, and remember to leave plenty for the pollinators.

 Caution

The leaves are toxic. Make sure you have this species, as some milkweeds are poisonous. There are a small amount of cardioactive glycosides in the root, which isn't an issue for most folks but could negatively interact with those who are taking heart medications.

> **HERBAL PREPARATIONS**
>
> Fresh root tincture is considered best, but the dry root tincture and decoction are also quite effective.

poke

Phytolacca americana

PARTS USED root, fruit

A very powerful lymph mover for swollen glands, tonsillitis, and more.

How to identify

Poke is a giant native weed, growing up to 10 feet tall and sometimes almost as wide. The stems get to be purplish as they get bigger, and the alternate leaves can be a foot long, oval, and entire. There are often a few large stalks coming out of the same root, and they branch toward the top to form racemes of white flowers that become clusters of purple berries.

Where, when, and how to wildcraft

Poke grows from Canada to southern Florida and west to Kansas and mid-Texas. It could be that it earned its common name because it keeps poking up everywhere.

Though it is the root or berries that are used for medicine, the very young shoots can be enjoyed as an edible, cooked in two or three changes of water; the resulting poke salat was first made famous by Elvis Presley singing about Poke Salad Annie (just kidding . . . it was actually Tony Joe White).

The fruit matures from August through October and can be picked as soon as the berries are ripe and purple. The toxicity is mostly in the seeds, so the berries can be mashed in the mouth or mashed up with a spoon but

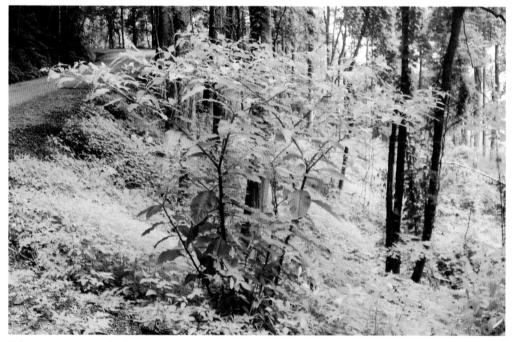

Poke is a common sight throughout the Southeast, but as big as poke gets, it's not a shrub.

[187

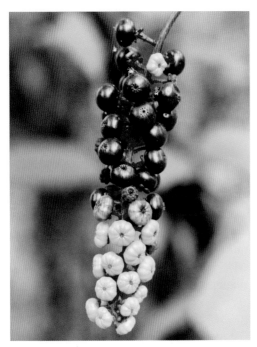

The purple berries of poke make a less intense preparation than the roots but are still strong medicine.

the tonsils, though I'm not sure how to do this without inducing a gag reflex. But it works.

Though mostly used for acute infections with swollen glands, it can also be used internally and topically for chronic swollen lymph glands, especially if they are hard and painful, and for mastitis and breast cancer. The breasts have a lot of lymph tissue running through them, so breast health issues are often treated with lymphatic herbs. It is good to be aware that even though there is a long tradition of using this plant topically, it can cause redness and irritation in some people, in which case discontinue and use gentler herbs.

Both roots and berries have been used as part of cancer formulas, though they should be combined with other herbs under the direction of an experienced herbalist. The root especially should not be used lightly, see caution section for possible side effects.

definitely not blended—you don't want to break open those seeds. Luckily they are as slippery as flax seeds.

To dig the roots you'll need a big shovel. The roots can be as thick as a man's thigh, and they go deep. Be careful as you dig; they break easily.

Medicinal uses

This is a potent lymph mover and a heroic remedy, meaning that the effect is strong and too much will cause side effects. The root especially is very potent and should be used only by people who know what they're doing; the berries are considered much safer.

Both parts strongly move lymph fluid and are great herbs for acute swollen lymph glands, as in tonsillitis or pharyngitis or even minor cases of strep throat. For bad sore throats the tincture can even be painted on

Future harvests

This is an abundant weed, no worries here.

Caution

Larger-than-recommended doses can cause nausea, vomiting, or diarrhea, as well as a migraine-like headache and general not-funness. More than that can cause coma, and some deaths have been reported. Sometimes the topical application of roots or the infused oil can cause skin irritation, which goes away when the application is discontinued.

> ### HERBAL PREPARATIONS
>
> Tincture the berries fresh 1:2 at 95% and use 5–30 drops, but start low and work up. The root is more intense and can be tinctured 1:2 at 95% alcohol and used in doses of 1–5 drops.

prickly ash

Zanthoxylum clava-herculis, Z. americanum
PARTS USED bark

A circulatory stimulant useful for poor circulation, arthritis, and pain.

How to identify

Two *Zanthoxylum* species occur in the Southeast, southern prickly ash (*Z. clava-herculis*) and northern prickly ash (*Z. americanum*). Both are spiny trees with compound leaves, but they need to be differentiated from another common but unrelated spiny tree, devil's walking stick (*Aralia spinosa*).

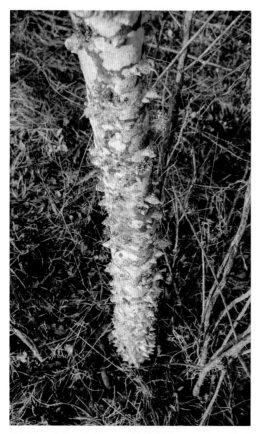

Prickly ash has lighter-colored bark and spines that over the years turn into triangular corky nubs.

Both prickly ash species are pinnate with 5–11 leaflets (northern prickly ash) and 7–15 leaflets (southern prickly ash) per leaf. Devil's walking stick has much larger leaves because it is 2- to 3-times pinnate, the leaves fanning out as they divide and divide more. And although prickly ash trees sometimes form stands, devil's walking stick commonly forms thick thorny stands on wood edges.

Prickly ash trees (aka toothache trees) have a peculiar look to them as they grow older—what start as thorns on the trunk turn into corky pyramidal outgrowths on older trees. But the thorns on the leaf stalk stay sharp, mostly paired in the northern species and sometimes paired, sometimes single in between leaflets in the southern species. Northern prickly ash tends be shorter, usually only about 10 feet high; southern prickly ash grows to 20, occasionally 50 feet. Southern prickly ash also has thicker leaves. Leaves of both species are slightly toothed to entire and are more pointed than those of black locust trees, which are also spiny.

Prickly ash is a member of the citrus family (Rutaceae), related to lemons, oranges, and rue. When the leaves are crushed, they release a wonderful aroma that is reminiscent of limes.

Where, when, and how to wildcraft

Southern prickly ash is more common in the Southeast, along the entire Atlantic coast, across Florida, through the Gulf states to

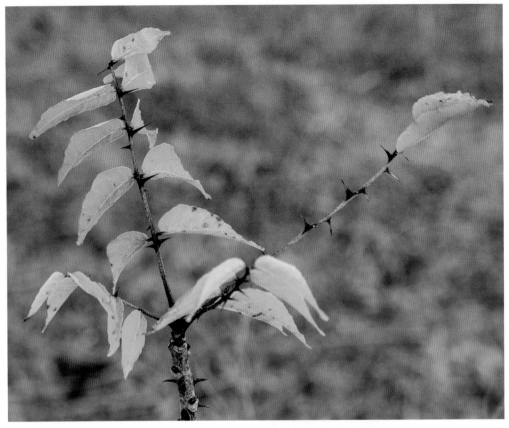

The new leaves of prickly ash are pinnate and have thorns in between the leaflets.

eastern Texas and heading north into Louisiana as far as Arkansas and sporadically into Mississippi and Alabama.

Northern prickly ash is more abundant in the northern Midwest but goes as far south as the Virginia mountains and Kentucky, and occasionally pops up in other southern states.

The tree starts leafing out in February, and it's easy enough to prune a few branches from spring through early summer. A burlap sack (such as what coffee roasters have) is great to carry these thorny sticks back home without getting bled. Once home, strip the bark for medicine (see page 000). The outer bark is thin and doesn't need to be separated from the more medicinal inner bark.

Medicinal uses

Prickly ash is an unparalleled native herbal remedy with a long history of use. It is a warming circulatory stimulant, and most of its benefits derive from this power—its use for arthritis, the immune system, weak digestion, and of course cold hands and feet. It is also a good herb for specific types of pain when taken internally or for tooth pain when swished.

Its aromatic and bitter flavors stimulate digestion. Chewing the bark strongly stimulates salivation—technically a sialogogue, but prickly ash is more of a "droolagogue" by my standards. This ability to stimulate secretions can make it a great ally for people with dry mouth and insufficient digestive secretions, either chronically or because of drugs like beta-blockers or chemo.

Really, anyone with slow digestion and low secretions could benefit from this herb, and it could also help flatulent dyspepsia—farting because the food is just taking so long to get through the digestive tract. Just don't use it if there's already a lot of stomach irritation or inflammation (heat); in that case, you would need something more calming and soothing, not stimulating.

Its circulatory-stimulating property is stronger than that of ginger but not so hot and dispersing as cayenne. Ginger warms up the body internally and is great for being out in the cold too long, while cayenne is so dispersing that it ends up cooling off by stimulating the body to "sweat off" the extra heat. This is the reason why people in hot climates eat spicy food (I know you've been wondering!). Prickly ash is more internally warming and is very useful for those with chronic cold hands and feet, including conditions like Raynaud's disease. It also has been used for intermittent claudication, muscle pain, and cramping from low blood flow after exercise.

This same property makes it useful for chronic joint pain. Arthritis is traditionally treated using both blood movers and blood cleansers. This is because blood slows as it moves through the joint capsule: it's harder to run in curves than in straight lines. As it slows it can deposit toxins, just like debris can pile up in places where a river slows. An example of this would be how, in gout, the excess uric acid builds up in a joint.

It stimulates not just blood circulation but also lymph circulation. This is why it is found in traditional formulas for colds as well as in formulas for cancer, Lyme disease, or STIs. This would never be the main herb in the formula but something added to the formula to increase its efficacy.

Prickly ash is also a good pain remedy, especially for neuralgic pain like sciatica, or shooting pain. The bark can be chewed or the tincture diluted and used as a mouthrinse to help with tooth pain while simultaneously stimulating circulation in the gums.

Prickly ash is a great herb to have in your apothecary or around the house—a great example of a heating herb that doesn't overdo it.

Future harvests

Prickly ash is a fairly common tree along fencerows in some places, and it can form stands. As always when gathering from trees, prune branches judiciously and spread out your harvesting on one tree and in the stand.

HERBAL PREPARATIONS

Prickly ash is mostly used in tincture, the fresh bark 1:2 at 95% or the dried bark 1:5 at 50%. The bark doesn't last long dried and is best within a year of harvest.

Ambrosia artemisiifolia, A. trifida
PARTS USED leaves

One of the best herbs for allergies—for treating them, that is.

How to identify

Two species of ragweed occur on the East Coast. They don't even look related, but both can be used for the same medicinal purpose. Great ragweed (*Ambrosia trifida*) is a big plant with either ovate toothed leaves or leaves divided into 3 round lobes at the end, vaguely reminiscent of a sassafras (though of course it is an herb, not a tree). Common or annual ragweed (*A. artemisiifolia*) is smaller and has divided leaves. When crushed, ragweed has no strong smell; it just smells like a green plant.

The little flowers are nothing—hardly noticeable except that there's a ton of them when they do flower in late summer through fall. Unlike goldenrod, they are wind-pollinated, so don't need to attract insects with colorful petals.

Where, when, and how to wildcraft

Gather in mid-summer when tall but before flowering. The pollen from flowers is what causes the allergic reaction and honestly it shouldn't be a problem in tincture, but better safe than allergic. Cut the whole plant before

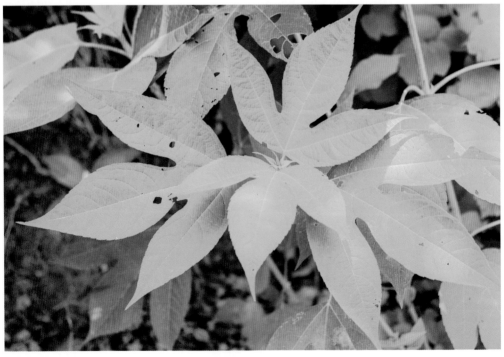

Great ragweed is a common weed of meadows, old fields, and disturbed areas.

flowering, and use the leaves and maybe some of the stalk where it is tender.

Both species grow throughout the Southeast and across the continent. They are common and abundant along roadsides, in fields, meadows—really you'll find them just about anywhere with a bit of sun. So they're easy to find, easy to harvest—just make sure the area hasn't been sprayed.

Medicinal uses

You ask, "What could ragweed possibly be good for?" It's good for allergies! No, really. It works to help allergic reactions. And it really works.

This sounds like homeopathy, but it's not. For some reason the leaves of this plant are great at mediating many kinds of respiratory allergies. I've seen it work for hay fever, cat allergies, dust allergies, anything that has a Type 1 IgE-mediated histamine response. It doesn't seem to work for food allergies or poison ivy, because those work through different mechanisms. I did see it help with hives once.

I can't explain why it works, but it really does. It is drying, astringent, and helps dry up excess mucus, but other herbs do this too, including yarrow, elder flower, and catnip. And yet they don't have quite the same effect on stopping the allergic reaction as this plant does.

Ragweed combines well with tincture of fresh nettle leaf for acute allergic reactions and is superabundant, maybe even too abundant for some. Which makes it an excellent replacement for the much less common but more well-known eyebright. Sometimes the common weeds are good substitutes for the uncommon popular herbs.

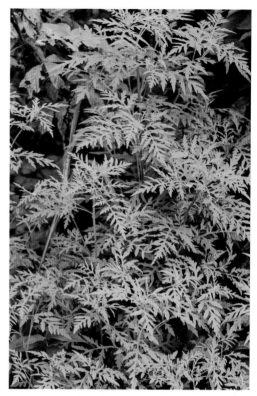

The leaves of common ragweed are quite different but the flowers are the same, and both ragweeds can be used the same way.

Future harvests

There is no worry about running out of ragweed. Ever.

Caution

If someone is very allergic to ragweed, it might be a good idea to take 1 drop of tincture first to make sure there's not a reaction.

HERBAL PREPARATIONS

Tincture or tea, fresh or dry. I usually tincture the leaves fresh.

---

raspberry

Rubus idaeus, R. occidentalis

PARTS USED leaves

A tasty tea that makes a great uterine tonic, especially during pregnancy.

How to identify

Blackberries and raspberries are both in the same genus and can look similar, but it is important to differentiate because they are used very differently for medicine. The two raspberry species listed here are the ones most commonly used, but other less common or cultivated raspberries could possibly be used as well.

The easiest way to tell the difference is by the fruit. Both groups have fruits that are actually clusters of smaller fruits on a base, or receptacle as it's officially known. Raspberries have fruits that peel off the receptacle like a thimble or a cap, whereas in blackberries the receptacle stays inside the fruit. This is true no matter the color of the fruit, which explains how we can have

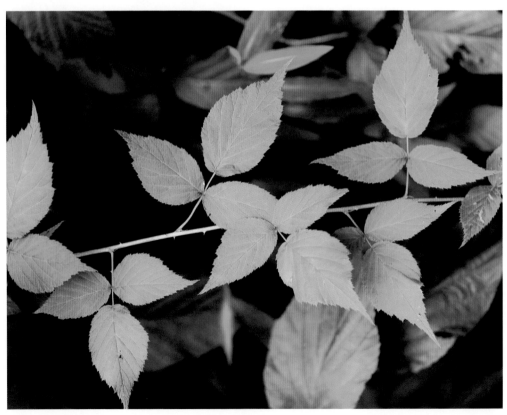

Although red raspberry is more famous as a medicinal, black raspberry, shown here, is more common in the Southeast and is also stronger.

black raspberries. Also raspberry flowers have white petals that are shorter than the green sepals, whereas the petals of blackberry flowers are longer than the sepals. For more on differentiating the two groups, see the blackberry entry.

The common red raspberry (*Rubus idaeus*) can be either native or introduced and is the official species used in herbal medicine, though I slightly prefer the black raspberry (*R. occidentalis*). Red raspberry has green canes that turn brown and woody with age; black raspberry has reddish canes that are glaucous, meaning they have a white bloom that can be rubbed off.

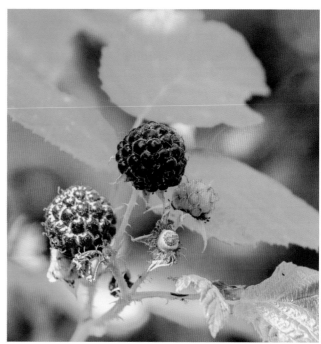

Despite the color, this is a black raspberry, not a blackberry.

Where, when, and how to wildcraft

All in all, these plants are easy to find. Even though red raspberry is the species in most books, black raspberry is much more abundant in the wild throughout the Southeast and is just as strong if not stronger. Both grow in fields, meadows, and yards—I've frequently had black raspberry come up in my yard where I haven't mowed, so I transplant them into a patch to make a berry vineyard.

The best time to harvest the leaves is during the summer when the plants are fairly large but before the end of the season when they start getting ragged-looking. Traditionally they aren't harvested after the first frost.

It's easy enough to harvest a large amount by wearing gloves and clipping whole leaves into a basket, then trimming the individual leaflets off at home; this is usually done after drying, when the leaflets can be easily broken off. The stems have more thorns, which is why they should be trimmed—or be prepared to wear gloves when making the tea.

Medicinal uses

Raspberry leaf is one of the classic tonics for the uterus; it is especially helpful for second- and third-trimester mothers, preparing them for childbirth. But plants don't see gender, and it can just as easily be used as a prostate tonic.

There are two ways that uterine tonics can work—either indirectly by affecting the hormones that affect the uterus, or by more directly affecting the physical structure of the uterus. This herb is one of the latter; it has a direct effect on the uterine lining.

Raspberry leaf has constituents that both relax the uterine muscle and tighten and tone the uterine lining, leading to easier birth and fewer menstrual cramps. The flavonoids in the leaf nourish the cells lining the uterus, making for a healthier endometrium.

For all these reasons, this herb can be used long-term to help prepare for birth; it also relieves menstrual cramps and other pelvic pain. Additionally, it has been used for morning sickness during pregnancy, sometimes in combination with peppermint.

Though it is often written about as a women's herb, it is just as useful for men with a similar tissue state. In other words, because it tightens and brings more tone to tissue, it can be used for prostate issues with lax and overly relaxed tissue tone. Think of someone who spends most of his day sitting, rarely exercises, and has a few extra pounds. This would be more for a boggy enlarged prostate like in BPH than where there is a lot of inflammation and heat, as in prostatitis. Overall, a great tonic when used over a period of time, and a nice-tasting tea.

Cultivated raspberries can also be used, though they are considered less effective.

Future harvests

Both these species are native but fairly abundant and can be harvested without much fear of damage to the stand.

Caution

Be aware that this tea can be drying when used over a long period of time.

HERBAL PREPARATIONS

The most common preparation is an infusion of the dried leaves, steeped for 15–20 minutes. A long infusion will bring out more of the tannins and won't be as tasty. It is sometimes tinctured, dry 1:5 at 50%, but the infusion is a better preparation.

red clover

Trifolium pratense
PARTS USED flowers

A common weed that cleanses and nourishes the blood.

How to identify

Despite the name, red clover is actually more purplish red. The closely related (but not medicinal) crimson clover (*Trifolium incarnatum*) is more bright red. Red clover is more common in the wild; crimson clover is a common cover crop and often found wild near planted fields.

Look closely at a flower head, and you can see it is actually a mass of dozens of tiny pea-shaped flowers. Red clover has round flower heads, whereas crimson clover's are elongated and conical.

The leaves are always in 3s, with a white chevon on each leaf. The related white clover (*Trifolium repens*) has smaller leaves, a paler chevron, and smaller and of course white flower heads.

Where, when, and how to wildcraft

Red clover can be found most anywhere that gets mowed only a few times a year,

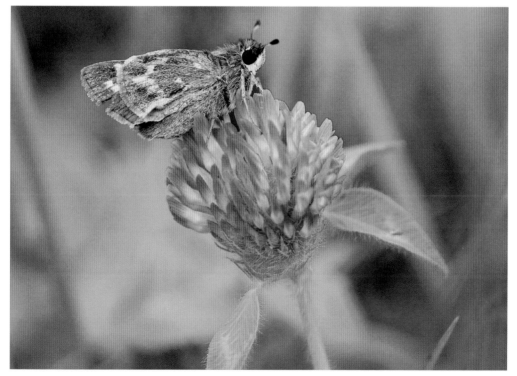

Red clover flowers fill fields and meadows for much of the summer, but make sure to pick ones that are more red than brown.

whether that's a woodland meadow or the edge of someone's yard. Though it is found in every U.S. state, it is less common in the Deep South.

It starts blooming in late spring and continues through late summer, but the blooms seem a little brighter earlier in the year, before it gets too intensely hot out. The easiest time to harvest a large amount is to wait a week or so after a meadow or pasture has been mowed and all the red clover bounces back and starts flowering again all at once. That way you won't have to pick through old brown flowers.

Another thing about picking these—when harvesting, pinch off the flower stalk just below the flower instead of grabbing the flower itself. This saves the flower from being bruised, which will cause it to oxidize and turn brown fairly quickly. Pinching off at the stem will assure your dried red clover flowers are still as beautiful and purple as when you harvested them.

Medicinal uses

Red clover is both gentle and very powerful, a perfect metaphor for herbal medicine. It is gentle enough to be eaten as is or in a salad, but powerful enough to be used in cancer formulas. It cleanses the blood, provides nutrients, and also makes a good lung tonic.

Red clover is a great alterative, working well to increase the body's ability to clear toxins. It also has some good micronutrients, making it a useful and tasty addition to a mineralizing tea, such as nettle and oatstraw.

Red clover has a specific action on the lymphatic system, much like violet leaves do, and the two make a nice combination when that's needed. It has a long history of being used internally and topically for breast health, as the breasts are full of lymph vessels. It has been used both to prevent breast cancer and to prevent its recurrence.

What is less known about red clover is that it is also a great lung tonic. The Eclectics used it for irritated cough, even for whooping cough. It nourishes the lung fluids but also helps clear out excess fluids deep in the lungs by its action on the lymphatic system, thus helping excessive coughing by removing the source of the irritation.

It can also be used topically for many kinds of wounds, and it even has some tradition of being used topically for cancer.

Future harvests

No worries about overharvesting this common and abundant European plant. Anyhow, we use only the flowers.

Caution

This plant does contain some phytoestrogens, and there is currently some controversy around using phytoestrogens in estrogen-dependent cancers. I wouldn't say don't use it, but I will say to do your own research.

HERBAL PREPARATIONS

Flowers dried for tea, or used fresh as a tincture for internal use or as an infused oil for topical use.

red root

Ceanothus americanus
PARTS USED root

A powerful lymph-moving herb deserving of more attention.

How to identify

Red root (aka New Jersey tea) is barely noticeable except when it's in flower. The plant itself is 1–3 feet high with tough green upright stems. It looks like an herbaceous plant but is in fact a shrub since the green stems stay upright and alive through the winter, producing more leaves the following year.

The leaves are simple, alternate, ovate, just barely toothed, and the only thing that distinguishes them are the 3 main veins coming from the leaf base. Since this is not a characteristic that jumps out at you from 10 feet away, the easiest markers for finding the plant are the bottlebrush tufts of white flower clusters in early to mid-summer.

An interesting sidenote: red root is one of the few plants outside of the pea family (Fabaceae) that can fix nitrogen in the soil. The richly red-colored roots have exterior white clusters that form a symbiosis with nitrogen-fixing bacteria.

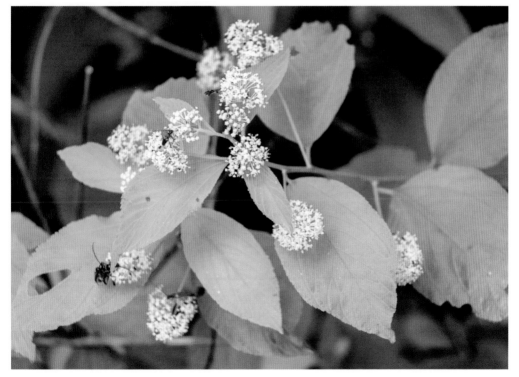

If you don't catch red root in flower it is almost impossible to find it, so keep an eye out for those bottlebrush flowers.

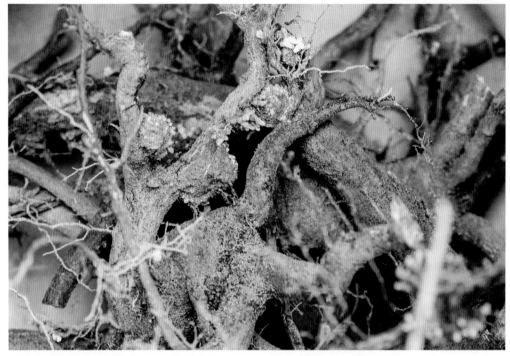

The root of red root is notorious for its toughness; often pruners, loppers, or even, yes, a hatchet might need to be deployed.

Where, when, and how to wildcraft

This is allegedly a common plant throughout the Southeast, though "locally abundant" would be more appropriate, for it grows in scattered stands. Usually when you find some, you find a lot. It prefers sandy or rocky soil and likes some sun and dryness, so it can be found on trail edges and into the woods a bit. Look for it next to trails or in open areas in pine-oak woods where you might also find hawthorn and sourwood when you look up and striped pipsissewa and greenbrier when you look down.

The best time to look for it is when it flowers in mid-June to late July, because otherwise you're going to have a hard time finding it at all. Dig the roots in fall after the flowers die back, or in winter if you can find those straight green stems. Which goes to show a wildcrafting adage—sometimes the best time to harvest a plant is not the best time to find it. Harvest when you see a good amount of plants, not one or two plants growing by themselves.

Medicinal uses

Red root is well loved among herbalists but little known in commercial herbalism because it doesn't treat a disease state so much as it improves a formula it is part of. As a strong lymph mover, it occupies a unique niche and would be a hard herb to replace.

Red root is my favorite herb for moving lymph, hands down. You've got a sore throat, even tonsillitis? Bring it on. Got some mucus, runny nose, and swollen glands? Add a little echinacea and red root just might do the trick. It is common in immune formulas not because it directly stimulates immunity or is antimicrobial, but because of its action on the lymph.

Herbalists pay much more attention to the lymph system than mainstream medicine; we are less focused on pathogens and have a greater appreciation of host resistance. The lymph vessels parallel the blood vessels and are the overflow storm drain of the body fluids. Once the fluid from the blood leaves the capillaries, only about 90% can get reabsorbed into the veins. The other 10% gets sucked up by the lymph system, where it stops at lymph node "check points" to get picked through. These nodes and lymph glands are major stations for the immune system, because this is where an antibody response to an infection first begins.

What's nice about red root is that it is halfway between a tonic and an acute herb. Cleavers, violet, or red clover would be too gentle for an acute infection; an herb like poke would be too strong for most common problems. Red root fills the niche nicely or it can be combined with the aforementioned herbs.

Red root has a long history of use for sore throat, tonsillitis, coughs, even cold sores. The Eclectics also used it for spleen enlargement and sometimes even as an adjunct herb for the liver. Since the breasts are masses of lymphatic tissue, this is a great herb for fibrocystic breasts, mastitis, and breast cancer (as part of a larger formula and protocol).

And because it improves fluid drainage from areas, it can also be used in formulas for stubborn growths, such as uterine fibroids or enlarged prostate (combined with stone root) or as part of a larger formula for tumors, benign or otherwise.

Future harvests

Red root tends to grow in stands, but it is a slow plant—slow to germinate, slow to grow, slow to spread. So harvest only when you find an abundant stand and then not more than one out of every five plants.

HERBAL PREPARATIONS

Start by chopping up the roots. This is not as easy as it sounds, since this shrub has a reputation for having one of the toughest roots out there. Best bet is to use good-quality pruners or even loppers for the big chunks. Once you've got it in chunks, make a tincture or glycerite with the fresh root, or dry to make a decoction.

The leaves, though not medicinal, make a tasty tea reminiscent of black tea (hence an alternative common name, New Jersey tea).

reishi

Ganoderma tsugae, G. curtisii, G. sessile
PARTS USED whole mushroom

Transformative and healing medicinal mushrooms for the immune system and for the spirit.

How to identify

In the United States, these mushrooms are best known as reishi, their Japanese name, but most mushroom books refer to this group as varnished conks. Several species occur in the Southeast; all are tough shelf mushrooms, meaning they grow out of the side of a tree like a shelf, and all have a shiny look on the upper surface as if they've been coated with varnish (hence yet another common name, varnished shelf mushroom).

They are typically yellow to red to reddish brown on the upper surface and white and smooth on the underside with many small dots or pores.

This combination makes the genus fairly easy to identify, but what's harder is to tell which species you are looking at. If it is growing on a hemlock then you have *Ganoderma tsugae* (aka Appalachian reishi, hemlock reishi, hemlock varnished shelf mushroom). If it's growing on a hardwood

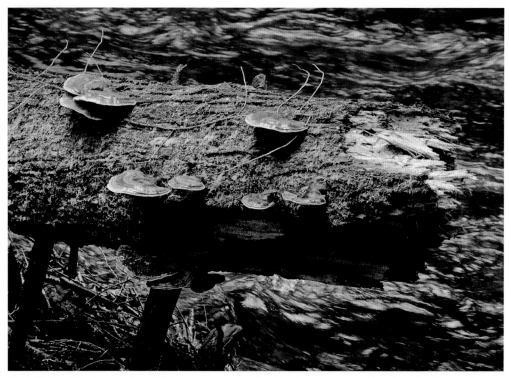

The sight of these powerful shelf mushrooms is the silver lining on the tragedy of the dying hemlocks.

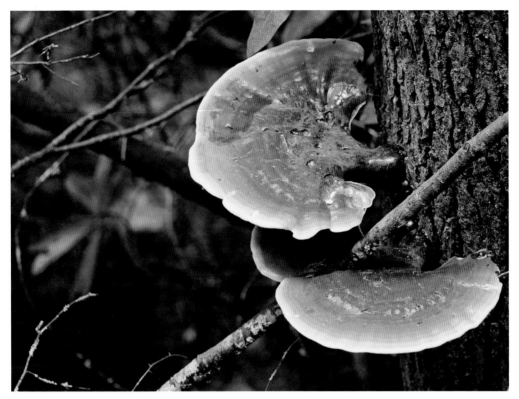

The white around the edge is the growing part of the mushroom; if harvested after the whole cap is red, then the mushroom will have time to produce spores.

like oak or maple it could be one of several species, the most common of which are *G. curtisii*, which has a noticeable stalk where it attaches to the tree, and *G. sessile*, which is stalkless, growing like a fan directly out of the tree. Sources list up to 10 *Ganoderma* species for the Southeast, but these three are the most common, and as far as we know all are equally useful, even though none has as long a history of use as the official Asian species, *G. lucidum*, which is itself now being split into several different species.

Where, when, and how to wildcraft

The hemlocks that grow in the Appalachian mountains from Pennsylvania through northern Alabama are dying a slow death because of the wooly adelgid. As hemlocks are one of the most abundant conifers in this area, this is having a huge impact on the ecosystem.

The small silver lining to this ecological tragedy is that as the trees die they can become host to the Appalachian reishi, which grows only on hemlocks. These sprout as white bumps in the spring, becoming red and shiny as the summer goes on, with a white growing edge that disappears as the fruiting body matures.

Best practice is to wait until late May or June, when the whole mushroom is red or at least has only a small white growing edge, before harvesting; this gives time for the mushroom to make spores and reproduce. But don't wait too long! Harvest it when the underside is still white and before it gets moldy or eaten by pleasing fungus beetles (yes, that's really what they're called). This is an annual mushroom, and by July the mushrooms are usually too funky to harvest. Other *Ganoderma* species may be annual or perennial, but none are as abundant as the Appalachian reishi these days.

The best way to harvest is to use a sharp knife and cut the fruiting body of the mushroom near where it meets the tree so as not to disturb the mycelium inside of the tree body itself. Chop when fresh if you want to have any chance of chopping it.

Medicinal uses

Reishi does several incredibly useful things. It does an amazing job of supporting the immune system; it is deeply calming for the nervous system; it's a powerful adaptogen and a mild heart tonic. Any of these alone would make for powerful medicine, but the combination in one medicinal substance is amazing.

All these mushrooms contain polysaccharides that are potent immune modulators. We use the term "immune modulator" instead of immune tonic to reflect that they create balance in the immune system and don't just stimulate more activity. This means that they can be used for people who are immune depressed or have chronic immune deficiency symptoms (as with cancer and AIDS patients) as well as for overactive immune reactions, such as seasonal allergies and autoimmune conditions (along with assessing for possible food allergies).

Reishi is also calming and nourishing for the nervous system. In Chinese medicine, ling zhi (as it is known) is said to nourish the blood of the heart, which helps ground the spirit. This makes it particularly useful for insomnia with dream-disturbed sleep,

especially if someone feels deficient or "too tired to sleep." I've also used it for insomnia after emotional trauma or PTSD.

This blends well with its adaptogenic activity to help nourish and balance the nervous system and adrenals. Like all adaptogens, it helps create better endurance for stressful circumstances, giving a certain "grace under pressure," one might say.

Overall, it is a good tonic herb for any depleted or overly stressed person who is getting sick more often, or having anxiety, depression, or insomnia.

Future harvests

The main thing is to wait until the mushrooms are old enough to produce spores before harvesting. As word of this medicine spreads, it is being overharvested in some areas, so please harvest with care, leaving plenty to reproduce. *Ganoderma tsugae* in particular has been overharvested and is often picked when too young and mostly white, before it has produced spores. Wait until there is very little if any white edge to the cap, and the reishi is more likely to have reproduced.

HERBAL PREPARATIONS

Chop the mushroom up when fresh into cubes 1–2 inches across, then dry. The most traditional way to use these is as a decoction, simmering a good handful in a quart of water for 20 minutes, or up to 2 hours or more. But then that decoction can be concentrated and frozen, or preserved with alcohol. In small amounts, this also makes a great addition to stock or broth. Just don't overdo it, or the bitter may overpower the other flavors.

Smilax spp.
PARTS USED root

Powerful but slow- and long-acting blood cleanser.

How to identify

The genus *Smilax* is easy to identify, even if it can be challenging to figure out which of the many species you have. The genus has two basic groups: species that are tough woody vines with long straight thorns, and those with no thorns and vines that die back each winter. The species used for medicine (*S. bona-nox*, *S. rotundifolia*, *S. glauca*, *S. pumila*) are all in the former (thornier) group.

There are other thorny plants out there. But raspberries, blackberries, and roses are all shrubs (or sometimes ground-trailing vines) with long spreading canes, not climbing vines. Also their thorns are generally curved, not triangular and sticking straight out as in sarsaparilla. The thornless species could be confused with wild yam, but wild yam leaves are whorled at the base before becoming opposite and then alternate and

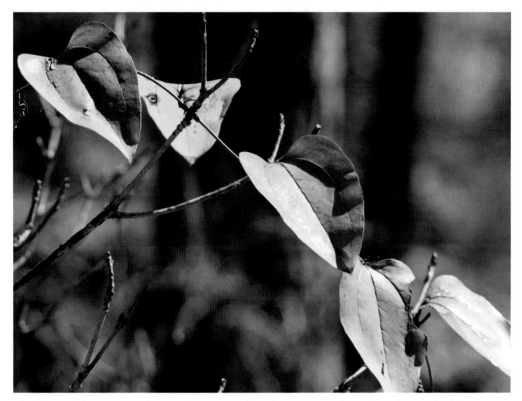

The sarsaparillas (aka greenbriers, catbriers, sawbriers) so common throughout the woods of the Southeast are excellent substitutes for the imported "true" sarsaparilla (aka zarzaparrilla, tu fu ling).

have 7–13 main veins instead of just 3.

Note that the common name sarsaparilla (sass-par-IL-la) usually refers to the Caribbean and Central American species. Since some of the North American plants can be used similarly, I am taking some liberty with the name, but several 19th-century herbal books also used native North American *Smilax* species as equivalents for the Central American and Caribbean species and used this same name, so it is historically accurate.

Also note that wild sarsaparilla has some overlap of usage. See the entry on that plant in this book.

Where, when, and how to wildcraft

One or another sarsaparilla grows throughout our region, and the aforementioned species are the ones most commonly used traditionally for medicine. They are common in shaded woods, trailsides, edges of meadows—really just about anywhere.

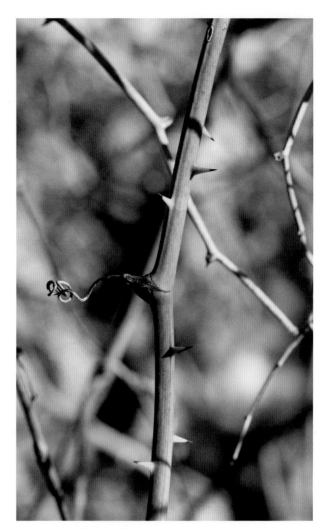

The sarsaparillas used for medicine all have thorns.

Though plants are all too easy to find ("Ouch!"), it is a challenging root to dig and chop. Trace back the vine to find the root, then cut the tops off a foot above the ground and move the vines away so you don't get an unwanted piercing. Dig down until you figure out which way the root runs and then trail it along with a good soil knife and a lot of patience. Like most roots, it is best harvested in the fall or, secondarily, the early spring. But plants are easily found in winter and can be harvested then if the ground isn't frozen.

Medicinal uses

Sarsaparilla is the poster child for the herbal category of blood cleansers. It is a slow, gentle tonic herb that, taken over time, can have a powerful effect on cleansing the body of toxins while also having the added benefit of reducing inflammation. This makes it a great herb for healing the gut and treating chronic joint pain and chronic skin conditions. It even has a place in Lyme disease protocols; whether this is from an antimicrobial effect, a beneficial effect on the gut, or as a general anti-inflammatory and blood cleanser is still up for debate. One of the early uses of this plant by Europeans was to treat syphilis; though it's not used that way now, it is interesting to note that the pathogen behind Lyme disease is a spirochete, the type of bacteria that causes syphilis.

In holistic herbal medicine, both chronic skin disease and arthritic conditions are treated by clearing the body of toxins that might be "gumming up the works." Sarsaparilla has a long tradition of helping with osteoarthritis and rheumatoid arthritis, as well as for helping hot, red, and irritated skin conditions, such as psoriasis, acne, and eczema. This beneficial effect is compounded by the anti-inflammatory effect of the saponins in the root.

It also has a beneficial effect on the gut and has been used by some herbalists for leaky gut syndrome and general poor digestion. It seems to bind bacterial toxins in the gut, which would contribute to its anti-inflammatory effects as well as taking some pressure off the liver and kidney detoxification pathways.

Last but not least, sarsaparilla helps balance hormones. Though the specifics are a little vague, it does have a traditional use for low testosterone, including as an aphrodisiac. Herbalist Aurelien Cardinal uses it to increase uptake in androgen receptors for trans folks, and Eric Yarnell uses it as a hormone modulator in all kinds of people.

This is a very useful plant. Just remember that it works slowly, and its real potency unfolds after weeks or perhaps months of consistent use.

Future harvests

It's hard to imagine these vines being over-harvested. They are abundant, universally disliked, and take a long time to gather. All the same, they are native plants and provide wildlife habitat, so treat them with respect.

HERBAL PREPARATIONS

Most commonly used as a dry root decoction, but it also works as a tincture. The roots can be fermented into a soda or alcoholic beverage, like beer or mead. Sarsaparilla combined with sassafras was the original root beer, which was originally a health drink! Oh, how far we have fallen.

sassafras

Sassafras albidum
PARTS USED root bark

A blood mover and blood cleanser that tastes like root beer.

How to identify

Sassafras is a small tree, usually 5–20 feet tall, rarely to 50 feet. The trunk never goes straight up like a tulip poplar or a pine, but bends gently as it rises, with most of the leaves in the upper third of the tree.

The leaves are distinctive: some are football-shaped, some mitten-shaped with 2 lobes, and some are 3-lobed, looking like a ghost from a Charlie Brown Halloween special. This is a pretty unique characteristic, with only a couple look-alikes. Great ragweed can have entire and 3-lobed leaves, but it is an herb, not a tree, and its leaves are opposite. Mulberry also bears variously shaped leaves on the same tree, but sassafras has more roundedness to its leaves and smooth margins.

All parts of the tree are aromatic, and the leaves are moist and tasty.

Where, when, and how to wildcraft

Sassafras occurs from southern New York to central Florida and west to eastern Texas. It is common throughout the Southeast, tending to like somewhat acidic soils with some pines and oaks mixed in, or even hickories, and is found in many different

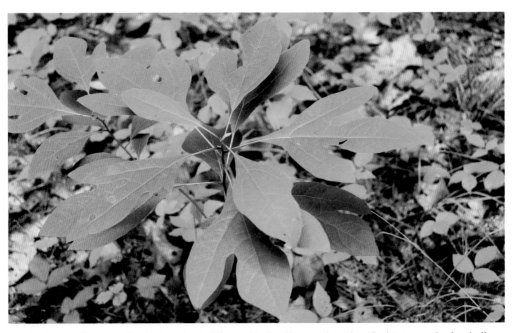

This baby sassafras tree already has the 3 different kinds of leaves that identify this tree—the football, the mitten, and the ghost.

environments from flat land up into the mountains at medium elevations.

Usually roots are harvested in the fall, but tradition holds that the best time to gather them is spring. I don't know why that is, but there must have been a reason. Dig the roots by following out a runner, maybe even using a mattock to unearth the root and pruners or even loppers to cut the root at the tree base. With larger roots, use just the bark; smaller roots can be used as is.

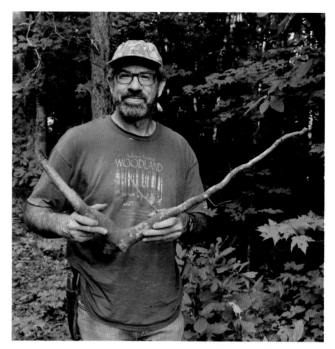

I'm getting cheesy with a long sassafras root I just harvested—the longer section was running lateral to the ground.

Medicinal uses

Sassafras is a relative of cinnamon, and it is a warming blood mover as well, but it is also a blood cleanser. This combination of cleansing and moving the blood makes it useful for a number of different conditions, from chronic skin conditions to joint problems.

Sassafras was actually the original export from the American colonies, even before tobacco—mainly because it was thought or hoped that it could cure syphilis.

Future harvests

It's not uncommon to find large stands of sassafras, so always look for abundance. When digging, think about ways to thin the stand by taking one of two trees that are growing too close to each other, thus giving the other tree more space to grow and thrive.

 Caution

There is some concern about the constituent safrole, but it seems to be dangerous only when it is concentrated into an essential oil. The tea is totally safe, and the tincture is pretty safe too because there is so little safrole in there.

HERBAL PREPARATIONS

The root bark is most commonly used as a decoction but can also be made into a tincture, 1:3 fresh or 1:5 dry. It also makes a great fermented soda, mead, or most traditionally, a root beer.

saw palmetto

Serenoa repens

PARTS USED fruit

A nourishing anti-inflammatory for the respiratory system and for genitourinary issues, notably BPH.

How to identify

These are shrub-sized palm trees (palmetto means "small palm"). The leaves are palmate and the whole plant is usually less than 6 feet tall. The long petioles that support the leaves are armed with sharp spines, which will tear up the legs of anyone foolish enough to wade through a colony of saw palmettos in shorts.

Although the spines are the main difference, saw palmetto also looks different from the other major shrub palms, principally dwarf palmetto (*Sabal minor*), in that its palm fronds are stiffer and a darker green. Looking more closely, saw palmetto petioles stop abruptly at the start of the leaves and are "squared off," whereas dwarf palmetto has a petiole that tapers into the leaf, forming a narrow V shape.

Where, when, and how to wildcraft

Saw palmetto grows from the southeast-ernmost tip of South Carolina south across

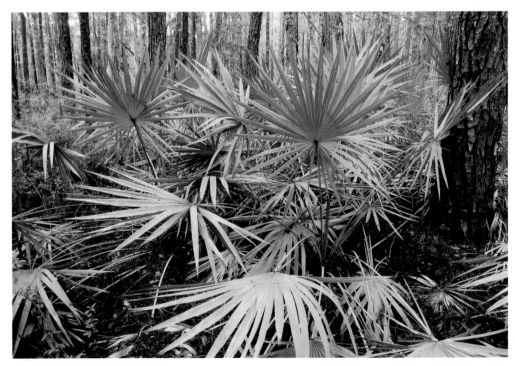

Thickets of saw palmetto are a common sight from Beaufort, South Carolina, south through Florida and west along the Gulf to Texas.

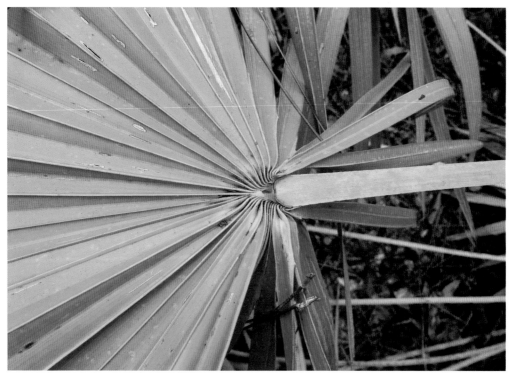

Saw palmetto petioles stop abruptly at the start of the leaves.

Florida and west along the Gulf Coast to just barely into Louisiana. It spreads mostly by underground stolons, forming large stands. The hard part is finding it when the berry, the only medicinal part, is ripe.

In Florida it can go to fruit at almost any time, but August and September are the best bet for ripe berries. When ripe they are purple-black, oval, and oily, very much resembling a large olive, and coming from a long stalk extending from the base of the plant to form a panicle of berries. Harvest as many as you see; be aware that they are oily enough to stain a harvesting bag, and they have a musty blue cheese kind of smell that is not the most appealing. They can be used fresh or dry.

Medicinal uses

Saw palmetto is known first and foremost as an herb for enlarged prostate. It is an interesting plant in that it both nourishes the sexual organs but also moves and clears inflammation. This combination of building and clearing, as well as its specific hormonal effects, makes it helpful for a number of uses. It was also traditionally used for lung issues.

It is one of the first remedies to think of for an enlarged prostate such as in BPH (benign prostatic hyperplasia), a noncancerous overgrowth of prostate tissue which can cause urinary tract issues. BPH is thought to be caused by an excess of DHT, a breakdown product of testosterone that is itself also a strong androgen. Saw palmetto inhibits 5-alpha-reductase, the enzyme that converts testosterone into DHT. This action seems to help reduce an enlarged prostate, especially when combined with nettle root and perhaps stone root or wild hydrangea. But the anti-androgenic effect also seems to help women with PCOS (polycystic ovarian syndrome), possibly through a similar hormone-blocking mechanism.

The fruit has a traditional use as a nourishing herb for the pelvic organs, especially in older and depleted people. But even as it nourishes, it also reduces inflammation and irritation in the genitourinary tract and has been used for interstitial cystitis, uterine fibroids, and even for urinary tract infections.

Although less commonly used for respiratory symptoms these days, saw palmetto has a history of being used for chronic coughs, asthma, and laryngitis. It may just have the same properties of nourishing while being anti-inflammatory in the lungs as it does in the genitourinary system.

Future harvests

This is an incredibly abundant plant where it grows and only the fruit is used, so there's no problem for future generations. The berries are eaten and loved by many wild animals, so leave some behind.

HERBAL PREPARATIONS

Tinctured dry 1:5 at 75% alcohol, or fresh 1:2 at 95% alcohol. Can make a decent infusion, and the funky flavor can easily be covered by other herbs.

self heal

Prunella vulgaris
PARTS USED aerial

An antioxidant internally and a wound-healer externally.

How to identify

Self heal (aka heal all) is a robust upright plant, 1–1.5 feet tall, with entire (occasionally slightly toothed) oval leaves. Like other plants in the mint family, it has opposite leaves, a square stem, and irregular flowers, but unlike many other mints it has no aroma.

The flower heads of self heal can be found in yards and fields or out on trails in the woods.

The stem itself can also be green or purple, or sometimes purple just at the leaf nodes.

The blue-purple flowers have a white lower lip and are in a tight head at the top of the stalk, unlike some related and similar-looking plants (e.g., ground ivy) that flower along the stem and have leaves in between some flowers. The leaves are usually 2–3 inches long, larger than the deadnettles and henbits (*Lamium* spp.).

Where, when, and how to wildcraft

The plants usually come up in late spring, flower in early summer, and then keep flowering through early fall. It can be harvested whenever the plant is in full flower, or you can harvest leaves earlier for first aid purposes. The same plant is used in Chinese medicine; they wait until the leaves wilt and the plant goes to seed to harvest it, so maybe there is some medicine in the seeds that Western herbalists are missing.

This is a common plant of yards, meadows, fields, and trails. Interestingly, it is considered both native and Eurasian; some botanical nomenclature recognizes two different varieties of the same species, though to be honest the differences are minute and hard to notice, so this book treats self heal as one species.

It grows abundantly in our region as far south as the Florida panhandle. It's a fairly easy plant to spot when in flower, as long as you're looking down at the ground.

Medicinal uses

Though mostly used in the United States as a simple first aid remedy or a flower essence, self heal is actually a subtle and powerful anti-inflammatory, antioxidant, and generally cooling herb for the whole body.

It is a great herb for first aid since it is so abundant and easily found, whether in yards or in the woods. Being both astringent and antioxidant, it has a long history of use applied topically to heal wounds and skin ulcerations. And those same properties of helping tissue to heal have also led to its being used for mouth and gum problems, including bleeding gums, as a gargle or rinse. The 16th-century herbalist Gerard said of self heal, "There is not a better wound herbe."

This herb is a powerful antioxidant, having more rosmarinic acid than rosemary itself! This could be why it is such a great herb for chronic inflammation and acute wound healing, especially when wounds are hot, red, and painful. It can also be used for gastrointestinal issues such as chronic diarrhea, hemorrhoids, and mild internal bleeding. It's even shown some positive effect against herpes viruses.

In Chinese medicine, self heal is a primary herb to "clear heat," which I interpret as helping calm the inflammatory process that causes the body to heat up. It is especially used for liver fire rising up to the head—red, painful, and swollen eyes or headaches with irritability and dizziness. But it also has the ability to dissolve accumulations so has been used for swollen glands, lipomas, or even goiters. It's been used in cancer formulas to treat tumors as well as for hyperthyroid and hypertension.

One of the more popular flower essences, it is said to increase one's tendency to want to take care of oneself. Herbalist Lupo Passero adds some to her formulas to increase client's desire to actually take the medicine that will be good for them.

This all-around wonder-herb is vastly underappreciated in Western medicine and deserves much more attention than it's received.

Future harvests

This is an abundant plant that can survive occasional mowing. Cut only the top half of plants when harvesting, and they're bound to come back.

HERBAL PREPARATIONS

Topically it can be used as a fresh leaf poultice or made into an infused oil or salve. Internally it can be made into an infusion or a tincture, fresh 1:2 at 95% or dry 1:5 at 50%.

shepherd's purse

Capsella bursa-pastoris
PARTS USED aerial

A common weed useful for internal bleeding.

How to identify

This small plant could easily be mistaken for bittercress (*Cardamine* spp.) or other spring mustard family weeds—until one sees the heart-shaped seedpods. The plant is hardly noticeable, growing 1–2 feet high, but it does grow in abundance where found.

The leaves are mostly basal, oblong, and lobed like other mustards; the few stem leaves are long, alternate, and linear. After the plant flowers and then goes to seed, the basal leaves may wither and disappear. The flowers are tiny and white with 4 even petals. As the plant elongates into seed there remains a cluster of white flowers at the tip as the heart-shaped seedpods form along the length of the stem. It's nigh-on impossible to positively identify this plant without seeing a seedpod.

Where, when, and how to wildcraft

In the Southeast, this is a plant of early to mid-spring; further north it is more of a summer plant. But if you miss looking for this plant in March or April then you've missed your chance for the year. It is found in every U.S. state, though more abundant in some than others.

Harvest the whole aboveground plant—leaves, flowers, and seeds, clipping underneath the basal leaves.

Medicinal uses

Shepherd's purse has a long reputation for stopping bleeding, but it's important to be specific because there are different kinds of bleeding. It doesn't do a great job applied

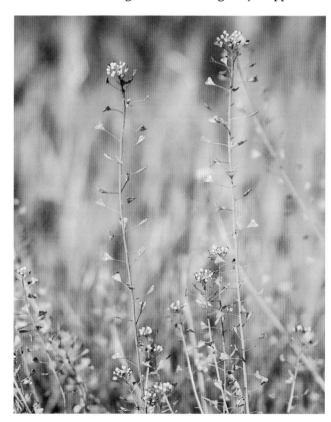

Each spring brings a handful of small weeds in the mustard family, sheperd's purse among them.

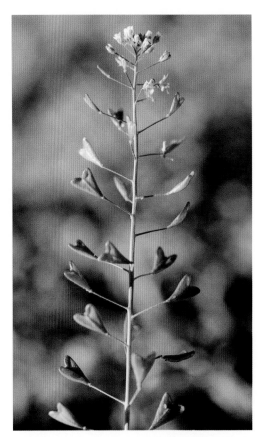

But only shepherd's purse has those heart-shaped seedpods.

topically (use yarrow for that), but it is good for passive hemorrhage, a slow and leaky internal bleeding. Think of it as a remedy for bleeding stomach ulcers (after seeing a doctor), dangerously excessive menstrual bleeding, or postpartum hemorrhage. I have heard from midwives not to use it until after birth, or you risk causing hour-glass contractions.

Well known for stopping bleeding, this herb also has another excellent use—it helps the kidneys clear uric acid. This makes it extremely effective for gout, especially combined with nettle and cleavers, where a buildup of uric acid in the body leads to intense pain in one joint of the body, often the big toe.

Future harvests

It's a weedy annual, harvest as much as you want. Leave some to make seeds for next year.

HERBAL PREPARATIONS

Tincture of fresh aerial plant, 1:2 at 95% alcohol, or fresh glycerin extract.

skullcap

Scutellaria lateriflora, S. incana
PARTS USED aerial

This is one of the best herbs for the entire nervous system, being both calming and nourishing, helping with pain, anxiety, and insomnia.

How to identify

Although about 25 species of skullcap occur in the Southeast, only a few are used and only one is official: mad-dog skullcap (*Scutellaria lateriflora*). The other one I use is downy skullcap (*S. incana*). Other species might be useful but have not yet been tried. Some species are infrequent to rare, so harvest only plants that are common in your area.

All skullcaps are in the mint family (Lamiaceae), and besides lacking a smell they have all the other botanical characteristics of

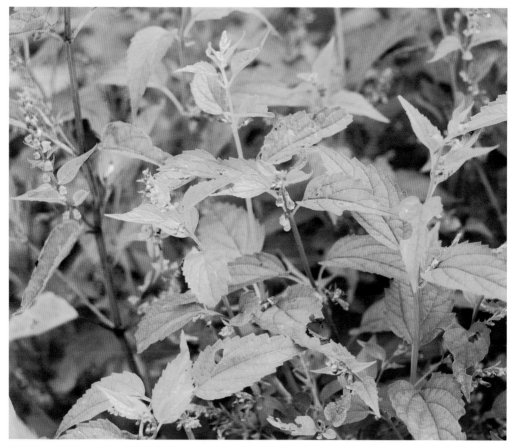

Mad-dog skullcap, the official skullcap of the Southeast, doesn't grow tall and carries its small blue flowers on one side of the flowering stalk.

that family, namely square stems, opposite leaves, and irregular flowers. What makes this genus unique is the helmet-shaped flowers and seed heads that swoop up in front like a pope's hat (hence the common name). They have slightly toothed leaves, except for *Scutellaria integrifolia*, which has entire (smooth-edged) leaves.

Mad-dog skullcap is a thin, slight plant with small blue flowers, growing 1–2 feet high; it is so small, it is easy to walk by without noticing it. Downy skullcap is a larger, more robust plant, 2–3 feet tall, with larger and showier flowers. Overall, it is much more noticeable.

Where, when, and how to wildcraft

Mad-dog skullcap prefers shade and can often be found next to creeks and streams in woods and in wetlands. It doesn't grow in water, but it does like damp areas that get occasionally flooded. Where it grows in the Southeast is a bit unpredictable; it is abundant in most of Virginia and much of Tennessee but almost nonexistent in the mountains of North Carolina, showing up again as far south and west as Louisiana and Arkansas.

Downy skullcap grows in a very different habitat. It likes drier areas and partial shade and is usually found where woods and meadow meet, both 10–15 feet into the woods and about the same distance into the meadow. Although abundant in the Blue Ridge mountains, it is only scattered across the rest of the Southeast.

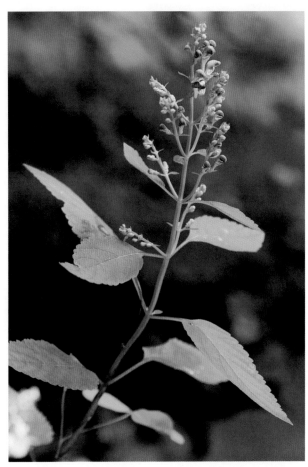

Downy skullcap, a taller plant with showier flowers, is more bitter than mad-dog skullcap and makes for a stronger sedative action.

For either plant, harvest the whole plant in middle to late summer when it is in full bloom or even when it is in seed. As long as the leaves still look good, it is OK to harvest. It's never really an abundant plant, so harvest with consideration. The whole plant of mad-dog skullcap can be used, but for downy skullcap, the tough woody stems should be sorted out and discarded.

Medicinal uses

Skullcap is a highly useful herb that belongs in everyone's apothecary. It is my favorite nervine, both calming and nourishing, making it a useful tonic for several different conditions, including anxiety, nerve pain, headaches, and even epilepsy.

By calming the nervous system, it seems to reduce pain signaling; so skullcap can be used for many kinds of pain, although it is most specific for nerve pain. It is my first choice for sciatica, spinal pain, or the kind of shooting pain that can indicate nerve pain, usually combined with St. John's wort.

It has a long history of being used for tics and tremors, even being used in the 19th century for epilepsy—what one might call "liver wind" in Chinese medicine, because it helps move qi that is "jammed up" and causing the tremors. For the same reason, it can be helpful for migraine headaches; for this use, it is best combined with blue vervain.

The combination of nourishing and calming can be perfect for certain kinds of insomnia, especially when people feel worn thin and exhausted, what I call a deficiency-type insomnia. Understanding the difference between insomnia from excess and from deficiency can be really helpful in treatment, especially for chronic insomnia.

Insomnia is mostly treated in Western herbalism as a condition of excess energy in the nervous system and so sedative herbs are used. But often in chronic insomnia the person's nervous system is exhausted and depleted, and they might feel "too tired to sleep." In this case, valerian and other sedative herbs won't help and might even make things worse. Herbs that nourish the nervous system will often work better—besides skullcap, I might also think of reishi and a good dose of magnesium. Mimosa bark could also be added if there is an emotional aspect to the insomnia such as trauma.

Finally it is a great herb for anxiety, either for acute anxiety attacks (though anemone is a stronger medicine here) or as a tonic taken long-term to prevent anxiety.

Future harvests

Skullcaps don't tend to grow in large stands, so harvest with care and leave plenty for future generations. Spread out your harvesting by walking between harvests. Also, be careful not to set off streambank erosion when harvesting along wooded creeks.

HERBAL PREPARATIONS

Fresh plant is the preferred form. Make into a tincture at 1:2, or use glycerin at the same ratio. You can also make a decoction of the dried herb (Light 2018).

skunk cabbage

Symplocarpus foetidus
PARTS USED root

A respiratory antispasmodic.

How to identify
The first hint of this plant each year is the alien-like flower that bulges out of swampy areas in January like a gnome periscope. Each low-growing spike of flowers is covered by a hooded spathe, much like other flowers in the Araceae, like Jack in the pulpit and calla lily. Curiously, it generates its own heat, which is why it can bloom in January and melt the snow around it.

The leaves come out later, directly from the root; they are large (1–2 feet long), flat, and vaguely cabbage-like. Despite the name, they are not edible—they contain calcium oxalate crystals, and the experience would be like chewing glass. The "skunk" in the name is pretty descriptive; a sulfurous odor surrounds these plants, and if you are in any doubt as to identity, break off a piece of leaf and take a good whiff. One sniff and you'll know if you have the right plant.

Where, when, and how to wildcraft
This is a more northern plant that extends its range down into Virginia and West Virginia, and barely into the mountains of North

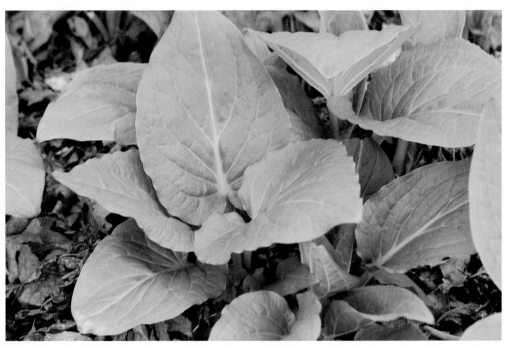

Yes, you would think the giant leaves would be hard to miss in swampy areas, but wait until you smell that skunky funk.

Carolina at the Virginia border. It is always found in swampy woods areas, like the flood-plain of a stream. In North Carolina, it is not uncommon to find it abundantly around Boone, for instance.

Because it likes to grow in the muck, it is a chore to dig. And messy. There is a taproot that reaches straight down and lots of side roots that shoot off horizontally. One plant can make a couple of quarts of tincture, and I haven't noticed any difference between the flavor of taproot and side roots. A good shovel is a necessity here. And a lot of patience and perseverance.

Medicinal uses

Skunk cabbage is first and foremost a smooth muscle antispasmodic, most notably for the lungs, where it was traditionally used for spasmodic asthma and whooping cough. It seems to also break up phlegm in the lungs and is a relaxing expectorant. It is also a bronchodilator and may be useful for some kinds of pain.

Mostly it was traditionally used for lung spasms. As both an antispasmodic and bronchodilator, it is very useful for spas-modic (not inflammatory) asthma—a smaller subset of asthma clients. But it is extremely useful for intense coughing fits, like one experiences in whooping cough. One of the classic indications is for coughing that's so bad it feels like you're going to throw up. Ironically, if you take too much of this herb you might throw up yourself.

This is a potent herb that should be used only by experienced herbalists, and only in low doses.

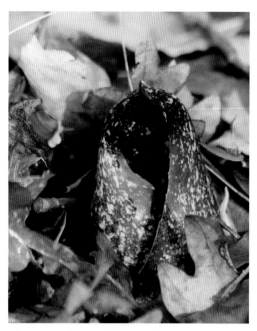

The strange flower of skunk cabbage rises out of the January muck, sometimes burning through the snow around it.

Future harvests

Skunk cabbage is abundant where it is found, forming solid patches covered over with its distinctive leaves. Don't pick if it is rare in your area or you are on the edge of its range.

Caution

Not for use during pregnancy or lactation. Use low dose only; larger doses may be emetic. Avoid if there's a history of calcium oxalate kidney stones.

HERBAL PREPARATIONS

Fresh root, tinctured 1:2 at 95%. This is an advanced herb recommended for skilled practitioners only. It is a low-dose botani-cal: 3–15 drops in water, 3 times a day. The undiluted tincture may irritate the mouth and throat.

slippery elm

Ulmus rubra
PARTS USED inner bark

A soothing herb for sore throat, acid stomach, and more.

How to identify

Though it can be a tall tree, slippery elm seems most noticeable when it is 15–20 feet high along roadsides and streamsides. The leaves are doubly toothed and come to a point at the tip; their base is uneven, as with all elms, and there are strong veins coming out laterally from the center vein. The leaves are on the larger side (larger than those of American or Siberian elm), sandpapery above and hairy beneath; the young twigs and buds are also rough hairy. This plant comes with a fun party trick—take a leaf and lay it flat on your palm, then slap it with your other hand. If the upper surface sticks to your hand, then it is definitely slippery elm.

Where, when, and how to wildcraft

It grows from New England south to the mountains of northern Georgia, west through Kentucky and Tennessee, and south through Arkansas and Louisiana. In all areas, it is being attacked by the same Dutch elm disease that is killing many of the American elms, so what was once an abundant tree is becoming far less common. Once the infection begins, there is nothing that can treat the tree, so you might as well harvest and use the medicine before the tree dies.

The leaves of slippery elm are widest toward the tip, strongly veined, and have large teeth on the edge—but that "drip tip" cinches the ID.

To harvest, trim off a branch and then take off the corky outer bark with a draw knife. Then sweep those away and angle the draw knife down a bit further to get strips of pure inner bark. I don't always take off the outer bark when debarking other trees, especially if the bark is thinner, but for slippery elm it does make a better end product. Slivers of inner bark seem to make the best tea.

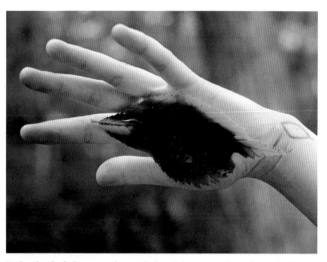

Pick a leaf of slippery elm and slap it (yes, you heard me right), and one side will stick to your hand.

Medicinal uses

The very name of this tree implies its medicinal use—the tea feels slippery in your mouth when you drink it, and that's exactly what it's used for. It treats sore throat, peptic ulcers, and pain on urination. It is soothing and moistening to many surfaces. It can also be used topically to hold a poultice in place.

This is one of the first herbs I think of for a sore throat from talking (or teaching) for too long, or just for general dehydration. The tea or the pastilles are wonderfully comforting and moistening for an irritated throat. They'll even help a sore throat during a cold, though they won't help fight the virus.

For the same reason, it can be helpful for any irritated condition of the digestive tract. It can be used for overly acidic stomach, peptic ulcers, or esophageal reflux. Look for symptoms like burning pain, irritation, and discomfort. If it feels more boggy than hot then the aromatic digestive herbs might work better. It can also help pain upon urination during a urinary tract infection.

An unusual but helpful use it to make a thick gruel of the powder as a food to help with dehydration from diarrhea or vomiting. I've seen it used at many large gatherings in the woods where diarrhea was a problem and people started getting dried out. Though this sounds symptomatic, dehydration from diarrhea is one of the leading causes of death in lesser developed countries.

Future harvests

Slippery elm has been overharvested at times, and Dutch elm disease is putting a lot of pressure on the remaining trees. So the best time to use them is if they are just beginning to get the disease, or if they are in a place where they need to get cleared anyway. Otherwise, most elms should be left to grow.

HERBAL PREPARATIONS

Slippery elm works best as a cold infusion—let the powder or bark strips sit in room-temperature water for a few hours then strain and drink. The hot infusion is medicinal but has more of a goopy texture. The powder can also be made into cough drops.

Solomon's seal

Polygonatum biflorum

PARTS USED root

A deeply healing and moistening herb that also helps tendons.

How to identify

Solomon's seal is a majestic plant that arches over like it's taking a bow. That itself is fairly distinctive, but a few relatives have a similar look. Solomon's plume (*Maianthemum racemosum*, aka false Solomon's seal) is the most common look-alike, but its flowers and berries are all in a big cluster (or plume) at the end of the main stalk; it also has more pleated, rougher-looking leaves with a bit more of a zig-zag to the stalk than Solomon's seal.

The plant itself can be fairly large, 3–4 feet long, with leaves alternating on the stem. The leaves have a blue-green tint to them, similar to the color of wild yam leaves, and they are softer and smoother than Solomon's plume, not hairy at all.

The main way to tell this plant is by the flowers, which dangle in clusters of 2–4 from

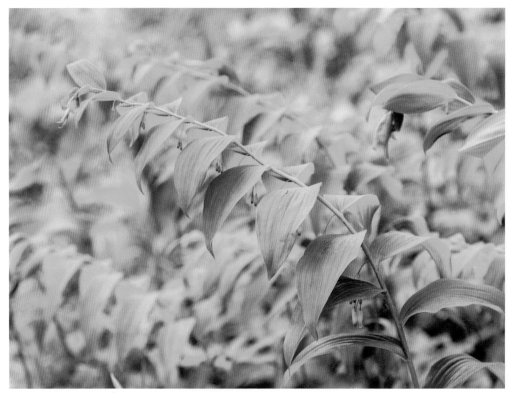

Solomon's seal has a soft appearance—it just feels softer and is more of a blue-green than Solomon's plume, not to mention the flowers run down the middle of the plant.

where the leaf meets the stem and then turn into blue berries by mid-summer.

Where, when, and how to wildcraft

This plant occurs throughout the Southeast as far south as northern Florida. It thrives in rich, wet woods and can sometimes be found along the sides of forest roads.

I prefer to harvest the roots of larger plants, in late summer or early fall. Because it comes up early in spring before the trees leaf out, Solomon's seal dies back earlier than other plants and once its leaves drop, it's almost impossible to find. The roots have rings on top from the previous year's stalk, each circle a king's "seal" to the imaginative; the age of a plant can be told by counting the rings.

Medicinal uses

I've always thought of Solomon's seal as a yin tonic that is deeply nourishing to the fluids of the body, but it is also a well-known remedy for tendon issues.

If you think about yin and yang as being the water and fire of the body, a yin tonic like Solomon's seal is good for people who are deeply dry. Not just dehydrated but with dry creaky joints, dry throat, dry skin—just generally lacking in moisture and oil. Thinking about the plant this way it's easier to understand the variety of its traditional uses—it can be used after recovery from a respiratory infection when the lungs are dried out from secreting so much mucus; it can be used for arthritis, specifically the arthritis of age, with a deficiency of synovial fluid making the joints dry and creaky. It's good for anyone who needs internal lubrication, so it could even be good for the dryness associated with menopause.

This same moistening aspect might be why it is so good for a variety of tendon issues. It has a nourishing effect on connective tissue and can be used internally and topically for tendonitis and carpal tunnel syndrome, or to help rebuild damaged tissue.

After a fracture, the bones actually heal faster than the tendons and ligaments around them, so Solomon's seal combined with gotu kola and horsetail is a good medicine to take a couple of months after breaking a bone; to support healing, be sure to also eat lots of blueberries, purple cabbage, and other richly colored fruits and vegetables.

Because as we grow older we all tend to get more dry, this root is also in some longevity formulas for people over 50 to help them maintain their spark. Overall, this beautiful herb is soothing and moistening to the whole body.

Future harvests

This plant is not as common as it used to be, so harvest with caution and respect. Harvest only from abundant stands and take only one out of six plants. Like black and blue cohosh and other woodland plants with rhizomes, the older root can be harvested and the front of the root with next year's bud can be replanted. Solomon's plume, which is more abundant and commonly found, should be explored as a potential substitute. Or one could use plantain or other moistening herbs.

HERBAL PREPARATIONS

Roots can be used in decoction, fresh or dry tincture, or topically as an infused oil.

Lindera benzoin
PARTS USED twigs, fruit

A warming remedy that stimulates digestion.

How to identify

Spicebush (aka Carolina allspice) is such a common understory shrub that the hard part isn't finding it, it's noticing it! The plant itself is not that distinctive, with many branches coming out of one base, and the leaves are oval and often slightly wider toward the pointed tip. It is much easier to notice in late summer and fall, when the female plants are filled with small red berries. Each berry has one large seed in it.

The flowers are tiny and yellow and bloom in March and April before anything has leaves on it, including this plant. There is also a distinctive aromatic smell to the leaves and branches, like a cross between cinnamon and

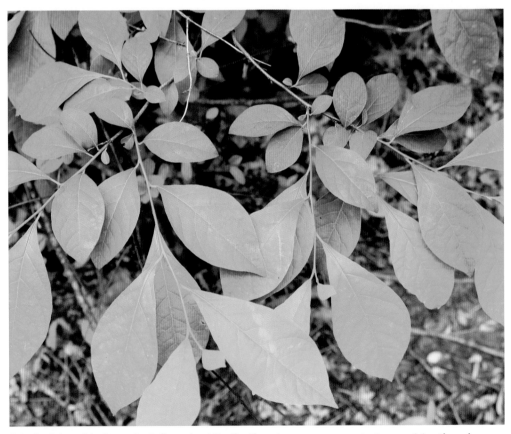

Spicebush is a ubiquitous shrub throughout the Southeast; as soon as you start recognizing those leaves, you'll see how common it is.

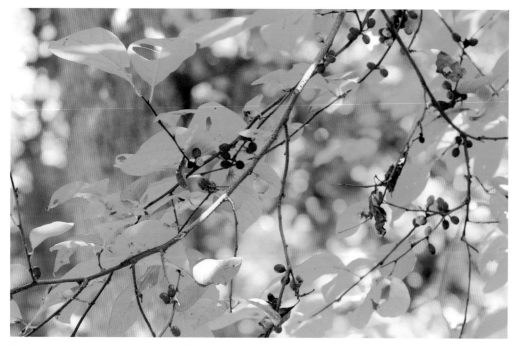

Each fall, spicebush develops the red berries that can be used as the namesake spice, Carolina allspice.

allspice—which makes sense, since this is in the same family as cinnamon and sassafras. The bark is smooth and gray, sometimes forming corky warts in age.

Where, when, and how to wildcraft

Spicebush is abundant throughout the Southeast down to the Gulf Coast and northern Florida. The twigs are best harvested in the early spring, ideally before the shrubs even have leaves on them, which means you need to find it by the flowers. Afterward is fine too, but by fall the twigs have lost most of their smell. They are lightweight, and so it takes a lot of harvesting to get a little bit of medicine. Luckily these shrubs are common and abundant where they grow. Oddly the smaller twigs are much more aromatic than the bark on older branches.

Harvest the berries in fall when they are red. It's hard to get them to dry well without a dehydrator.

Medicinal uses

This common shrub is not a powerful remedy, but it is both abundant and useful, so it's worth learning about. The twigs and the leaves smell strongly and wonderfully of allspice and make a tasty tea. This flavor is exactly what the medicine is—stimulating digestion, warming up the body, and helping sweat out a fever.

It has a deeply warming effect on digestion, less sharp than peppermint and more like dried ginger, though not as resinous. It helps stimulate a slow and sluggish digestion without being irritating to the digestive lining. Somehow it manages to just get things moving.

This same property, to get things moving and warm things up, makes it a decent herb to sweat out a fever. It might not be the first herb I would think of, but it's gently persistent, so would be good for someone with a frail cold constitution. This warming power can also help bring on a menstrual period that is late due to cold.

Future harvests

This native plant is often abundant but still should be harvested with appropriate care. Trim the branches as you would prune a fruit tree, taking branches that are overlapping other branches or that are getting shaded out.

 Caution

Contraindicated in pregnancy because of its moving potential. This is somewhat theoretical—but better to be safe.

HERBAL PREPARATIONS

Bark is mostly used as a decoction. Berries are mostly used as a condiment and substitute for allspice but make a serviceable infusion as well.

spikenard

Aralia racemosa

PARTS USED root, fruit

A warming and energizing tonic that nourishes and clears the lungs.

How to identify

This plant dies to the ground each fall and so is not a shrub, though it is often mistaken for one. Like black cohosh and other large, robust woodland plants, it sends out a stalk that forms a mosaic of numerous leaflets all on a plane, the better to catch the limited light of the deep woods. The leaves are 2- to 3-times pinnate, and each leaflet is heart-shaped at the base, fairly oval, slightly toothed, and comes to an elongated point at the tip.

Spikenard sends up a tall flower stalk with numerous umbels of white flowers in late summer; these ripen into purple berries by September. Each plant can be several feet across and in flower and berry can be 8 feet high.

Where, when, and how to wildcraft

It can be found up in the mountains along places where water runs—sometimes next to creeks up in a holler, but more often just the crease in the hillside where water flows

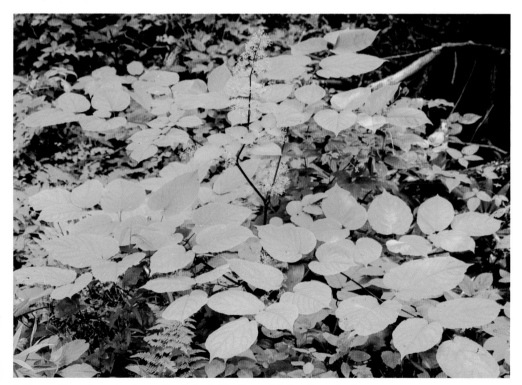

Spikenard is such a robust woodland plant, it's often mistaken for a shrub.

down during a heavy rainstorm. It can even be found on trailsides and old forest roads; it likes to have a bit more sunshine than the deep woods offer.

This plant grows in the mountains from New England south to northern Georgia and scattered across Tennessee and Kentucky to the Ozarks of northern Arkansas and Missouri.

Harvest the berries when purple in late summer, and the root in fall. You don't need much—one mature plant can provide a quart or two of fresh root tincture, so harvest it only where you see a decent amount of it.

Medicinal uses

Our native spikenard shouldn't be confused with the Old World spikenard that was mentioned in the Bible and is still used in aromatherapy. That plant is in the valerian family; this one is in the ginseng family.

They have a similar smell but aren't at all the same medicinally.

This plant has some chemistry in common with ginseng, containing ginsenosides that make it a good qi tonic and adaptogen. But there are also a lot of resins in the root (the berries even taste resinous, like the smell after blowing out a candle). These resins act as expectorants to help break up phlegm in the lungs, and they make the plant a little too moving and heating for the standard definition of adaptogen.

The roots make a great remedy for those with low energy and weak lungs—for example, someone who chronically gets bronchitis and lung infections, or has just quit smoking and has a lot of gunk to get out of their lungs. It is also a great remedy to use after a lung infection has passed and someone still has phlegm in their lungs but no energy to cough it up and out.

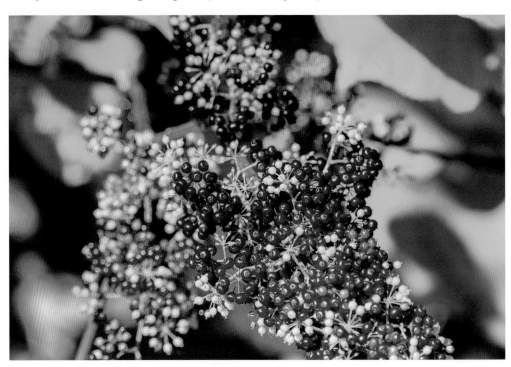

Spikenard's purple berries are a tasty and energizing treat in September and October.

It can be used somewhat like ginseng but has such a strong lung resonance that, again, it cannot be considered a pure adaptogen; but the berries have less resin and therefore make a better adaptogen, if that's what you want from the plant. The berries also make a tasty mead, in case you're interested.

This blend of strengthening the lungs while also stimulating expectoration makes it a fairly unique lung herb that can be used combined with angelica for acute bronchitis with lung congestion and fatigue, or to recover energy and eliminate residual phlegm after an illness has gone. This makes it a helpful plant to have around.

Future harvests

Spikenard is not very common, so harvest with great care and only when an abundance of plants are found.

HERBAL PREPARATIONS

Root or berries tinctured fresh 1:2 at 95%, or roots dry 1:5 at 50% alcohol. A syrup of either or both is probably the most traditional preparation. Be prepared to wash all your tools for the next few days: the sticky resin is almost impossible to get off. Rubbing alcohol seems to be the only thing that dilutes the resin, so keep a pint of that around before processing this plant.

St. John's wort

Hypericum perforatum

PARTS USED flowers

A nourishing and balancing herb for the entire nervous system, good for pain and depression.

How to identify

Many species in the genus *Hypericum* share the common name St. John's wort, but only one or two have medicinal uses. The official species used in herbal medicine is *H. perforatum*, an invasive plant from Europe. This species is bushy and branching but not woody, 2–3 feet high. The leaves are opposite, entire, and ovate, and the abundant flowers have 5 equal yellow petals that are deliciously sun-colored and smell vaguely like laundry soap.

More than two dozen *Hypericum* species occur in the Southeast, so make sure you

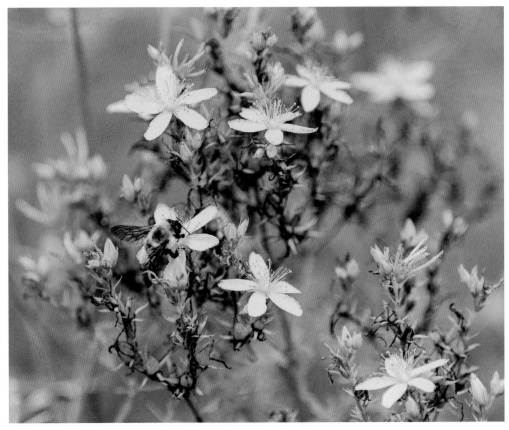

The European St. John's wort can fill North American meadows and fields with its bright sun-colored flowers.

get the right species. To make sure you have the right one, pick a leaf and hold it up to the sun. You should see tiny white dots, which are actually the oil glands of the plant. Then put a leaf on your palm and run a fingernail over it. It should leave a red line of that same oil, which contains the medicinal component, hypericin.

The only native species that might be medicinal is spotted St. John's wort (*Hypericum punctatum*), which also has tiny perforations in the leaf when held up to the sun, but the dots are black instead of clear. It forms small clusters, grows upright, and only branches at the top, whereas the European St. John's wort branches from the base. The native plant has larger leaves and smaller flowers.

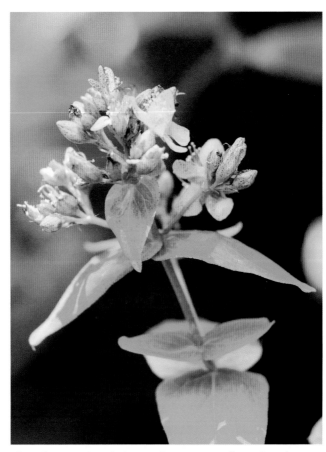

The only native St. John's wort that is potentially medicinal, spotted St. John's wort, has smaller flowers and larger leaves than the official species.

Where, when, and how to wildcraft

St. John's wort is a plant of the sun. The sunny yellow flowers bloom most prolifically on St. John's Day, the Christian holiday that celebrates the longest day of the year with the most amount of sunshine, so plan for a summer solstice harvest.

This European invasive is found in disturbed areas, growing in great swaths of yellow in places that receive full sun (open meadows, mountain balds, old cow pastures) in Virginia, West Virginia, and Kentucky south to parts of North Carolina and Tennessee, becoming less abundant further south.

For most of the continent it's a weed. It is illegal to grow in certain western states, and the Klamath beetle, which feeds exclusively on this plant, has been released to control it. Ranchers get concerned about this plant because ingestion of large quantities by cows can cause severe sunburn and even death.

Medicinal uses

It's best known as an herb for depression, bringing in the sunshine during dark times, but it's really a nourishing tonic for the entire nervous system. It is also an excellent first aid remedy for pain and bruises, which has been forgotten due to its current popularity as an antidepressant.

The primary way it works is by nourishing and calming the nervous system, which so many of us need these days. In the 19th century it was used with milky oat seed for neurasthenia (weakness of the nervous system); see the entry on oats for more on that.

Though this herb has had quite a ride as an antidepressant, it's not an herbal Prozac. All this hype about antidepressant herbs makes me wonder why antidepressants are some of the most prescribed pharmaceuticals in the United States. Not to say there aren't verifiable chemical imbalances in some people's brains, but before using a remedy to fix a disease called depression, we first need to look inside and find the roots of our melancholy—turn off the TV and spend a day alone in the woods! We must not simply accept the easy remedy as a cure-all without doing the soul-searching—St. John's wort just won't cover that up. The greatest causes of depression in our society are alienation and the ensuing loneliness, and not following our heart's true passion.

That said, think about St. John's wort for stressed-out depressed people combined with milky oat seed. Or to open up the shades and let the sun in for melancholy, combined with lemon balm. Also useful for seasonal affective disorder and PMS. Because it is a tonic, don't expect immediate results. Wait 2–3 weeks to begin feeling it and 2–3 months for full effect, but there may be some immediate effects as well.

St. John's wort also has a long history for first aid. The infused oil can be used topically for burns and slow-healing wounds, and it is especially good for nerve pain, from sciatica to spinal pain. For symptomatic relief of spinal pain, rub the oil on and take the tincture internally. Nothing will hold you over better until you get to the chiropractor.

Combine it with arnica oil for an all-purpose "trauma oil" for any kind of blunt trauma. Just don't use arnica on injuries that break the skin—it's too irritating; but St. John's wort by itself is OK.

This popular herb has been well researched, and in that research they found it interacts with certain drugs because it speeds up the liver's clearing of those drugs. The cool thing about that is that now we know that it is also an herb that clears toxins from the liver as well as drugs!

Future harvests

No worries about overharvesting this invasive European plant; we use only its flowering tops.

Caution

St. John's wort can stimulate the liver to clear some pharmaceuticals from the body faster, including the hormones found in birth control pills. So doublecheck herb-drug interactions with this plant. Some who take large doses can become more sensitive to sunburns (photosensitivity), even though the infused oil of the same herb can treat burns or sunburns.

HERBAL PREPARATIONS

The fresh herb is considered superior and is preferred for tincture or glycerin extract. To make the infused oil, bruise the herb (mash it in your hands) before putting it in a jar. It is the only infused oil that I leave in the sun to infuse.

Collinsonia canadensis
PARTS USED whole plant

An underused plant that helps move chronic stuck conditions.

How to identify
Big, toothed, opposite leaves with spikes of yellow citronella-smelling flowers are a dead giveaway. The leaves could be mistaken for wild hydrangea, which also has large, opposite, toothed leaves, but that plant is a shrub with woody stems and stone root is herbaceous. The leaves also look a bit like wood nettle, but that plant has alternate leaves and will give you a sting to remind you who's who.

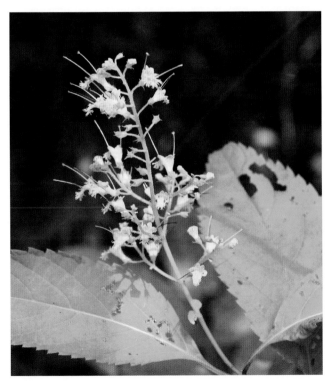

The flowering tops of stone root are a common sight in late summer forests, letting off a citronella-like smell.

Where, when, and how to wildcraft
This plant grows pretty abundantly in the woods. Though it emerges in April, it's usually easier to spot when in bloom in late summer. I often see great swaths of it driving through forests in August.

It grows from Maryland south to northern Georgia, mostly in mountains and the Piedmont, and west through Tennessee and Kentucky as well as some scattered locations in the Deep South.

You can harvest the whole plant when in flower—roots, leaves, and flowers. Or you can harvest leaves and flowers in late summer and come back for the root in October. Either way, I usually tincture the leaves and flowers in one jar and then set about washing and chopping the roots. When I give it to people, I blend the two equally.

Chopping the roots is not an easy task—there's a reason this plant is called stone root! Good pruners and maybe even loppers will help get it into small enough chunks to be usable.

Medicinal uses
This useful but lesser-known herb is usually one part of a larger formula. It is a deep and slow blood mover, especially for the pelvic area and for portal

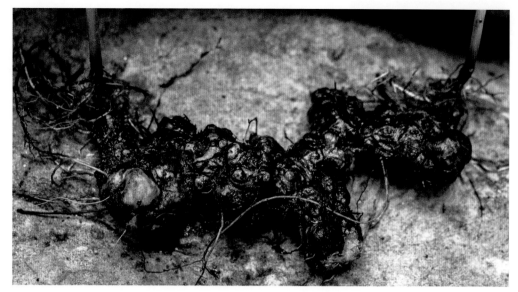

There is a reason for stone root's common name: the roots are often flat and hard as a rock.

congestion. Doing that, it helps break up accumulations in the body. It is also a vascular tonic because of its flavonoid content.

Stone root is an excellent tonic herb for hemorrhoids and varicose veins, especially combined with witch hazel tincture. It mainly works by opening up the portal vein, the vein which drains blood from the pelvic and abdominal areas, including freshly assimilated nutrients, and brings everything up to the liver for processing. When the liver gets overwhelmed or the portal vein backs up, it can cause congestion of the fluids and blood in the pelvis, which often shows up as hemorrhoids and varicose veins.

This can also show up as uterine fibroids and enlarged prostate: when fluids aren't being drained well from the pelvis, then waste products start accumulating and the tissue isn't as healthy—you get the stagnant pond effect. Stone root gets those fluids moving and so can reduce those types of growths. For prostate problems, such as BPH, it combines nicely with saw palmetto, and for uterine fibroids it pairs nicely with red root.

It is also considered an antilithic, meaning it can break up kidney stones. Combined with wild hydrangea and gravel root, it helps to both break up stones and get them moving out of the body.

Future harvests

It is fairly abundant where it grows, so it is not as great a concern as many other woodland plants.

HERBAL PREPARATIONS

Fresh 1:2 tincture of root and at a different time (if possible) the leaves and flowers combined.

sumac

Rhus glabra, R. copallinum, R. typhina
PARTS USED fruit, bark, root

A common scrub tree that is cooling and anti-inflammatory.

How to identify

All the sumacs are small scrubby trees growing up to 15 feet high with clusters of berries beginning in summer that persist through winter. The leaves are pinnate with 7–31 leaflets. Fragrant sumac (*Rhus aromatica*) has only 3 leaflets but wasn't used for medicine as far as I know.

The first thing to be aware of, and the most common question about sumac that I get, is how to differentiate the medicinal species of sumac from poison sumac (*Toxicodendron vernix*). Luckily, smooth sumac (*Rhus glabra*), winged sumac (*R. copallinum*), and staghorn sumac (*R. typhina*) are much more common than poison sumac and are easily distinguished from it. The two easiest ways to tell the difference are the color of the berries and the location. Poison sumac is the only species with white or yellow berries, and all the other safe-to-touch sumac species have red berries. Easy (when the berries are out).

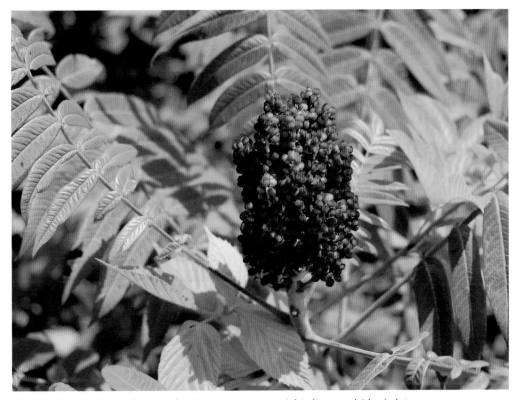

The red clusters of smooth sumac berries are a common sight along roadsides in late summer.

Also, in most of the country, poison sumac occurs only in true bogs; in some parts of the Deep South along the coastal plain, it can also be found in streamhead pocosins. Overall, you're not going to find it that often, but the rash is so intense that if in doubt, avoid it.

Where, when, and how to wildcraft

The sumacs written about here are found in meadows, roadsides, old pastures—wherever there's some disturbed areas where the forest is just starting to come back. They're common on many country roads as well, making them easy to find. I prefer to harvest them from meadows or small roads to avoid the pollution of busier roads.

Use a pruner to clip the whole cluster of berries from mid-summer through to frost after a couple of sunny days in a row. The rain will wash out some of the medicinal compounds, but they come back soon after. Traditionally the berries are harvested before the first frost, but in a pinch you could harvest later—they just won't be quite as strong.

Since there may be small insects living inside the berry cluster, you may want to submerge them in cold water for 5–10 minutes to let the bugs float to the surface. This will reduce some of the medicine, but it does make a more vegetarian end product.

The root can also be used and is dug in the late fall. Go for medium-sized trees in a stand of sumac, cutting the tops first with a saw and then digging down and around. The wood and roots are both surprisingly light and fragile.

Though there is some traditional use of the bark, I haven't used it myself.

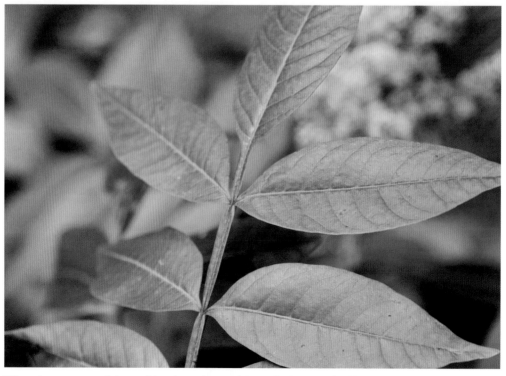

Winged sumac, one of the traditional species used, is easily distinguished by its winged leaf stalk.

Medicinal uses

The flavor of the berries is sour and astringent, and this indicates its use to cool and shrink inflamed tissues. It can be a refreshingly cooling drink on a hot day and in the same vein can be used to bring down an overly high fever.

Like many berries, sumacs are high in vitamin C and flavonoids, which are also good for the immune system and long-term health. This might in part explain why the fruit was used for respiratory health.

The berries and the roots have been used to cool off inflammation and irritation in the urinary tract, while the astringency helps create better tissue tone. The tincture or especially the tea can help with symptoms of frequent urination, or symptomatically for chronic irritation, such as in interstitial cystitis.

Sumac has also been used for passive ulcers anywhere in the digestive tract. This is probably a combination of its use as an astringent (closing up wounds) and the flavonoids speeding up healing and acting as a tissue tonic.

For the same reasons it can be used as a mouthrinse for apthous ulcers, gum disease, or other conditions where tissues in the mouth are damaged and boggy with poor circulation.

Future harvests

Sumacs are native but abundant throughout the Southeast, so there is little risk of harming the stands. If digging roots, dig trees at the edges of a stand, favoring trees that are growing closer together. In other words, think of it like pruning to help the survival of the remaining trees.

HERBAL PREPARATIONS

The berries can be tinctured fresh 1:2 at 95%, or dried 1:5 at 50%. Traditionally they were also infused in apple cider vinegar—just fill a jar with the berries and fill to cover them.

For a tasty drink, put one large or two small clusters in a gallon of water, loosely cover, and set in the sun for a few hours. You'll find out why one of the local names for sumac is lemonade berry.

Liquidambar styraciflua
PARTS USED bark, fruit, resin

A powerful antimicrobial, skin-healing herb that also helps respiratory infections.

How to identify

Sweet gum trees are tall, 60–100 feet high; leaves are conspicuously star-shaped, each with 5–7 sharp lobes pointing out like a starfish. It's hard to imagine another leaf that looks similar, except for possibly the Asian species of this genus which are planted in towns. The bark has a rough texture, sometimes with sticky resin growing in between the ridges.

The other striking feature of this tree are the "gum balls"—the abundant spiked hollow

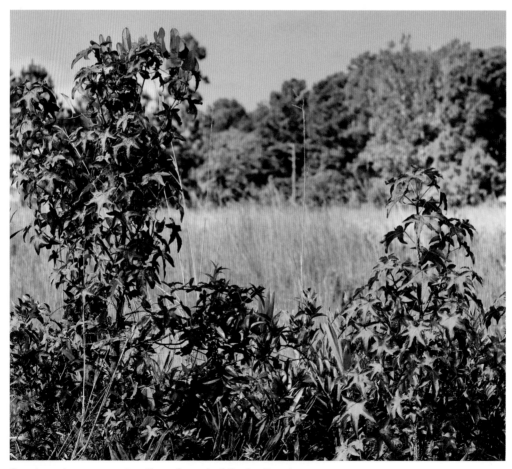

Sweet gum is a common tree through much of the Southeast.

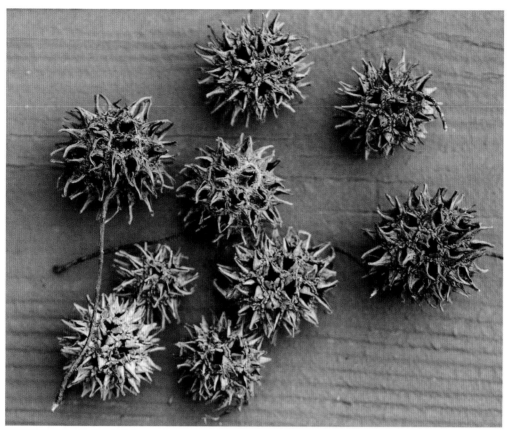

The spiked balls of sweet gum can be used for medicine—just try to avoid stepping on them barefoot when harvesting.

balls that pose a hazard to anyone walking barefoot underneath this tree. They are most reminiscent of a medieval mace.

Where, when, and how to wildcraft

This tree is usually found in abundance in places where it grows, often on roadsides and as a first-succession tree, though taller trees can hold their own in a later stage forest too. It grows in every state of the Southeast but is less common in the mountains, not growing much above 1,500 feet elevation.

Harvest the bark in the spring, the unripe fruits in the early fall, and the resin whenever you find it.

Medicinal uses

It's hard to believe how popular this herb was based on how little is written about it in modern herbal medicine. It is still very popular as a folk remedy, though, because it is incredibly common and incredibly useful for everything from coughs and colds to arthritis pain.

Much of its medicine comes from the antiseptic resin that runs through its veins. This resin, like the resin of pine trees, can be used topically as an antiseptic and antimicrobial—just what the tree is using it for. The resin (or gum) oozes out of wounds and slowly solidifies; it can be put on wounds right away or stored for later use. It can also be extracted into a liniment for that purpose. This antiseptic action has been used internally for sore throats, urinary tract infections, and diarrhea.

The resin makes a good expectorant, though not as strong and stimulating as white pine resin. It can still be helpful at breaking up mild lung congestion and getting the phlegm up and out, and it has a long history of use in the Southeast for coughs and colds. The combination of expectorant and antimicrobial is especially helpful.

Another species, *Liquidambar formosana* (lu lu tong), is used for pain in Chinese medicine. Its Chinese common name translates as "all roads open"—it is that good at opening the channels to get things moving in the body. All pain in Chinese medicine is thought to be from stagnation, and the Asian sweet gum balls are considered excellent to move both qi and blood. It is specific for low back pain and pain in the extremities but also for pain from injury. In general, Chinese medicine looks at resinous herbs for pain, whereas Western herbalism looks at resins as antimicrobials.

Will Morris talks about using lu lu tong to open up the diaphragm of people who are holding their breath because of nervous tension. Again, it comes back to the idea of opening things up to allow for better movement. This ends up having a relaxing effect, though it is not considered a nervine herb.

Indigenous people poultice the leaves topically for mild arthritis as well, according to Darryl Patton (2017). So there are still some similarities between the Chinese and our region's traditional use of these plants.

Future harvests

It is a native plant but can be found in profusion throughout the Southeast, so there is little worry of overharvesting as long as one

HERBAL PREPARATIONS

The slightly unripe sweet gum balls make a good decoction and can be dried and tinctured 1:5 at 50% alcohol. One might choose to put the balls in a burlap sack and rub it around well first to get the spines off so they don't cause injury later.

The resin can be used as is or preserved for later use. Though I've never tried it, there's no reason it couldn't make a great liniment for injuries.

The bark can also be harvested and used dried in decoction or tinctured fresh 1:2 at 95% or dried 1:5 at 65% alcohol.

is respectful of the tree.

Dipsacus fullonum (D. sylvestris)

PARTS USED root

A remedy for damaged tendons, low back pain, and possibly Lyme disease.

How to identify

Teasel is an unusual-looking plant. The leaves are poky and thistle-like, and the main stalk even more so. It is a biennial, so the first year it has just basal leaves, and the second year it puts up a flower stalk and then dies.

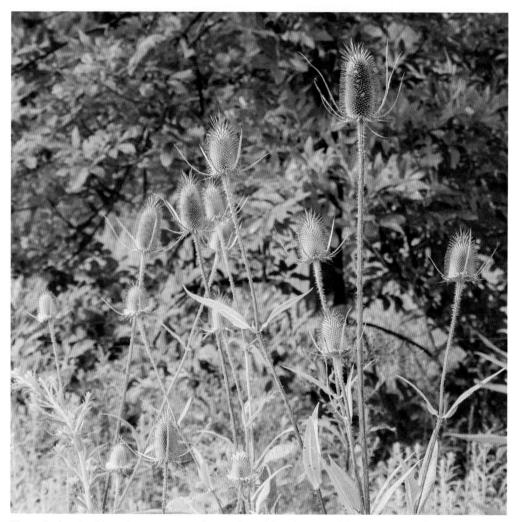

The spiky heads of teasel were once used to card wool, but the root of this noxious weed can be used for Lyme disease, among other things.

The leaves on the upper part of the flowering stalk sometimes grow together to form a cup that catches rainwater.

The flowers are strange prickly ovals with long thin bracts underneath. The purplish flowers start flowering in the middle of the head then continue flowering both up and down the flower head at the same time. The flower head is tough enough that it used to be used for carding wool.

Where, when, and how to wildcraft

This European weed is naturalized all along the East Coast from southern New England south to the North Carolina border, west into Tennessee and Kentucky, and off to Arkansas and Missouri. It is usually found on roadsides and waste places.

Make sure any plant you're considering rooting up is growing in a relatively clean place. Since it is a biennial, the root of plants that have gone to flower won't have as much potency, so it is better to harvest either in the fall of first-year plants or the spring of second-year plants before they take off. It's a decent-sized taproot, so a long shovel will be helpful to dig the root.

Medicinal uses

Teasel is another Asian species that is becoming weedy here but has a long history of use in traditional herbal medicine. Chinese medicine uses the root for muscle and tendon pain and even healing bones, but it is probably most well known in the United States as an herb for Lyme disease.

The Chinese use the closely related *Dipsacus asper* (xu duan) for pains and aches due to deficiency, especially pain in the lower half of the body—lower back, hips, and knees. It is also said to strengthen the tendons and bones and can be used for fractures and tendon damage resulting in swelling, pain, and inflammation. It can even be used topically for this effect. It also has the reputation of stopping a threatened miscarriage, possibly with bleeding. It could be a good herb for general soreness and pain in someone growing older and for osteoporosis. Herbalist William LeSassier first started using our American teasel as a substitute for the Chinese.

Later, Matthew Wood took this a step further and used teasel for Lyme disease. He's been using it this way since 1997 with positive results. It seems to have an action on the *Borrelia* spirochete specifically, drawing the spirochete that causes the infection out of the tissues and into the bloodstream so that the immune system can take care of it. This is most effective in low doses of tincture, as higher doses may cause a die-off that triggers a reaction, so please read up on this before attempting it yourself.

Not bad for a noxious weed.

Future harvests

This is an invasive weed, and it's fine to harvest as much as you want.

HERBAL PREPARATIONS

Dried root 1:5 at 40% alcohol. Or standard infusion.

Usnea spp.
PARTS USED whole lichen

A powerful antimicrobial.

How to identify

Usnea (aka old man's beard) is a lichen, a curious symbiosis between fungi and algae, with the fungal mycelium providing the structure and the algae wrapped around it photosynthesizing and providing the sugars. Some lichens grow on the ground, but usnea grows exclusively on trees, both alive and dead, forming branching dull green strands. It doesn't affect the health of the tree but uses it simply as a place to attach. Lichens in general are a sign of clean air; they won't grow in polluted environments.

The main indicator to identify usnea from other lichens is to look for a white thread in the middle of every tendril. Find a piece that's not too brittle, or get it wet if necessary, then gently pull a strand from both ends. If it is a true usnea, there will be a white elastic thread in the middle, surrounded by the sea-green algae.

Other related lichens may also contain usnic acid, one of the active constituents, and there are no poisonous look-alikes on the East Coast. The only poisonous look-alike is *Letharia vulpina* (wolf lichen), which grows

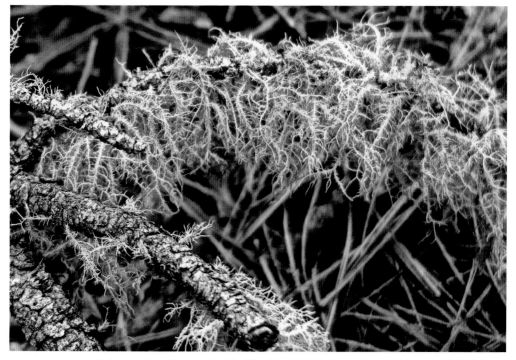

Usnea, a common lichen on branches, can be identified by the white thread inside the green sleeve.

in the northern Rockies, California, Oregon, and Washington, and it is a brighter yellow-green, not the dull green of usnea. It also lacks that central white cord that characterizes usnea.

There are many species within the genus, but lichen identification is outside the scope of this book and also somewhat immaterial, as all have similar constituents.

Where, when, and how to wildcraft

Usnea is best harvested from downed limbs on the ground; you'll often find these in good quantity after a spring rainstorm. Just strip off the bundles while trying to get as little as possible of the tree bark that it's attached to.

Good-quality usnea should still be green and somewhat flexible, at least when wet. If it is turning pink or orange then the fungal part is dying, and if it is crumbly brittle then it might be dead and should not be used.

Usnea can be harvested any time of year. You may have to go through your haul and pick out other lichens that were growing on the same tree, as well as any tree bark that made its way into your sack.

Medicinal uses

Usnea is the best-known medicinal lichen, sometimes touted as an alternative to the overharvested goldenseal for infections. Best known as an antibacterial, it has also been used as an antiviral by many herbalists, including some who used it during the COVID-19 pandemic with good results for the early stages of viral infection.

Like many herbs used for infections, usnea is bitter, cold, and dry. It has a long tradition of use for many kinds of respiratory infections, especially ones with thick mucus (catarrh). It works as a mild expectorant, and herbalist Will Morris says it opens the lungs and improves breathing, possibly by getting excess fluids out of the way.

It is also used for the genitourinary tract, and it is excellent for urinary tract infections; Bill Mitchell even used it as a diuretic as well as urinary antiseptic. It has a history of being used for sexually transmitted infections, both internally and as a pessary. The pessary can also be used for cervical dysplasia.

Finally, it is an excellent topical antiseptic, useful for wounds and staph infections. For this, the raw lichen can be applied directly or the tincture can be used. Although usnic acid is very oil soluble, it is best not to use oils and salves on open wounds as the oil can trap in bacteria. But for wounds that have healed over, the infused oil could be helpful.

Future harvests

Best practice is to harvest usnea only from downed branches, where it won't live long anyway, as opposed to taking from standing trees.

HERBAL PREPARATIONS

There are different opinions about the best way to prepare this. Usnic acid, the main antimicrobial constituent, is more alcohol and oil soluble, while the immune-modulating polysaccharides are more water soluble. And heat seems to help.

Some dry fry the lichen first before tincturing dry 1:5 at 70% alcohol, and some tincture as is, then put it in a water bath or bain-marie to heat things up delicately with the lid on loosely. But the important thing to be aware of is that alcohol is extremely flammable and can easily ignite, so a room temperature tincture is the safest way to go.

Viola spp.
PARTS USED leaves, flowers

*An abundant plant that cleanses
the lymph system and helps with a dry cough.*

How to identify
Little is known about which of the approximately 40 different species of violets that occur in our region are the best to use. The one thing that is generally agreed on is to use the ones with blue (occasionally white) flowers and only basal leaves. The violets that form a flower stalk and have yellow flowers are generally not used for medicine or food.

The leaves are heart-shaped, slightly toothed, and come to a sharp point at the apex with "earlobes" at the base of the leaf.

Similar-looking medicinals include liferoot and wild ginger. The leaves of liferoot (and other *Packera* spp.) are rounded at the apex and have more pronounced (but still shallow) teeth. Wild ginger has a rounded top as well, but has a smooth (not toothed) edge, and the whole leaf is wider.

Of course the cute little violet flowers are unmistakable and tasty—irregular flowers that sit like small butterflies on the extended flower stalk. Each has a nectar-filled spur pointing back to the plant that's visible when

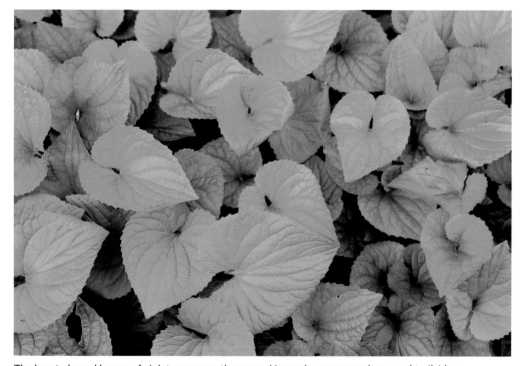

The heart-shaped leaves of violet can cover the ground in yards, open meadows, and trailsides.

you turn the flower upside down. Since there are some unfriendly look-alikes in addition to those just mentioned, the flower is the easiest way to make sure that you do actually have a violet in front of you.

There are so many species that I won't describe each one, but the most frequent violet, seen in fields, yards, and meadows throughout the Southeast, is the common blue violet, *Viola sororia*.

Where, when, and how to wildcraft

Violets are cosmopolitan. You can find them just about anywhere—in a yard in the city, in a suburban park, in a meadow or along a trail in the deep woods. Just make sure to harvest from a clean location.

Most violets bloom abundantly in mid-spring before trailing off to an occasional pop throughout the year. I generally harvest in spring and summer when the leaves are still soft and, ideally, flowers are present. To harvest, just pluck a few leaves and flowers as you amble through a patch without taking too many from any one plant.

Medicinal uses

Violets are one of those abundant and easy-to-use lymph movers, like red clover or burdock. They cool off inflammation and irritation, are moistening, and have been used for a dry cough. Like those other herbs, they are both gentle and powerful enough to be used in cancer formulas.

I think of violets first and foremost as a lymph mover. The lymph system is the storm drain of the body's fluids, helping return interstitial fluid from around the cells back to the blood. In the process, this fluid is examined by the immune system in waystations (lymph nodes and glands), to check in on what's happening downstream. If there is an

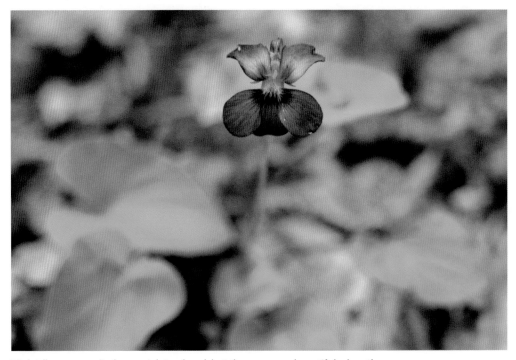

Violet flowers aren't always violet-colored, but they sure are beautiful when they are.

active infection or some other problem, fluids can get held up there and cause a swelling of that lymph node.

The lymph vessels themselves don't have an active pump in the way that the heart moves blood, so the motion of our muscles against the lymph is what pushes things along. Movement is the best lymph mover, but sometimes we need herbal support, too, and that's where lymphatic herbs come in—violet being one of several, including cleavers, red root, mullein, and poke.

Though each of these herbs has its own character and uses, they are all generally used for chronically swollen lymph glands, and in the treatment of cancers that use lymph vessels to spread. Violet is also specific for the breasts, where there is a lot of lymph tissue. As such, it has been used as a poultice for mastitis and in formulas for breast cancer prevention.

Violet leaves are also mucilaginous and helpful for the treatment of dry cough. Although plantain, slippery elm, and other demulcent herbs can help with dry cough, the lymphatic effect has a special place here. Mostly our lungs clear toxins by using tiny hairs (cilia) to push fluids and mucus up and out, combined with spasmodic compressions (coughing) when appropriate.

But when fluid is deep enough in the lungs, beyond the point where cilia exist, then the lymph system helps drain the excess fluid. This is why many lymphatic herbs are also considered positive lung herbs—violet, red clover, and even the classic lung herb, mullein.

One of the fascinating things about herbal medicine is that we have herbs like violet and red clover that are gentle enough to be used for food but powerful enough that, taken over time, they can treat something as big as cancer. Gently altering the body's environment for the better is a special paradigm, very different from using strong remedies to kill cancer cells.

Violet is not our most powerful herb, but it is abundant, easy to harvest, and very useful for home medicines.

Future harvests

Violets are native but abundant. They usually grow in patches, so just spread your harvest out, and the patch should bounce right back.

HERBAL PREPARATIONS

Tincture fresh, 1:2 at 95%. Make an infused oil of fresh leaves. Eat the flowers as tasty treats or decorate cakes and salads with them.

white cedar

Thuja occidentalis
PARTS USED leaves

An antifungal and antiviral herb that also helps with warts.

How to identify

Several evergreen trees are commonly known as cedars. On the East Coast, white cedar (aka northern white cedar, arborvitae) refers to *Thuja occidentalis* and eastern red cedar refers to *Juniperus virginiana*. Out west, red cedar refers to *T. plicata*. And even more confusing: none of these are the "true" cedar of the genus *Cedrus*. But that's less worrisome because those don't grow wild in the United States.

Looking at the leaves is enough to tell the two genera apart: plants in *Juniperus* have some flat overlapping scales but also some sharp needle-like leaves, whereas plants in *Thuja* have only the overlapping scales. Thuja leaves also all lie flat, so if you can easily press a branch between your palms, you're on the right track. And finally, thujas have tiny cones; junipers have modified cones that look like blue berries, though botanically they aren't berries at all.

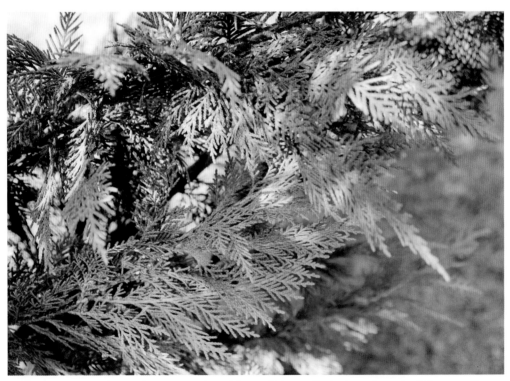

Whole branches of white cedar can be gathered for medicine; unlike juniper, the entire foliar spray lies flat without any needles.

Thujas appear columnar when seen from a distance, making it look as if they've been trimmed and manicured when they are actually just a wild plant.

Where, when, and how to wildcraft

White cedar can be found in the mountains of North Carolina and Tennessee, north through Virginia and West Virginia. It is also cultivated as an ornamental and planted by lumber companies after a cut.

Cedar leaves are evergreen and can therefore be harvested year-round. Clip small branches, fanning out the harvest and not taking too much from any one part of the tree. Then the green leaves can be trimmed off the branches in chunks and used as is for medicine.

Medicinal uses

White cedar is antiviral and antifungal, working slow and deep. It also helps topically with HPV and other warts. And like its cousin juniper, it is used for many urinary tract issues as well as for enlarged prostate.

When it comes to antivirals, white cedar is not fast acting, so it's better for lingering deep infections than acute upper respiratory infections. But for a lung infection that's gone on for a week (or a month), resisting all treatment, adding thuja to the formula can often help.

It is also a great antifungal and can be used for yeast infections, athlete's foot, ringworm, and other fungal issues, both topically and internally. It has a long history of helping to remove warts, both regular warts and genital warts (both are caused by HPV viruses).

Though the essential oil is sometimes used for skin warts, for genital warts it's better to use the infused oil or a wash of the tea. The infused oil or a salve made from that oil can be used for any fungal skin condition.

Thuja is also used for many conditions of the urinary tract. It improves the tone of the urinary tract and can help with incontinence from laughing or coughing, dribbling urine in the elderly, and enlarged prostate, whether due to BPH or chronic prostatitis; in the latter case, it would also help with any possible infection.

Future harvests

Harvesting a few branches here and there low on the tree won't harm the tree if it's established.

Caution

Because of its uterine-stimulating properties, not to be used during pregnancy. Not for long-term use; it contains thujone, which has cumulative toxicity. Most of the reported toxicity of this tree comes from the concentrated essential oil, though there have been reports of people having digestive upset after eating large quantities of leaves.

HERBAL PREPARATIONS

Tea, tincture, infused oil, salve, and pessary. Note that the tincture or tea will often cause a client to exclaim, "It tastes like Christmas!" regardless of their spiritual background.

Quercus alba
PARTS USED bark

A simple but very potent astringent for wounds and diarrhea.

How to identify
This is the classic oak, tall and slow-growing. It has a light-colored bark and alternate leaves and branches. The hairless leaves have 7–11 even lobes, which are rounded at the tip, not sharp-tipped like those of the red oaks.

Where, when, and how to wildcraft
White oaks are common trees of the entire East Coast down to very northern Florida. They are a monarch tree, powerful and noticeable in the midst of a forest or in a yard. They are most common in mature forests but can be found in places that have been cut if they've let the big trees stand.

Harvest the bark by cutting a few limbs with loppers in the spring. Then strip the bark off the limbs using a sharp knife. If you're lucky you can get the bark off in quills instead of having to whittle it off strip by strip.

Medicinal uses
White oak is a simple, powerful, and safe astringent. It is an excellent wound dressing and works well topically to dry up poison ivy rashes. It can also be used internally for

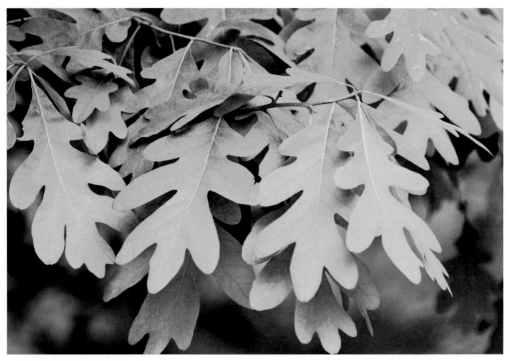

The round-lobed leaves of white oak.

diarrhea. The decoction works very well as a gargle for a sore throat, especially if there's excess mucus, or for bleeding gums.

Internally, it is usually used in combination with other herbs for all but the most serious diarrhea. It is somewhat antiseptic as well as astringent, but mostly it is not going to treat the cause of the diarrhea, just the symptom. So if there is an infection or parasite, be sure to also give herbs to treat that.

The decoction can be used for a runny and drippy nose, whatever the cause, although gentler herbs might be better to use first or in combination with this strongly drying herb. It could also be used in a neti pot but with the same warning, so as not to overly dry out the nasal passages.

Mostly I use it externally, either using the decoction as a wash for weepy poison ivy rashes, or in a salve for recent wounds. It helps stop bleeding and draws the edges of a wound together to make for faster healing, especially combined with plantain. It is also taken internally to stop bleeding in the digestive tract or applied topically in powder for bleeding hemorrhoids.

Future harvests

As long as you take just a few limbs off mature trees, it should be fine.

 Caution

Too much tannins inhibit digestion, so for short-term use only.

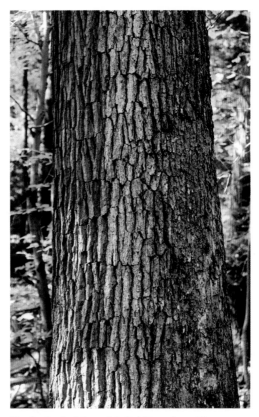

The bark of white oak is light in color, with strong ridges.

HERBAL PREPARATIONS

Tincture dried bark 1:5 with 50% alcohol and 10% glycerin to keep the tannins in solution. Can be made into an infusion to use as a wash topically (too astringent a tea to actually drink).

white pine

Pinus strobus

PARTS USED needles, bark, resin

A great expectorant for phlegm in the lungs, the resin is also an excellent antiseptic.

How to identify

People sometimes use the word "pine" to describe any conifer, but some of these cone-bearing plants are toxic or have medicinal properties that differ from the pines. Any plant in the pine genus can be used for pretty much the same medicine, but this might be very different from how juniper and white cedar are used, for example. What separates the pines from other conifers is their long needles, in bundles of 2–6. How long the needles are and how many are in a cluster help to determine which pine you are looking at. Sometimes looking at the characteristics of the pine cone can help, too.

Though many, if not most, pines have a tradition of use, white pine, the focus of this entry, has the most written about it. White pine needles are in bundles of 5 and are 2–4 inches long with a thin white stripe on the underside of each needle. The individual needles as well as the whole tree have a softness to them, and sometimes white pines get sculpted by wind and weather to look

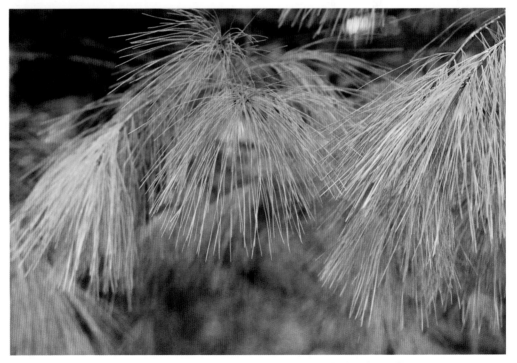

White pine has 5 needles per bunch and a white stripe down the back of each needle.

like a Taoist nature painting. The limbs form whorls around the main trunk.

There are about a dozen species of pine in the Southeast. Loblolly pine (*Pinus taeda*) has also traditionally been used for medicine. Its needles are longer (6–9 inches) than those of white pine and only 3 per cluster.

Where, when, and how to wildcraft

White pine is primarily found in the mountains and Piedmont from Virginia to Kentucky south to northern Georgia, middle Tennessee, and Alabama. Further south the loblolly pine takes over; it is abundant from eastern Texas through all the Gulf states to northern Florida, and north through the coastal plain to Maryland and Delaware. Again, any tree in this genus will work similarly, but these two are the most popular ones to use in the Southeast.

The needles grow year-round so can be harvested fresh in spring or fall and either used fresh or dried. As always, the bark is best and easiest to process in spring and early summer. Take resin from wounds in the tree during warm days, when it is loose and runny.

Pine limbs often get knocked down in the wind, so the best and easiest time to find them is to go to a pine thicket after a good spring storm and pick up the branches from the ground—just make sure they are recently fallen, no older than a couple of days for best results.

Clip the tips of the branches, which are full of needles; this is easier than picking off every bunch of needles. Then chop the small branches from the limb and use a knife to etch two circles in the bark about a foot apart, then a line connecting the two circles. Be sure to cut deep enough to start feeling the resistance of the heartwood, which will have a different texture.

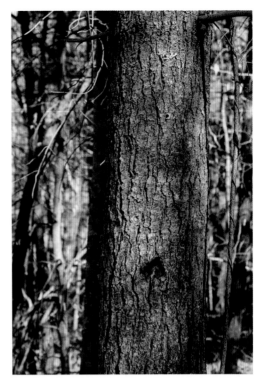

The bark of pine trees has a distinctive look and is often covered in white resin that acts as an antiseptic for the tree and for us.

Then get the knife under the edge of the bark along the line and start prying it up. Once you get that edge started, the rest should start peeling up and you can pull the cylindrical quill of bark off with your hands. If it's not easy, then you either haven't cut deep enough or the limb is older and the bark is dried. These quills dry well for later use in tea or cough syrup.

Cleaning up is a big issue. The sticky resin in the bark isn't easily removed from knives, saws, or hands. Soap and water works only to remove the dirt that was stuck in the resin. Rubbing alcohol seems to be the only thing that works, and every medicine maker needs to have a bottle of this around (and not just for impromptu hand sanitizer). Rubbing down everything involved in making pine medicine is a necessary part of cleaning up; wipe all tools (and hands) with a paper towel and then use soap to get the alcohol off. Otherwise it's going to be a sticky situation, so to speak.

Medicinal uses

White pine needle or bark is first and foremost a lung herb, opening up the bronchioles, killing microbes, and breaking up and moving out mucus. It is a stimulating expectorant, with the bark being stronger than the needles but the needles being much easier to come by. It is also antiseptic when applied topically and can be useful for arthritis.

As you might imagine from my name, I'm a little partial to pine medicine. But surprisingly, it is more commonly used in folk medicine than in modern herbal practice; you won't find it often on store shelves or in many formulas. Maybe it's like dandelion—too common for people to think about bottling and selling it. It has certainly been used throughout our region for years as a major medicine. It is a powerful, common, and yet often overlooked remedy for respiratory infections.

As with the many other resinous plants that help the lungs—spikenard, angelica, and white cedar, to name just a few—it seems that its sticky resins are what make white pine so good for the lungs. Since these aromatic resins are not very water soluble, the body tends to excrete them through the lungs, which is where they have their best effect, acting as both antimicrobials and expectorants. A nice combination, really—first killing microorganisms in the lungs and then stimulating the clearing of excess mucus that can serve as a breeding ground.

The straight resin can be picked off wounds in a pine tree and put directly on wounds as a waterproof antimicrobial bandage. A small ball of resin can be sucked on for a sore throat or lung issues, but don't chew it—it will stick to your teeth for hours!

In general, resins are used in Western herbalism as expectorants or antimicrobials, but in Chinese medicine they are used as pain relievers. Even things like myrrh and frankincense, which in European herbalism are used for skin and mouth infections, are used in Chinese medicine mostly to treat injuries. And so pines are used for helping with pain that's worse in cold and damp weather and to treat "fixed, deep pain in the joints with difficulty flexing or moving" (Chen and Chen 2012).

Future harvests

Most pines are pretty abundant, but still: harvest from trees that are abundant where you are looking. Avoid harvesting from any living pine that has been timbered and is only very slowly coming back. Harvesting blown-down limbs is always encouraged, and never ever harvest bark from a standing tree.

> **HERBAL PREPARATIONS**
>
> A short decoction for the needles or a longer decoction for the bark is a great tea. The bark makes an excellent cough syrup as well, decocted and preserved with honey or simple syrup. White Pine Compound Cough Syrup was an official remedy sold in the United States for decades, and its main ingredients were equal parts of white pine and wild cherry with small amounts of spikenard, poplar buds, and bloodroot (note—I would recommend leaving out the potentially toxic bloodroot).

white pond lily

Nymphaea odorata

PARTS USED root

An anti-inflammatory and circulatory stimulant for many genitourinary issues.

How to identify

This is a water-dwelling plant, related to lotus and other water lilies. A few of these species are similar-looking, and seeing the flower is the best way to differentiate them. White pond lily has beautiful white flowers with many petals that open wide in the morning and close in the late afternoon, and they have a lovely aroma, as the specific epithet suggests. Its leaves are round with a V-shaped notch and they float on the water, unlike those of some of their relatives, where the leaf is below the water or juts up out of it. They are a dull emerald green on top and usually reddish beneath with air pockets that help them to float.

Where, when, and how to wildcraft

Although it is found across the country, in our region it is mostly scattered across the

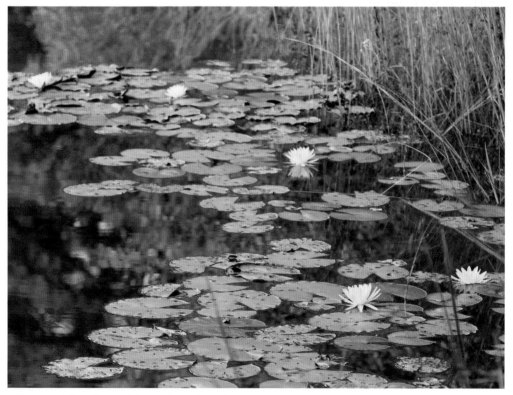

White pond lilies bloom at the surface of ponds.

coastal plain into the Piedmont, from Virginia to Georgia and west to eastern Texas, in ponds and lakes and even sloughs if there's enough water. It is found almost everywhere in Florida.

White pond lilies spread easily and can form large colonies; over centuries, they turn ponds into marshland as their leaf litter piles up on the bottom.

Harvesting the roots of this plant from the bottom of a pond is an adventure. Be aware that the kind of place this plant likes to grow is the kind of place that alligators like, and they aren't always evident at a glance

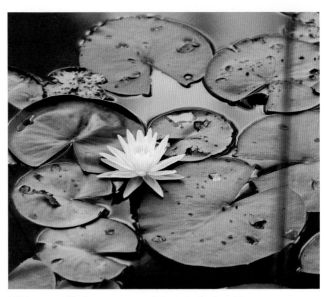

White pond lily leaves are reminiscent of a Pac-Man.

so do your due diligence. When you know it's safe, dive in and start digging. There's no way to dig this root without getting underwater, so take off your clothes and put on your swimsuit (if you choose). The roots run along the bottom and are held in place by a number of small rootlets, giving the whole root the look of a sea monster. Use a soil knife to cut these side roots and bring this monster up from the deep.

Medicinal uses

White pond lily is a unique medicine for the pelvic area and genitourinary tract that cools off hot inflammatory conditions while also increasing blood and lymph circulation to help move congestion. Because it is also astringent and antiseptic, it lends itself to a number of different uses, including some digestive issues.

Its main historical use is for irritated and congested conditions of the vagina and uterus. It was used for uterine and cervical cancers, both drunk and as a douche or suppository. Because it is also astringent, it can

be used for leukorrhea or excess menstrual bleeding from inflammation. It can be used for interstitial cystitis, which is a chronic inflammatory condition of the urinary tract, and for prostatitis with the same state.

In the digestive system, it is used for a similar tissue state where it manifests as gastritis, colitis, and diarrhea. It dries, tightens, and tones the mucosa of whatever system it is applied to and helps stem excessive discharge. Deborah Frances uses it when the pain is sharp, not dull and achy.

Future harvests

It isn't a common plant, but it can be locally abundant, so find places where it has formed large colonies and then harvest a few plants off the edge.

HERBAL PREPARATIONS

Tincture the fresh root 1:2 at 95% alcohol or 100% glycerin. Or use a strong decoction of the dried root.

wild cherry

Prunus serotina
PARTS USED bark

Nice-tasting remedy that relieves excessive coughing.

How to identify

Wild cherry (aka black cherry) is by far the tallest cherry tree, getting to be as much as 80 feet. It can be identified by its scaly "potato chip" bark that persists except on the oldest trunks, which still have rough horizontal lines revealing more reddish bark underneath. The young branches are also reddish. Break a twig or crush a leaf, wait 30 seconds, and then take a good whiff—you should get the "bitter almond" smell that is so distinctive of this genus.

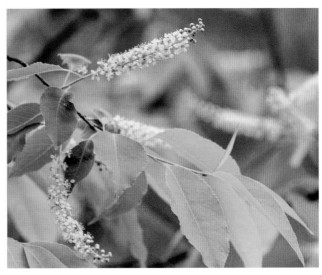

The bottlebrush flowers of wild cherry are a common sight in mid-spring throughout the Southeast.

The simple and alternate leaves are up to 6 inches long, and thin though not as thin as fire cherry (*Prunus pensylvanica*). Unlike fire cherry, they have blunt teeth, and the underside of the midrib has a line of small hairs.

Perhaps most distinctive are the bottlebrush flower clusters that appear in abundance in mid-spring, later turning into clusters of small purple bittersweet cherries. You never know how abundant this tree is until you see it, everywhere, during the blooming months.

Where, when, and how to wildcraft

Wild cherry grows from Canada to central Florida and west to Kansas, Oklahoma, and eastern Texas. It can be found in a wide variety of habitats, from rich cove forests to oak-hickory forests to disturbed areas. In mid-spring, when the trees are blooming, the bottlebrush flower clusters can be spotted along the interstate, roadsides, and in the woods.

Bark can be harvested in the spring after the flowers are finished, though the Eclectics said it is best harvested in the fall. Some say that the potentially toxic cyanogenic compounds are highest during flowering, but others (Kiva Rose, for one) say it just makes stronger medicine. Experiment and see what works best for you.

Prussic acid (aka prunasin), a type of cyanogenic glycoside, is what make the leaves and bark smell like bitter almond. It is responsible for both the medicine and the potential toxicity of the plant. Notice the resemblance between "cyanogenic" and "cyanide"? It's not a coincidence—if fermented then cyanide can be produced, so make sure to use this plant either completely fresh or dry it thoroughly and quickly.

This is not just a theoretical concern—horse people hate this plant because branches fall off easily in a storm and into a corral, where the horses then eat the wilted leaves, get cyanide poisoning, and occasionally even die.

The easiest way to harvest this plant is to keep track of where the trees grow, then visit the day after a windstorm and pick up recently downed branches—luckily we use the bark not the leaves. The best bark is considered to be from the medium-sized branches, not the twigs or the older tree bark.

Medicinal uses

Wild cherry is one of the best remedies to stop excessive (hectic) coughing by relaxing the nervous irritability in the lungs. For the same reason, it can be used for irritability in the digestive tract.

There are several different types of remedies for coughs—stimulating expectorants make it easier to cough up phlegm, relaxing expectorants open up the bronchioles and relax resistance to the cough, and demulcents physically soothe the tissue, like a balm, to reduce the irritation.

Wild cherry works differently, not by physically soothing the tissue but by relaxing the nerves that are sending the signal of irritation to the brain so that the brain doesn't react to an irritant by trying to cough it out. It's really working as a nerve sedative, like a milder version of peach, which is in the same genus. It works very well most of the time, which is why cough drops were traditionally made from wild cherry and are still cherry-flavored (though who knows if there's any actual cherry left in there anymore?).

If wild cherry isn't strong enough to stop a cough and help someone get to sleep then there are stronger remedies such as black cohosh or skunk cabbage that could also work, but it's always worth starting with a gentle remedy like wild cherry first.

Just as it works on the lungs, it works to help allay inflammation in the digestive tract that is causing irritability and possibly even diarrhea, while simultaneously stimulating digestion and appetite. It also has some action to help calm the heart and can be used for palpitations and a rapid excited pulse.

Future harvests

This is an abundant tree where it grows, fast growing and easily reproducing. So as long as you don't harm the tree you're harvesting from, you're good.

Caution

Not for use during pregnancy. The bark contains cyanide-like compounds, and since some amount of these compounds remain in the medicine, it is best not to use this long-term.

HERBAL PREPARATIONS

Heat can destroy wild cherry's medicinal compounds, so it is best taken as a strong cold infusion or perhaps as a hot infusion. It can be tinctured fresh 1:2 at 95% alcohol, or 1:5 at 60% alcohol and 10% glycerin. It also makes a great cough syrup, made by taking a strong cold infusion and adding half as much honey as there is tea. Adding some brandy will help keep it shelf stable but isn't necessary if you plan to use the syrup within a month or two.

Geranium maculatum

PARTS USED root

A powerful astringent for the urinary and digestive tract.

How to identify

Wild geranium is a prolific woodland plant with palmately lobed leaves and 5-petaled magenta flowers. At a certain point each spring, trails and roads in the woods will be lined with these bright flowers. After pollination, the fruit extends into a long pod that splits in two, like an open crane's bill.

Wild larkspur (*Delphinium tricorne*), a poisonous look-alike, has very similar leaves, though its flowers are completely different, looking more like a wizard hat and beard with a spur on the back. The differences between the two are subtle, but wild geranium's leaves are usually divided into 5 somewhat even lobes that are regularly and coarsely toothed. Larkspur leaves can be in 5 lobes (sometimes more, sometimes less), and the teeth are irregular and mostly at the far edge of the leaf instead of along it. If you don't know these plants and can't find them in flower, it is highly recommended that you do not pick wild geranium, as you may have its deadly poisonous look-alike.

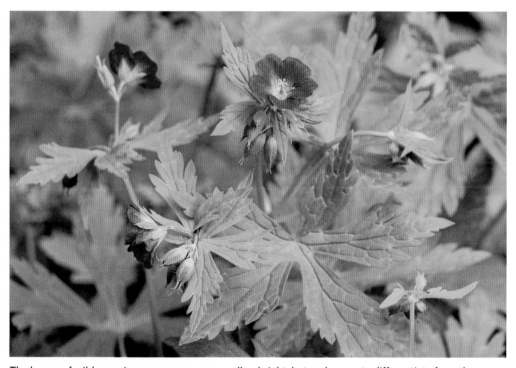

The leaves of wild geranium are a common woodland sight, but make sure to differentiate from the poisonous wild larkspur.

Also, don't confuse wild geranium with its close relative, Carolina geranium (*Geranium carolinianum*), a common weed of meadows and gardens.

Where, when, and how to wildcraft

Wild geranium grows from southern New England and New York south to middle Georgia and Alabama and west into northern Louisiana. It is a common plant of meadows, trails, roadsides, and open woods, occasionally into the woods as well.

It blooms abundantly in the spring, and that's the best time to find it and make a positive ID. This is also the best time to dig this root, as harvesting in the spring means not harvesting the afore-mentioned poisonous look-alike, but note: the tannins in the root are highest in spring, lower in fall. It is not a big root, and you won't need anything more than a soil knife to dig it.

Medicinal uses

This is a simple but strong astringent for internal use, whenever an astringent is needed. It is specific for many conditions of the digestive and urinary tracts.

It is a great herb for urinary incontinence, whether from age or after pelvic surgery, or whenever there is a lack of tone in the gen-itourinary system. It seems to tighten and tone the trigone sphincter, and combining it with some pelvic floor muscle exercises will help a lot.

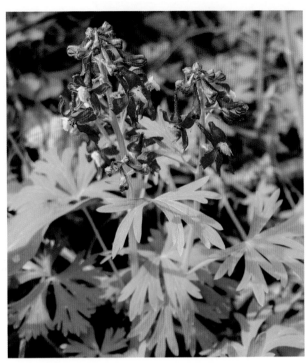

The leaves of wild larkspur, a deadly look-alike, are danger-ously similar to those of wild geranium, though its flowers are markedly different.

It is also used for any kind of ulceration or damage to the digestive tract, including peptic ulcer, ulcerative colitis, and diver-ticulitis as part of a formula. It is also used for chronic diarrhea (along with assessing food choices).

Future harvests

Harvest this woodland native only where it is abundant, and never take more than one out of four plants.

HERBAL PREPARATIONS

Mostly used as a tincture, fresh 1:2 at 95%, or dry 1:5 at 50% alcohol with 10% glycerin to stabilize the tannins.

wild ginger

Asarum canadense

PARTS USED root

A hot herb—unrelated to true ginger;
this spicy-tasting root is used for colds with chills.

How to identify

Plants are often found in decent-sized patches, maybe 20–30 feet across. The leaves are deciduous, pubescent, and grow in pairs. They are heart-shaped and basal (only), so could be mistaken for other plants—for example, liferoot and the more common violets.

Unlike liferoot, the leaf margin is entire (not toothed), and unlike the violets, the tip of the leaf is rounded (in violets, the tip comes to a point). One other characteristic of this family is the unusual shape of the base of the leaf—whereas in violets the two "earlobes" meet, in wild ginger, a straight line runs across the base of the leaf between the two lobes.

Hexastylis, another genus in this family, is more common as one travels further south; all its various heartleaf species (aka little brown jugs) have thick evergreen leaves, whereas the wild gingers have softer leaves that persist only through the warm months. It is possible that some *Hexastylis* species could be used for medicine, but both the use and toxicity are still up for debate.

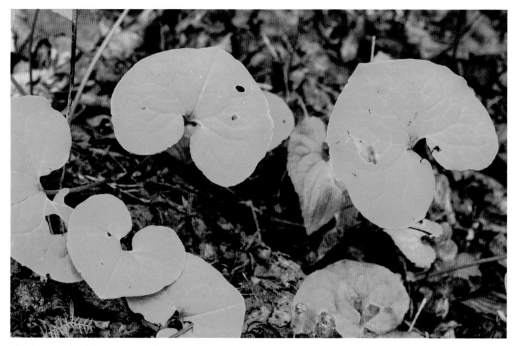

The leaves of wild ginger usually grow in pairs.

Where, when, and how to wildcraft

Abundant in the Northeast, less so in the Southeast, but it can still be found at 3,000 feet and above as far south as North Carolina and northern Georgia, then at lower elevations up through Tennessee, Kentucky, Virginia, and West Virginia.

Wild ginger is usually found in patches in rich soil in the deep woods. Be aware of where you harvest; this is an uncommon plant in some places and should be protected, not harvested. But if you find a good amount of it, you can dig up some roots from around the edge of the patch, being careful not to disturb the other plants. The roots are close to the surface and easily dug up by hand. Don't harvest much because you won't need this plant often.

Medicinal uses

This plant has a very specific medicinal use. It is used, as is the related species in China, for a cold or flu with lots of chills and body ache. It is used only short-term and only for this specific presentation—not a commonly used herb, in short, but always fun to see in the wild, and I will occasionally dig up half an inch of root just for a spicy nibble.

This is not an antiviral herb, as far as I know; it is used for upper respiratory infections with a sense of cold and dampness to help warm things up and get things moving. It could even be used for a low-grade fever as long as the person is feeling more cold and chilled. It might even help bring a temperature up if needed to sweat out a cold.

The heating nature of this root also helps break up thick stuck phlegm in the head and chest, though deeper herbs would be needed if the phlegm was coming from bronchitis or pneumonia. But it could be used for a sinusitis with thick white phlegm.

It is also used for the body ache one gets during a cold or flu. It is not really a pain reliever; it most likely acts on the antiviral immune system chemicals (cytokines) that cause the body pain. Basically it is used to get things moving and is even used in China for chest pain from stagnant qi.

Future harvests

Although more common down through Virginia to Kentucky, it is less common into North Carolina and Tennessee and should be harvested there with caution and awareness.

Caution

Not safe in pregnancy and not for use longer than a week at a time. There is debate about wild ginger's toxicity. It contains aristolochic acid, which can harm the kidneys when taken over a period of time. Some herbalists say that it is fine because it is only taken for short periods of time anyway. But Lisa Ganora (2009) says that even though it contains only small amounts of aristolochic acid, its regular use should probably be avoided (especially during pregnancy/lactation).

HERBAL PREPARATIONS

Mostly used as a fresh root tincture, 1:2 at 95%. But could also be dried and used in infusions or decoctions.

wild hydrangea

Hydrangea arborescens, H. cinerea

PARTS USED root

A useful plant to break up kidney stones and relieve urinary tract irritation and inflammation.

How to identify

Wild hydrangea is a small shrub, usually 3–4 feet high, occasionally to 6 feet, with woody bark that starts peeling as it ages like a sycamore tree (hence its other common name, seven barks). The current-year stems on the upper part of the plant are usually green, so look halfway down the plant to see if it is woody, as stone root and wood nettle have similar large leaves, though wood nettle leaves are alternate, not opposite.

It flowers in June and July—rounded heads of small white fertile 5-petaled flowers with a few large sterile flowers around the outside for the purpose of drawing in pollinating insects. The cultivated hydrangeas have exaggerated this by selecting for plants that have only the infertile flowers, giving them that snowball effect. I don't suggest using ornamental hydrangeas for medicine, and besides, most cultivars likely derive from different species.

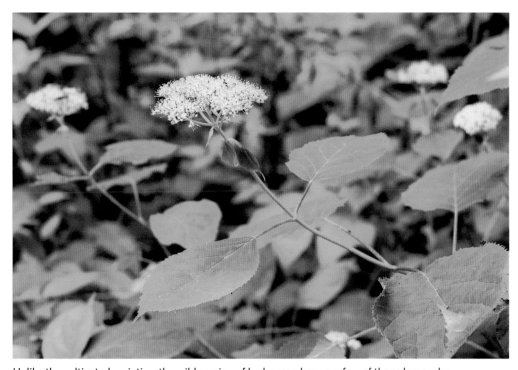

Unlike the cultivated varieties, the wild version of hydrangea has very few of those larger showy infertile flowers.

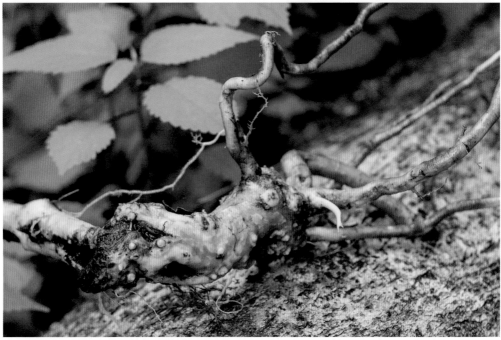
The root, the medicinal part of wild hydrangea, is as tough as one would expect from a shrub.

There are actually two species of wild hydrangea, and both can be used for medicine. The leaves are large, oval, toothed, and opposite. The leaves of smooth hydrangea (*Hydrangea arborescens*) are smooth and green underneath, the only hairs being on the midrib; ashy hydrangea (*H. cinerea*) has white or gray undersides to its leaves. The latter plant also has more of the showy sterile flowers.

Where, when, and how to wildcraft

Wild hydrangeas are found from Massachusetts and Pennsylvania south to mid-Georgia and the Florida panhandle, and west to Arkansas and sporadically Louisiana. They prefer rock outcrops and seem to be most abundant along forested mountain creeks and seeps. They seem to really like streambanks in the shade.

Harvest in the fall. The roots are tough but not too hard to dig, just hard to chop. Because they do tend to grow on streambanks, be careful when harvesting not to cause erosion of the bank—so, best not to harvest on steep areas.

Medicinal uses

Wild hydrangea is probably best known as a remedy to eliminate kidney stones or gravel (small stones), but they are also a great anti-inflammatory for irritation of the urinary tract.

It doesn't seem to break up stones so much as it facilitates their movement out of the body. For this purpose it can be combined with other antilithic herbs like stone root and gravel root, with a demulcent like plantain added to protect the urethra from damage.

Even though it doesn't break up stones, regular use seems to prevent stones from forming in the first place. And once someone gets one kidney stone they are prone to get more.

In my practice I have used it more often as a urinary tract soother than for clients with kidney stones. It has a wonderful ability to soothe and calm hot and irritated conditions of the kidneys, bladder, and urethra, so I have found it useful as part of a formula for interstitial cystitis. In that condition a person feels like they have a chronic UTI, but urinalysis shows no sign of infection. The chronic irritation causes the tissue of the bladder to swell, which triggers the feeling that we have to pee; this causes a frequent desire to urinate, but not much urine is passed. This is the same thing that happens in a UTI, but there the infection is causing the swelling.

For the same reasons, it can be helpful for prostatitis with painful urination.

Even though wild hydrangea is not commonly used or readily available in commerce, it's a good herb to have on hand for any irritation or inflammation in the urinary tract, whether or not there's an infection.

Future harvests

These native woodland shrubs are abundant enough and not commonly used, so sustainability is not as much of an issue as it sometimes is. Just be sure not to cause damage that would trigger streambank erosion. And as always, harvest from abundant stands.

HERBAL PREPARATIONS

To work with the kidneys and urinary tract, it is typically made as a decoction and also works well as a tincture, with the dose being put in water before taking it.

David Winston (2013) recommends soaking the roots in room temperature water for several hours before bringing it up to a boil. This seems to hydrolyze the constituents for best extraction.

It can also be made into a fresh root tincture, 1:2 at 95%, or dry root tincture, 1:5 at 50% alcohol.

wild sarsaparilla

Aralia nudicaulis

PARTS USED root

An overlooked tonic herb that is both an adaptogen and a blood cleanser.

How to identify

This species is not to be confused with the botanically unrelated "true" sarsaparillas of the genus *Smilax*. This plant is in the ginseng family, and the leaflets are actually shaped a lot like American ginseng, but they are arranged pinnately, not palmately. In other words the leaflets grow on either side of a leaf stem, like pieces on a feather, and not all from one point. It is also 1–2 feet tall, a bit larger than your average ginseng plant.

The plant flowers in mid-spring; the flower stalk comes up from the root and is short and barely noticeable, usually being overshadowed by the leaves. It is usually found in small stands, but isolated individuals can be found as well.

Where, when, and how to wildcraft

Though this plant is abundant in some parts of the Northeast and upper Midwest, in the Southeast it is found most abundantly in the mountain areas of Virginia, West Virginia, North Carolina, and Tennessee. Be careful harvesting on the edge of its range, where it might be more rare.

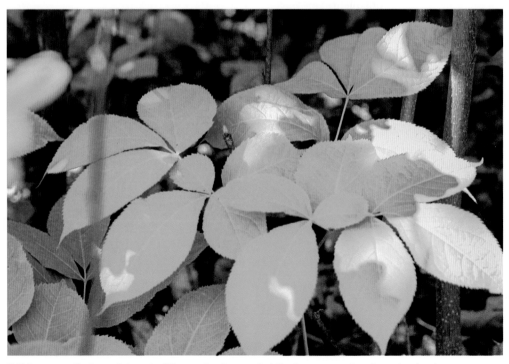

Wild sarsaparilla is reminiscent of its cousin ginseng, but the leaves are pinnate, not palmate.

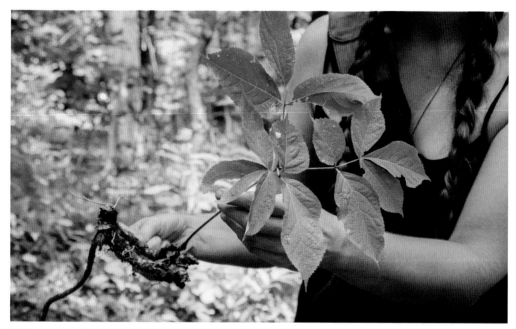
Wild sarsaparilla root, unearthed. Both the taproot and the runners can be used for medicine.

It is a stand plant and should be harvested only where you see several plants together. Both the taproot and the runners can be dug in late summer and fall using a soil knife.

Medicinal uses

Though it is often lumped in with spikenard, which is in the same genus, or with the unrelated sarsaparilla, this herb deserves its own entry. Though not a powerful plant, it is useful and a nice one to have around. It is a gentle adaptogen and qi tonic as well as an alterative, and I think of it more for home and kitchen use than for outright disease states.

It's never really been a major medicine in clinical practice. A reference I found in one old medical book dismisses it as a home remedy used as a syrup for recovery after a long illness. But to me that makes it perfect as a tonic and describes one of the ways to use it.

What makes it ideal as a recuperative herb is its dual ability to clear out toxins from the blood while simultaneously creating more energy as an adaptogen. Wild sarsaparilla acts similarly to sarsaparilla, though with a little less of the blood-cleansing properties and maybe a little more of the adaptogenic properties.

Future harvests

There are areas where this is an abundant understory plant and places where it's rare. Be aware of where in the plant's range you are before harvesting, as there are other herbs that can do similar things. Harvest only from abundant stands

HERBAL PREPARATIONS

Typically prepared as a decoction or a syrup; it can also work as a tincture.

wild yam

Dioscorea villosa
PARTS USED root

A balancing hormonal herb and antispasmodic.

How to identify

Wild yam is a unique-looking plant that is related to the true yam (not the sweet potato variety called yam in the United States) but is definitely not edible. It is a small woodland vine that rarely grows longer than 5–8 feet. The leaves are heart-shaped with conspicuous curved veins; they are whorled toward the base of the plant, then become opposite, then alternate higher up on the stem. Some thornless *Smilax* species could be confused with wild yam, but none have whorled leaves.

The related cinnamon vine or air potato (*Dioscorea polystachya*) is an invasive Asian plant; though its leaves look somewhat similar, they are more elongated and opposite, and the whole vine can grow up to 60 feet long. Perhaps the most conspicuous characteristic of it are the small round tubers dangling from the leaf axils.

Where, when, and how to wildcraft

This plant grows in wet woods or on trails and tolerates both rich and acidic soils. It

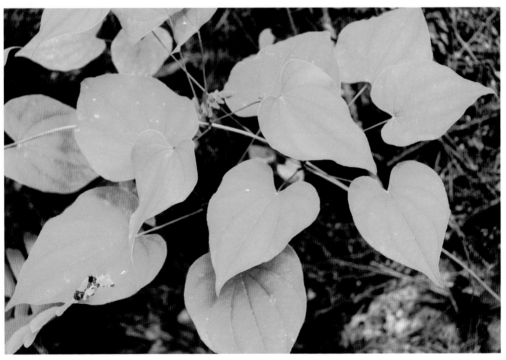

Wild yam forms short vines with bluish green leaves that are heart-shaped and have strong veins that curve toward the tip.

occurs from southern New England west to eastern Minnesota, south to the Florida panhandle, and just barely over the border into Texas.

Harvest in fall after the nights start getting cold, but don't wait too long as the leaves fall off earlier than most other plants. Dig the roots delicately. As with many woodland plants, they are actually rhizomes and run lateral to the ground. Cut the root tendrils holding it in the ground and harvest the main rhizome body. It's fine to use the rootlets for medicine too, but there's not a lot to them so don't worry about getting every little bit.

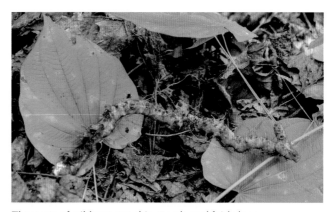
The roots of wild yam are thin, tough, and fairly long.

Medicinal uses

Wild yam has two main uses—antispasmodic and hormone balancer. To be clear, it is not a precursor to progesterone in the body, nor is it a contraceptive. Progesterone and other hormones can be synthesized from wild yam, and the first birth control pills were made from the Mexican wild yam, which is perhaps where this reputation came from. When you see wild yam creams with progesterone on a store shelf, the progesterone has been synthesized from wild yam in a lab, but that's not something home herbalists can do or that will happen inside our body. That said, the root does balance estrogen and progesterone in the body, probably because of its content of diosgenin and other triterpenoid saponins.

Perhaps because of this hormonal effect, it has a protective effect on pregnancy. I once gave it to a woman who was having contractions and pain in the sixth month of her pregnancy and was afraid she would lose the baby. After taking it consistently for a day, the contractions stopped; she took it for two more days and was able to go full term with a healthy daughter.

This plant also has an amazing ability to stop spasms of the smooth muscle, which is the type of muscle found in our internal organs. It can be used for menstrual cramps (uterine spasm) combined with black cohosh or black haw. It combines well with fringe tree for the pain of passing gallstones, and with wild hydrangea to help with kidney stones. It is also a great herb for the colonic spasms that occur in IBS and Crohn's disease, and Michael Moore used it for the intestinal spasms that accompany dysentery.

Future harvests

Wild yam is increasingly overpicked in our area. Spend a couple of years getting to know the area; harvest only when you find a lot of this plant, and even then only sparingly. It is not uncommon, but the individual roots don't weigh much, so it's not as abundant as it seems.

HERBAL PREPARATIONS

Fresh tincture is the best, prepared 1:2 at 95% alcohol. The dried root tincture can be made at 1:5 at 60% alcohol.

willow

Salix spp.

PARTS USED bark

The original aspirin, willow bark relieves pain and inflammation and reduces fever.

How to identify

There are many species of willow in North America and not all are medicinally useful. The ornamental weeping willow seems to have absolutely no medicinal value, for example.

The most abundant wild willow in the Southeast is black willow (*Salix nigra*), which grows into a fairly tall tree, up to 50–60 feet high, though it can reach 100 feet, making it the largest willow in the eastern United States. The bark is deeply furrowed, and the leaves are very long and thin, maybe 10 times as long as wide, and often have a slight curve. The back of the leaves is smooth and about the same color as the top surface, which differentiates it from some other willows.

Where, when, and how to wildcraft

Willow is always found near water, often on the sides of creeks and rivers in flat areas. When driving through farmland in the country, you'll sometimes see winding lines of trees cutting through the fields—these are often willows, shading a creek or branch.

Harvest the branches in spring or early summer, when the sap is still rising. The branches break off easily and can sometimes even be gathered after a spring windstorm from the ground. Use only a recent fall, nothing over a day old, or it will be hard to peel the bark off; as long as the leaves are green, the medicine is still present.

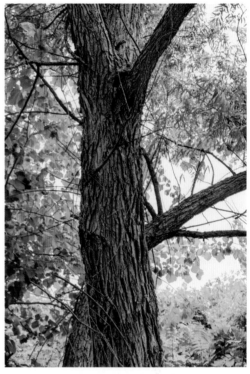

Black willow, the most abundant willow in our region, has deeply furrowed bark.

Alternatively, once you've trimmed some of the limbs off living trees using loppers or a folding saw, strip the bark off (see page 000). Remember to never cut bark off of a living tree; it is always better to cut limbs and then strip the bark off of them.

Medicinal uses

Willow bark does many of the same things that aspirin does—which makes sense

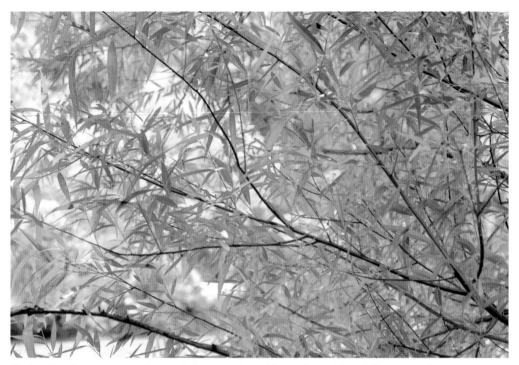
Black willow leaves are even longer than most other willows, often with a slight curve to them.

because it is willow that inspired aspirin in the first place. Although gentler than aspirin, it is a great pain reliever, anti-inflammatory, and fever reducer; however, it does not thin the blood and prevent clotting like aspirin does.

Salicylic acid was first isolated from willow in the early 1800s, when chemists examined the bark to figure out why the plant helped with pain. When the acid on its own proved to be too hard on the digestive tract (in the plant it is bound to a sugar as salicin, so not a problem), an acetyl group was added and voilà, aspirin was born. Turns out the acetyl group tends to prevent clotting, so an additional benefit (if looking for a blood thinner) or danger (if not wanting to die from bleeding stomach ulcers) was born. Willow does much of what aspirin does without the anticoagulant effect.

By reducing inflammatory reactions, willow can help alleviate mild to moderate pain.

It seems particularly useful for headaches, arthritis and other joint pain, and pain from acute injuries.

Future harvests

This is an abundant tree so a very sustainable harvest. Harvest from medium to large trees, spreading out the trimmings so they're not all on one side of the tree. Prune branches that are growing close together for better future tree health.

Caution

Do not use if you are allergic to salicylates and aspirin.

HERBAL PREPARATIONS

Tincture fresh 1:2 at 95% or dried 1:5 at 50%. Infusion works well too.

---

witch hazel

Hamamelis virginiana
PARTS USED leaves, twigs

Astringent and tonic for the blood vessels.

How to identify

This understory shrub never gets much higher than 10–15 feet. Instead of one main trunk, it will have several shooting out in different directions, the branches splaying out, zig-zagging, and generally doing their best to catch what light there is in the forest.

The leaves are just plain wonky—every leaf is a bit different. They have an uneven base, are irregularly wavy margined, and can even be different shapes, some more rounded and some more oval. It flowers in the fall and forms hard capsules by the spring.

Where, when, and how to wildcraft

This is a common shrub of wet woodlands from Canada to central Florida and west just over the line into Texas. Once you know what you're looking for, it's not hard to find, and usually when you find one, there are others nearby.

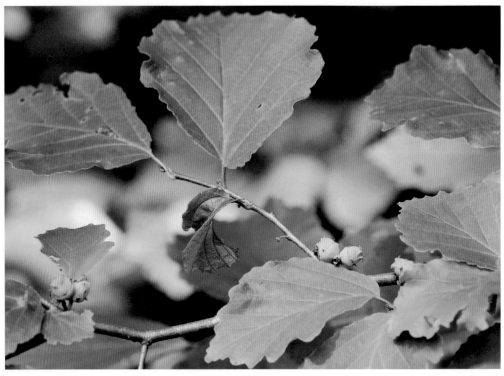

There's no other way to say it—witch hazel leaves are just wonky, off-kilter, and each one is a little different.

Harvest the slender twigs and leaves from late winter through early summer, and chop the twigs whole into your medicine. Michael Moore preferred to use fresh leaves.

Medicinal uses

Yes, this is the same witch hazel that is in the product sold in pharmacies across the country, but a tincture will be much stronger than that weak commercial product. This tree can be used as an astringent for the respiratory and digestive tract, but it seems to have a specific tropism for blood vessels, aiding varicose veins and hemorrhoids and helping stop internal bleeding. It gently moves stuck blood with its aromatics while tightening up the tone of the blood vessels, so it can also be used for sore or strained muscles.

There are a lot of astringent herbs out there, but witch hazel is particularly good for improving the tissue tone of blood vessels. In spider veins and varicose veins, the veins that are returning blood from low in the body start to lose tone, and a certain amount of "backflow" that results gives the veins a purple and swollen look. The extract taken internally and the liniment used topically can really help improve the strength of these blood vessels and tighten them up. For the same reason, it is an excellent herb for hemorrhoids—it can even be applied directly to pads created for that condition.

Traditionally, witch hazel has been used for internal bleeding of a passive character (that is, from slow leaky conditions), not from active damage. It can be used for bleeding ulcers, ulcerative colitis, blood in the urine, and even coughing up blood. It is very important, however, to point out that any internal bleeding should be checked out by a qualified health practitioner, as it could indicate a serious condition.

Finally, there is a reason our parents kept witch hazel in the medicine cabinet—it is a soothing and healing application for sore muscles, muscle strains, and joint sprains. The combination of aromatics to get the blood moving combined with astringents to tighten up the tissue help with many of these conditions. It is also effective used topically on burns, combined with a few drops of lavender essential oil.

Future harvests

This is often an abundant understory shrub, so as long as you harvest with care, there shouldn't be a problem. Harvest from older specimens and prune it like a fruit tree, taking a branch that overlaps another, for instance. Ask yourself—how can I trim this shrub to make it healthier?

HERBAL PREPARATIONS

Leaves and twigs can be tinctured fresh 1:2 at 95% alcohol, or made into a liniment by extracting in isopropyl alcohol or vinegar for topical application.

Pedicularis canadensis
PARTS USED aerial

An herb that helps relax tight and tense muscles.

How to identify

The leaves are almost fern-like, though not so much as the western species of this genus. Most of the leaves are at the base of the plant, though a few grow up the flowering stalk. Plants are easy to miss until they bloom in April and early May, each "beak" of a flower in various dark shades of yellow and red, borne in elongated clusters. Being under a foot high, you could still miss wood betony, but plants do tend to grow in big patches, which makes it easier to spot.

This is our region's only *Pedicularis* species. There are many more out west, and some consider the Rocky Mountain species *P. groenlandica* to be stronger. Don't confuse it with the "other" wood betony, the European *Betonica officinalis*, which is used somewhat differently in herbal medicine.

Where, when, and how to wildcraft

This low-growing woodland plant sometimes pops up on and near trails. It is most abundant in Virginia south to northern Georgia

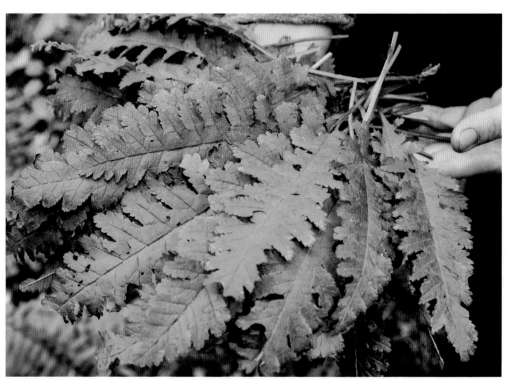

With wood betony, the leaves alone make strong medicine.

and west through Kentucky and Tennessee to Arkansas and Louisiana. It is sporadically abundant, so harvest only when you find a good-sized stand.

The best time to gather the plant is April and early May. Use all aboveground parts—the flower head and basal leaves. A few seeds in there won't hurt either. The leaves persist through September and are still plenty medicinal, so if you miss the flowering window then that's the second best time.

An important note about harvesting wood betony—it is a hemi-parasite. Even though it is green and contains chlorophyll, it is partially parasitic on nearby plants. So be careful what plants are growing within 5 feet of what you're harvesting, and make sure there's no poison ivy or other toxic plants.

Medicinal uses

This is one of my favorite herbs for relaxing muscular tension. I have massage therapist friends who give it to their clients before a session to loosen them up, or chiropractors who use it so that the adjustments will hold better and stay longer instead of getting pulled back out of place by tight muscles.

What's nice about it is that the effect is at the muscular level and doesn't affect consciousness—in other words, it won't make you drowsy or happy or especially agreeable to suspect business deals involving "prime land" in Florida. It simply relaxes muscle tension, affecting just the peripheral nervous system, not the central nervous system.

As such, this herb can be used for tension headaches, for sore back from spending the whole day leaning over a field weeding, or just for achy sore muscles from overuse. For a little extra power, combine it with black cohosh. You can also use it as an infused oil or salve, by itself or combined with valerian or arnica, and adding some essential oils of wintergreen, camphor, or some such.

An herb definitely deserving of more attention.

Future harvests

Even though it is locally abundant, harvest this plant gently. There aren't many flowers in early spring for pollinators in the woods, so it is beloved by bees.

HERBAL PREPARATIONS

I typically make it as a fresh leaf and flower stalk tincture, but it could also be dried for a simple infusion. The dried leaves also make a pleasant and relaxing smoke.

Achillea millefolium

PARTS USED leaves, flowers

Yarrow is a widely useful plant that can stop bleeding, stimulate digestion, and help with viral infections.

How to identify

Yarrow grows 1–3 feet high with white flowers in a flat-topped cluster and finely divided, feather-like leaves. Because this could also describe Queen Anne's lace (*Daucus carota*), there are some easy ways to differentiate the two. Look closely: yarrow flower stalks are attached up and down the stem in a corymb, rather than coming from one point on the stem as in an umbrella (umbel) like Queen Anne's lace. When seeing the two plants together the difference is more obvious, but when first starting out they can seem very similar. They are, however, in different plant families: yarrow is in the aster family (Asteraceae) and Queen Anne's lace in the parsley family (Apiaceae).

Yarrow grows in stands; some plants will have tufts of just basal leaves, others upright stems with alternate leaves.

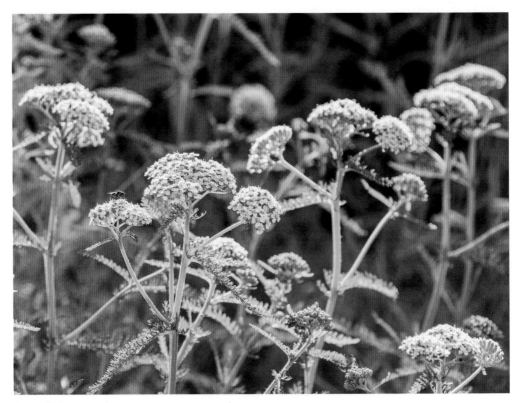

A stand of yarrow plants on a sunny summer day.

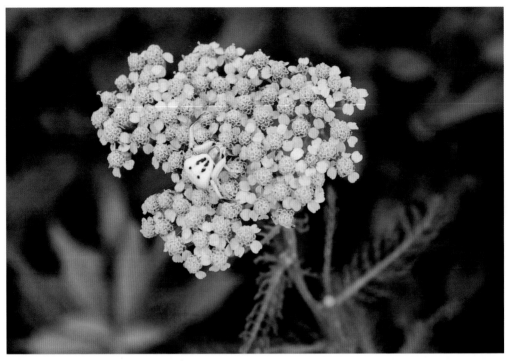

Looking closer, it's easy to tell the difference between yarrow flowers in the aster family and umbellifers in the parsley family.

Where, when, and how to wildcraft

This is a circumboreal plant if ever there was one—it grows in every U.S. state and every Canadian province. If you find an open meadow that gets mowed once or twice a year, you're likely to find yarrow. If you don't mow your yard for a few weeks, you might find some yarrow. From yards to alpine meadows to roadsides, this is an abundant plant. There's even some debate about whether it is native or an invasive plant from Europe.

Harvest when it is in full bloom and the inside of the flower heads (the disk florets) are more fresh and yellow than old and brown. This could be anywhere from early summer through early fall. Clip the plant low to the ground and either strip the leaves and flowers when fresh or dry it by hanging upside down and then strip.

Medicinal uses

Herb teachers, myself included, often tell their students to get to know 10 to 20 herbs well before expanding their knowledge. This is one of those herbs. It is a bit of a jack-of-all-trades that does a lot of things well.

This plant has actions on at least three major systems—the liver (bitter tonic and bile decongestant), the urinary tract (anti-septic and diuretic), and the cardiovascular system (flavonoid-rich capillary tonic, lowers cholesterol, lowers blood pressure). And beyond that, it is also an emmenagogue, diaphoretic, and hemostatic. So this plant is a handy one to have around for many occasions. It has so many uses that, ironically, it's often not used because it is impossible to pigeonhole.

Perhaps its most vibrant effect is on the liver and digestive system. Just tasting this herb can stimulate both appetite and liver function. The bitter taste stimulates the vagus nerve by reflex, increasing digestive secretions and improving assimilation of food. Many traditional systems of medicine associate the liver with the emotion of anger, and I have seen this herb help move anger that's been held in too long.

It has seemingly contradictory effects. Topically, it stops bleeding. Internally, it serves as an anticoagulant. How does one plant have such opposite effects? There are different mechanisms of action, but let's just say the mechanism of blood clotting is extremely complicated and one herb can sometimes have contradictory effect. It is interesting to note that in Chinese medicine, herbs that stop bleeding are categorized as "blood movers," of which this would be one.

As for the urinary tract, I've seen some UTIs healed using only yarrow. The Eclectics used an infusion for irritation of the urinary tract and suppressed urine. Whenever you want to treat the kidneys, bladder, or urethra, tea does seem like the most logical way to get it there, but I've also seen tincture given in water work.

The infusion or the tincture in hot water is a great diaphoretic to sweat out a fever. The traditional European treatment for fevers was to drink a hot tea of equal parts elder flower, yarrow, and mint, then take a hot bath, then wrap up like an enchilada and fall fast asleep. Most will wake up and the fever will be gone! Just don't try this with a seriously high fever, because a fever can cause serious problems when it gets too high.

Future harvests

No worries. Yarrow is an abundant plant with a strong root system, so as long as we don't disturb the roots, it will come back even after being mowed. Just be sure to leave enough flowers for pollinators and other wildlife.

HERBAL PREPARATIONS

Fresh leaf and flower tincture or dry as tea. Flowers have more of the sweating property, leaves more of the blood-clotting property, but are otherwise equal. You'll need the tea for the diuretic or the diaphoretic effect, but the tincture dropped into hot water also works just fine.

Rumex crispus, R. obtusifolius
PARTS USED root

A liver tonic that helps assimilate iron

How to identify

Two plants can be used as yellow dock: *Rumex crispus* (curly dock) is the official species, but *R. obtusifolius* (broad-leaved dock) can be used the same way. Both species have long leaves that are much longer than wide, dock being an Old English word for any broad-leaved plant. The unrelated burdock also has large leaves, often even larger, but it has a white underside and "earlobes" at the base of the leaf, whereas yellow dock is green on both sides. Mullein has large oval leaves, but it is very fuzzy; yellow dock is smooth. All these are biennials, having a rosette of basal leaves one year to store up energy in the root, and then the second year using up that energy to erect a flower stalk.

Yellow dock puts up its flowering stalk in mid to late spring, which is a reddish stalk with few if any leaves on it, and small pyramid-shaped flowers that become pyramid-shaped seeds; the seeds resemble buckwheat, which makes sense because they are in the same family.

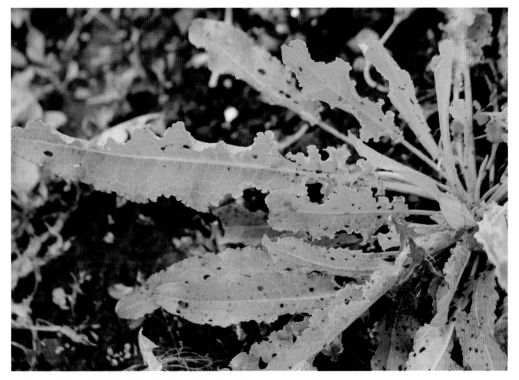

Curly dock, the official yellow dock species, has thinner leaves with wavy margins.

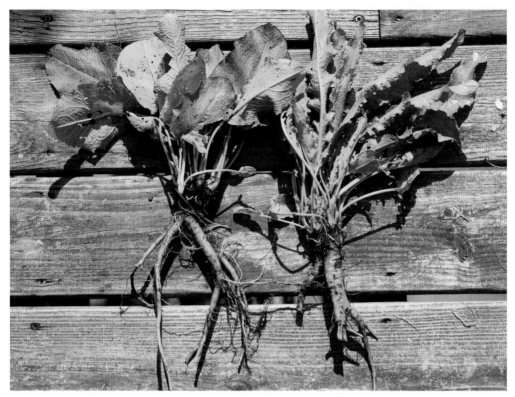

The roots of both broad-leaved dock (left, in this side-by-side comparison) and curly dock can be used as medicine.

Curly dock's leaves have wavy margins and are more narrow than those of broad-leaved dock. Also the seeds of broad-leaved dock have 2 or 3 small teeth on each edge of the pyramid; curly dock has smooth-edged fruit.

Where, when, and how to wildcraft

One or the other species grows up and down the East Coast and in almost every state. Both are found in every yard, meadow, and field where they can take hold. They grow on roadsides, sometimes even out of concrete. Broad-leaved dock becomes less common in the Gulf Coast states.

Dig the roots in the fall of the first year, when there are only leaves coming out of the ground, or after winter but before the flower stalk gets too big. If gathered much after

that, the root gets to be woody and tough and lacking in any medicine. Don't gather roots that are growing in water runoff as they aren't nearly as yellow and are also lacking in medicinal action.

The roots go straight down, so a good trenching shovel that is long and thin will come in handy.

Medicinal uses

Yellow dock is a moderately strong liver tonic and mild laxative, and it helps the body assimilate iron more easily. Even though like many liver tonics it is yellow, it does not contain berberine like some of these other herbs do. Because of its tonic effects on the liver, it can also be used for chronic skin conditions, particularly psoriasis.

Yellow dock tastes bitter, and that in part is why it works. It's a bit more bitter and so a little stronger than dandelion and burdock, and it is also more drying than those herbs. This liver-stimulating property might be why it is a laxative: it stimulates bile flow, and bile is the body's natural laxative.

For a long time yellow dock root was thought to contain large quantities of iron. But that has since been disproven, and it seems instead that it helps the body assimilate iron better by helping the transference of ferritin into the liver from the gut. So, if taking yellow dock for anemia, make sure to combine it with iron-rich herbs like nettle or iron-rich foods like blackstrap molasses, apricots, or raisins.

Herbalists usually treat skin conditions with liver herbs, and yellow dock has a particular usefulness in psoriasis, possibly because that condition is often associated with constipation and other digestive issues. And because it is drying, it can be used for weepy skin conditions as well.

Future harvests

This is a common invasive weed—harvest plenty, and there will be more.

HERBAL PREPARATIONS

Yellow dock is most commonly used as a tincture, fresh roots 1:2 at 95% alcohol, and dry roots 1:5 at 50% alcohol. It can also be made into an iron-rich syrup by decocting the roots and adding blackstrap molasses.

yellowroot

Xanthorhiza simplicissima

PARTS USED root

*An abundant herb on waterways, it is
a bitter tonic, liver cleanser, and antimicrobial.*

How to identify
Yellowroot (aka shrub yellowroot) is indeed a small shrub. Its woody stem grows straight up, rarely branching, to 2–3 feet high. The leaves all burst out of the very top of the plant at different angles; they are divided into 5–7 leaflets, each of which is sharply toothed. The inner bark is green-yellow, and the flesh of the root is intensely yellow.

Where, when, and how to wildcraft
Yellowroot is most abundant in the mountains but can be found to some extent throughout the Southeast, invariably within

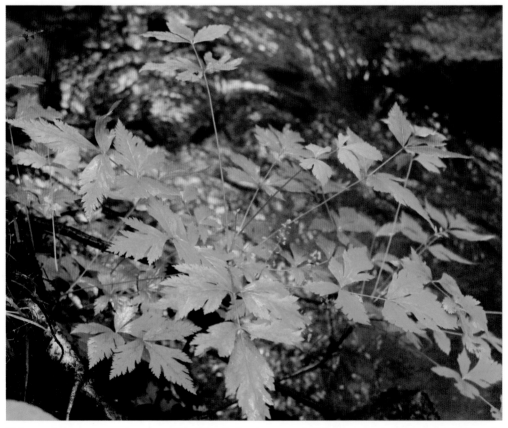

Yellowroot always seems to grow within 10 feet of a stream, and all the leaves are clustered at the top of its woody stem.

10 feet of a creek or stream. It forms large colonies with its runners, sending out roots that are only pencil-thin but can be many feet long. Be careful harvesting, as those lateral runners help keep streambanks in place and prevent erosion.

The root can be dug almost year-round but is considered best in the fall. Because the roots are so thin it takes a long time to harvest any kind of quantity, so be prepared. But there is always a stream nearby to wash them in, so that's a plus.

Medicinal uses

This plant contains the bitter yellow alkaloid berberine, the same antimicrobial, antifungal, and antiviral chemical found in barberry and goldenseal; it is used in much the same way as those herbs, although it is not quite as strong. The traditional use of the plant, however, was a bit more specific for mouth ulcers and liver problems.

Chewing on a bit of the root can really help mouth ulcers, canker sores, and even stomach ulcers—maybe because the berberine helps to kill some of the *H. pylori* bacteria that contribute to ulcers.

Thanks to its bitter taste, it also makes a great digestive bitter, stimulating the appetite before a meal and improving digestion, especially the digestion of fats and proteins. To this end, it combines well with dandelion, gentian, or burdock.

More than just bitter, yellowroot's main traditional use was as a liver and gallbladder tonic. It could be used as a general tonic for a sluggish liver or a tendency to form gallstones, specifically for indigestion after eating fats. It was also said to have some effect on diabetes.

It's a good herb to have around, more as a bitter tonic than as an antimicrobial, in my opinion. We can't tell everything about a plant just based on its chemistry, after all.

Future harvests

Although this plant can be locally abundant, harvest it gently to keep the integrity of the streambank ecosystem.

HERBAL PREPARATIONS

The traditional use is to cut the root into pencil-sized sticks and keep in a canning jar to chew on when not feeling good, and these sticks can still be found at local markets in the country. It can also be made into a tincture fresh 1:2 at 95%, or dry 1:5 at 50%.

Melilotus officinalis
PARTS USED leaves, flowers

A good remedy for point-specific pain.

How to identify

This is a tall plant in the pea family, up to 6 feet high, with thin straight stalks that branch up and down the plant and leaves divided into three. The flowers are in multiple spikes of small pea-shaped yellow flowers, making it look like a big yellow flag on roadsides in early summer. It contains coumarins, and so any part of the plant, when crushed, should smell like fresh hay or mowed grass.

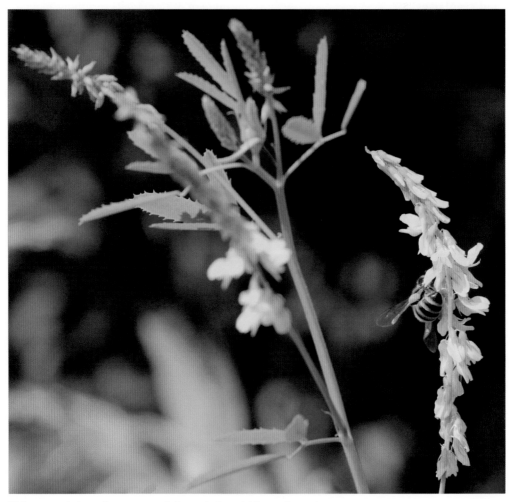

Yellow sweet clover is a common tall weed of roadsides and meadows.

Where, when, and how to wildcraft

This is a major plant of roadsides, untended fields, and disturbed areas, just about anywhere from coast to coast. It is abundant and weedy. Harvest throughout the summer, but plants are considered to have the best potency when first flowering in June. Harvest the whole plant, and then strip off the leaves and flowers to make the medicine.

Medicinal uses

Though this isn't a commonly used medicine, yellow sweet clover is a good one for some specific kinds of pain. It is also a mild blood thinner and can help with capillary congestion.

It is particularly indicated for point-specific pain that is boring or stabbing. I have used it for eye pain, sciatica, neuralgia, ovarian neuralgia, or other unexplained pain that doesn't fit into a specific category. It opens things up and gets things moving, so it is good for people who feel cold or deficient, or when there is a stuck feeling causing the discomfort. Coldness and soreness upon touch are a good indication for this remedy, which combines nicely with prickly ash for this kind of pain.

Future harvests

This is an invasive weed; no worries about overharvesting.

Caution

Because of its mild blood-thinning properties, do not combine with blood-thinning pharmaceuticals.

HERBAL PREPARATIONS

Tincture either fresh 1:2 at 95%, or dry 1:5 at 50% alcohol.

---

yucca

Yucca filamentosa

PARTS USED root

An anti-inflammatory for muscle and joint pain.

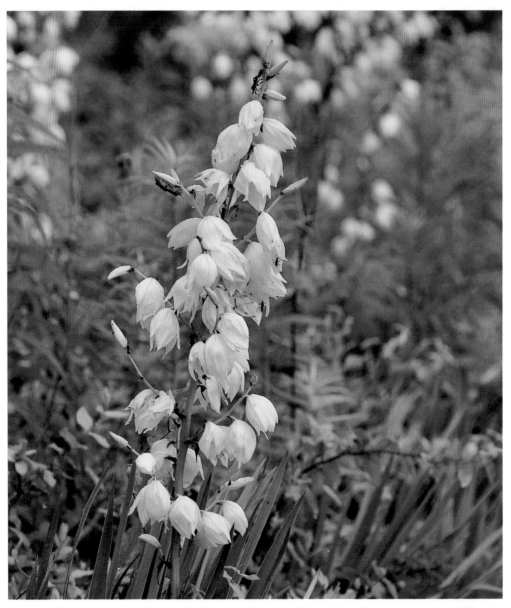

The white flowers are a real show stealer, but the long, tough, sharp-pointed leaves are unmistakable too.

How to identify

Yucca (aka Spanish bayonet) is eye-catching, with a unique-looking evergreen rosette of 1- to 2-foot-long leaves arising from the ground. Leaves are stiff and come to a sharp point, and there are frayed threads coming off their edges. Of the species in the Southeast, *Yucca filamentosa* is the most common and abundant, but any of the yuccas can be used similarly, including those grown as ornamentals.

The flower stalk shoots up in early to mid-summer like a 6-foot-tall flag pole of large white 6-petaled flowers. Before flowering, the stalk looks like nothing so much as a monster asparagus, to which it is related. After flowering, the flowers are replaced by round green capsules with strong lines running down the fruit.

Note that this is an entirely different plant from yuca or cassava root, which is in a different family and is the plant more often used as an edible; yucca too is edible, though not nearly as tasty.

Where, when, and how to wildcraft

Yucca grows somewhere in every state of the Southeast. Although perhaps not as abundant as the yucca plants in the Southwest, in our region it is often found in part sun and sandy soil, especially on the coastal plain and Piedmont but up in the mountains in some places, too.

The root is a deep taproot, and the spine at the tip of the stiff leaves is expert at piercing skin. So the best bet, once you find a yucca that you can dig, is to trim back the leaves and then switch back and forth between a digging fork to loosen the soil and a trenching shovel to dig down deeper. The root itself is thick and waxy, and one plant will usually yield several quarts of extract.

Medicinal uses

Yucca is a simple plant with a simple use: it is a great anti-inflammatory. This is due to the abundance of saponins in the root, which also make it useful as a natural soap or shampoo.

It is most commonly used for osteoarthritis or rheumatoid arthritis to reduce inflammation in the joints; it is also used for inflammation in the digestive or urinary tracts. For joint pain it can be used internally, or the roots can be mashed to make a poultice and applied externally.

This is a plant that does one thing but does it well. Considering how abundant it is in some places and how common inflammatory conditions are, it's a great plant to know.

Future harvests

This native plant is fairly hardy, but it is not abundant in some places. Make sure there is a good amount of yucca around before harvesting.

HERBAL PREPARATIONS

Yucca extracts well in both alcohol or water, or can be dried then powdered and put in capsules. The root decoction can be drunk or used in a bath. The tincture is made 1:2 fresh at 95%, or dry 1:5 at 50%.

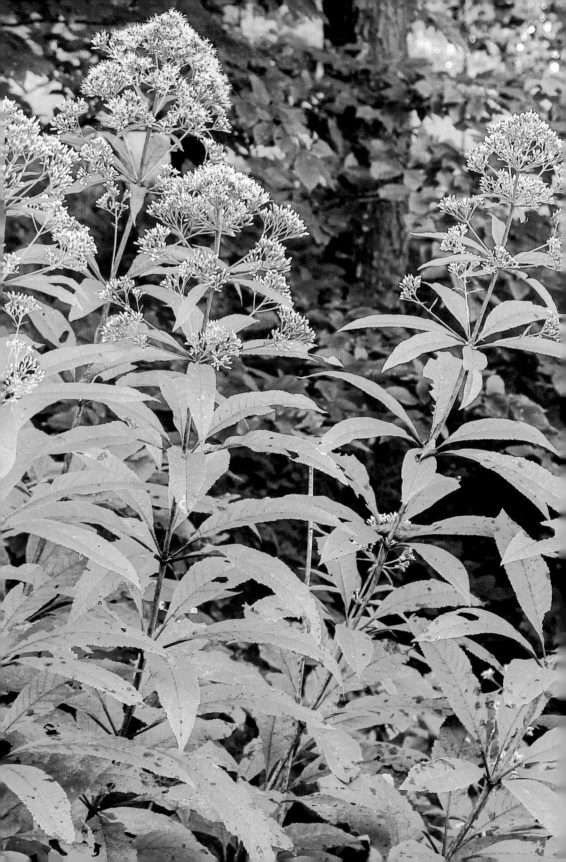

BIBLIOGRAPHY

Alfs, Matthew. 2003. *300 Herbs: Their Indications and Contraindications*. OTBH.

Chen, John, and Tina Chen. 2012. *Chinese Medical Herbology and Pharmacology*. Art of Medicine Press.

Dass, Vishnu. 2013. *Ayurvedic Herbology East and West*. Lotus Press.

Easley, Thomas, and Steven Horne. 2016. *The Modern Herbal Dispensatory*. North Atlantic Books.

Felter, Harvey Wickes, and John Uri Lloyd. 1898. *King's American Dispensatory*, 18th ed. Ohio Valley Company.

Ganora, Lisa. 2009. *Herbal Constituents*. Self-published.

Gardner, Zoë, and Michael McGuffin. 2013. *Botanical Safety Handbook*, 2nd ed. CRC Press.

Howell, Patricia Kyritsi. 2006. *Medicinal Plants of the Southern Appalachians*. BotanoLogos.

Kimmerer, Robin Wall. 2015. *Braiding Sweetgrass*. Milkweed Editions.

Lee, Michele E. 2017. *Working the Roots*. Wadastick Publishers.

Light, Phyllis D. 2018. *Southern Folk Medicine*. North Atlantic Books.

Moore, Michael. 1989. *Medicinal Plants of the Desert and Canyon West*. Museum of New Mexico Press.

———. 2003. *Medicinal Plants of the Mountain West*. Museum of New Mexico Press.

———. 2011. *Medicinal Plants of the Pacific West*. Museum of New Mexico Press.

Patton, Darryl. 2017. *Mountain Medicine*. Little River Press.

Pole, Sebastian. 2012. *Ayurvedic Medicine*. Singing Dragon.

Porcher, Francis. 1863. *Resources of the Southern Fields and Forests*. West and Johnston.

Priest, A. W., and L. R. Priest. 1982. *Herbal Medication*. L. N. Fowler & Co. Ltd.

Rogers, Robert. 2011. *The Fungal Pharmacy*. North Atlantic Books.

Tilgner, Sharol Marie. 2009. *Herbal Medicine from the Heart of the Earth*. Wise Acres.

Weakley, Alan. 2019. *Flora of the Southern and Mid-Atlantic States*. University of North Carolina at Chapel Hill.

Winston, David. 2013. *Herbal Therapeutics*. Herbal Therapeutics Research Library.

INDEX

A

abortions, 69
abrasions, 112
Achillea millefolium, 278–280
acidic stomach, 223
acne, 53, 97, 207
aconitic acids, 142
Acorus americanus, 90–92
Acorus calamus, 90–92
acquired immunodeficiency
    syndrome (AIDS), 204
Actaea pachypoda, 65–66
Actaea podocarpa, 65
Actaea racemosa, 64–67
Actaea rubra, 65–66
adaptogens, 79–80, 105,
    124, 126, 169, 171, 204,
    230–231, 268–269
adrenal exhaustion, 172
Aesculus flava, 83–84
Aesculus hippocastanum, 83
Aesculus pavia, 83–84
Agrimonia gryposepala, 34–35
Agrimonia parviflora, 34–35
Agrimonia pubescens, 34–35
agrimony, 18, 34–35, 166
air potato, 270
Albizia julibrissin, 158–160
alcohol, 25–28, 30, 148
allantoin, 183
allergies, 48, 53, 60, 92, 94,
    127–129, 169, 179,
    192–193, 204, 273

"all roads open", 242
Alzheimer's disease, 44–45,
    144, 154
Ambrosia artemisiifolia, 192–193
Ambrosia trifida, 192–193
American barberry, 51–53
American elm, 222
American ginseng, 80,
    124–126
American stinging nettle,
    168
American teasel, 243–244
amor seco, 59
analgesic, 47, 114
anemia, 169, 171, 283
anemone, 36–38
Anemone, 36–38
Anemone caroliniana, 37
Anemone quinquefolia, 36–37
Anemone virginiana, 36
angelica, 20, 39–42, 92, 166,
    185, 256
Angelica, 39–42, 79
Angelica archangelica, 41
Angelica atropurpurea, 40–41
Angelica sinensis, 41
Angelica triquinata, 39–42
Angelica venenosa, 40–41
angelico, 79–80
anger, 77, 107
anise, 118
annual ragweed, 192–193
anorexia nervosa, 92, 118

Antabuse, 148
antibacterials, 52, 114, 140,
    185, 246
antibiotics, 50, 53
anti-cancer agent, 73
antidepressants, 160, 233–234
antifungals, 52, 71, 73, 131,
    185, 251
anti-inflammatory, 35, 47, 97,
    122–123, 134–135, 138,
    140, 143–144, 166, 207,
    210, 212, 214, 237, 257,
    266, 273, 288–289
antimicrobials, 51, 53, 55, 60,
    130–131, 140, 143–144,
    166, 200, 205, 240–242,
    245–246, 256, 284–285
antioxidants, 122–123, 144,
    213–214
antiparasitics, 52–53, 71, 140
antiseptics, 27, 47, 49, 60, 128,
    135, 145–146, 181, 241–
    242, 246, 253, 254–256,
    258, 279
antispasmodics, 67, 68–69, 77,
    116, 148, 156–157, 176,
    220–221, 270–271
antivirals, 52, 78, 81–82, 110–
    112, 130–131, 139–140,
    148, 185, 246, 250–251,
    264, 285
anxiety, 37–38, 86, 162, 176,
    179, 204, 219

aphrodisiac, 80, 207
Appalachian reishi, 202
appetite, 41, 92, 118, 260, 280, 285
apple cider vinegar, 169
appreciation, 15
apricots, 283
Aralia nudicaulis, 268–269
Aralia racemosa, 229–231
Aralia spinosa, 189
arborvitae, 250–251
Arctium minus, 87–89
arnica, 277
arteriosclerosis, 152
arthritis, 41–42, 89, 112, 190–191, 207, 225, 241–242, 256, 273, 289
Aruncus dioicus, 65
Asarum canadense, 263–264
Asclepias tuberosa, 184–186
ashy hydrangea, 265–267
aspirin, 272–273
assimilation, 35, 107, 146, 280
aster, 56, 87, 107, 278
asthma, 42, 67, 156, 166, 185, 212, 221
Astilbe biternata, 65
astringents, 26, 34–35, 55, 60, 61, 63, 86, 129, 141–142, 146, 166, 181, 183, 193, 214, 239, 252–253, 258, 261–262, 274–275
athlete's foot, 251
attention-deficit/hyperactivity disorder (ADHD), 45
autoimmune conditions, 86, 204
Avena sativa, 170–172
Ayurveda, 44, 92, 125, 133

B

bacopa, 43–45, 123, 133
Bacopa caroliniana, 43–44
Bacopa monnieri, 43–45
balm of Gilead, 46–48
balsam poplar, 46
bam'a'gil, 46–48
bamgilly, 46–48
baneberry, 65–66
baptisia, 49–50
Baptisia tinctoria, 49–50
barberry, 51–53, 75, 107, 131, 181, 285
bark processing, 23–24
Bass, Tommie, 176
basswood, 151
bayberry, 54–55
bearsfoot, 56–58
bee balm, 12
bee stings, 183
beggar ticks, 59–60
Bell's palsy, 103
benign prostatic hyperplasia (BPH), 169, 174, 196, 211, 236, 251
berberine, 52–53, 282, 285
Berberis canadensis, 51
Berberis thunbergii, 51–52
Berberis vulgaris, 51–52
beta-asarone, 92
Betonica officinalis, 276
bidens, 59–60
Bidens, 59–60
Bidens alba, 59–60
Bidens pilosa, 59–60
Bignonia capreolata, 104–105
bile, 53, 107, 109, 116, 118, 131, 279, 283
birthwort, 150
bittercress, 215

bitters, 53, 117–118, 146, 162, 279–280, 283
blackberry, 18, 20, 61–63, 194, 205
black cherry, 259–260
black cohosh, 22, 64–67, 75, 260, 271
black haw, 67, 68–69, 135, 271
black raspberry, 194–196
"black salves", 73
blackstrap molasses, 283
black walnut, 18, 53, 70–71
black willow, 272
bladder, 53, 267, 280
bleeding, 142, 214, 215–216, 244, 253, 258, 275, 280
blood circulation, 42, 75, 89, 122–123, 135, 138, 146, 150, 162, 190–191, 209, 235–236, 242, 258, 275, 280
blood cleansing, 107, 112, 146, 181, 198, 206–207, 209, 269
blood issues, 86, 171–172
blood pressure, 67, 97, 108, 138, 148, 152, 176, 279
bloodroot, 16, 72–73
blood sugar, 53, 108, 131, 148
blood thinner, 273, 287
blueberry, 138, 225
blue cohosh, 15, 74–75, 150
blue vervain, 76–78, 176
blue violet, 246–247
boarhog, 20, 79–80, 185
boneset, 78, 81–82
Borrelia, 244
boswellia, 47
brain fog, 91–92
brain injuries, 144

brain stimulation, 45, 133
Brazilian vervain, 77
breakbone fever, 81
breast cancer, 188, 198,
    201, 249
breast health, 198
broad-leaved dock, 281–283
broken bones, 82, 133, 144, 225
bronchitis, 41, 156–157, 166,
    185, 186, 230–231
bronchodilator, 80, 221
bruises, 112, 160, 233
buckeye, 18, 83–84
bugleweed, 85–86
Buhner, Stephen, 60
burdock, 21, 87–89, 148, 248,
    281, 283
burlap bags, 22
burn-out, 172
burns, 112, 234, 275
bush clover, 49
buttercup, 75
butterflies, 134, 184
butterfly weed, 185
butternut, 70
bypass pruners, 21

C

calamus, 90–92, 118, 157
calcium, 142, 169
Camellia sinensis, 26
camphor, 277
Campsis radicans, 104
cancer, 114, 144, 154, 183, 188,
    191, 198, 204, 214, 249
canker sores, 97, 285
cannabis, 18
capillary congestion, 287
Capsella bursa-pastoris,
    215–216

Cardamine, 215
Cardinal, Aurelien, 207
cardiovascular system, 279
carminative, 103
Carolina allspice, 226–228
Carolina geranium, 262
Carolina water-hyssop, 43–44
carpal tunnel syndrome,
    103, 225
catnip, 81, 93–94, 193
cattail, 90
Caulophyllum thalictroides,
    74–75
cayenne, 191
Ceanothus americanus, 199–
    201
Cedrus, 250
Centella, 132–133
Centella asiatica, 132–133
Centella erecta, 132–133
cervical dysplasia, 131, 246
chamomile, 94, 152
chemotherapy, 118
chicory, 106, 108
chiggers, 20
childbirth, 174, 195–196
Chimaphila maculata, 180–181
Chimaphila umbellata, 180–181
Chinese angelica, 41
Chinese ginseng, 125
Chinese hawthorn, 138
Chinese medicine, 12, 41, 47,
    77, 79–80, 89, 92, 107,
    125, 139, 140, 144, 148,
    154, 159, 172, 186, 204,
    214, 219, 242, 244, 256
Chionanthus, 115
Chionanthus virginicus, 115–116
chlorophyll, 119
cholesterol, 118, 138, 279

chronic fatigue syndrome (CFS),
    57–58
chuan xiong, 79
Cicuta maculata, 39
Cimicifuga racemosa, 64–67
cinnamon, 209
cinnamon vine, 270
circular thinking, 120
circulatory stimulants, 42, 55
citrus, 189
cleavers, 95–97, 169, 201,
    216, 249
clematis, 98–99
Clematis terniflora, 99
Clematis virginiana, 98–99
clothing, 20
cloth shopping bags, 22
colds, 41, 60, 80, 82, 92, 97,
    111, 140, 164, 186, 228,
    241, 264
cold sores, 201
colitis, 55, 258, 262, 275
collagen, 138, 142
Collinsonia canadensis, 235–236
colon, 71
common horsetail, 141
common ragweed, 192–193
compound leaves, 18
congestion, 55, 112, 164
congestive dysmenorrhea, 150
congestive heart failure, 138
Conium maculatum, 39
connective tissue, 133, 138,
    142, 225
constipation, 89, 118, 283
Convallaria majuscula, 20
Cook, Frank, 11
coronary artery disease, 148
corpse plant, 119
cotton, 69, 100–101

coughs, 92, 157, 183, 186, 198, 212, 221, 241, 248–249, 260
COVID-19 pandemic, 246
cow parsnip, 20, 40, 102–103
crab apple, 136
crampbark, 69
Crataegus, 136–138
crimson clover, 197
Crohn's disease, 271
crossvine, 104–105
curly dock, 281–283
cyanide, 260
cyanogenic glycoside, 259–260

D

dandelion, 21, 41, 106–109, 118, 283
Datura stramonium, 20
Daucus carota, 278
deadly angelica, 40–41
decoctions, 26, 30
decongestant, 92, 164, 279
dehydration, 63
Delphinium tricorne, 261
demulcents, 146, 166, 183, 186, 249, 260, 266
dengue, 81
dents de lion ("lion's teeth"), 106
depression, 160, 204, 233–234
dermatitis, 116
devil's walking stick, 189
diabetes, 108, 285
diabetic retinopathy, 123
diaphoretics, 78, 81, 129, 179, 279, 280
diarrhea, 23, 35, 55, 63, 140, 148, 214, 223, 242, 253, 258, 262
Diervilla, 139

digestive issues, 41, 138, 289
digestive system stimulation, 53, 89, 92, 94, 107, 117–118, 125, 152, 162, 164, 183, 190–191, 207, 227, 258, 260, 262, 279–280, 285
digestive tract infections, 131
digestive tract tonifying, 35
digging fork, 20–21
Dioscorea polystachya, 270
Dioscorea villosa, 270–271
diosgenin, 271
Dipsacus asper, 244
Dipsacus fullonum, 243–244
Dipsacus sylvestris, 243–244
disturbed mind, 159
diuretics, 60, 97, 108, 129, 142, 146, 166, 169, 246, 249, 280
diverticulitis, 71, 262
dock, 87
dogwood, 12
dong quai, 41
downy skullcap, 217–219
drawing poultice, 183
dust allergies, 193
Dutch elm disease, 222
dwarf palmetto, 210
dwarf stinging nettle, 168
dysentery, 140, 271

E

Easley, Thomas, 105
eastern red cedar, 145, 250
echinacea, 81, 92, 97, 200
eczema, 53, 97, 207
edema, 97, 108, 129
elder, 18, 81, 110–112, 193, 280
electric kettles, 26

emetic, 156
emmenagogue, 101, 279
emotional issues, 37–38, 179
enlarged prostate, 169, 196, 201, 211, 236, 251
epilepsy, 78, 219
Epstein-Barr Virus, 57
Equisetum arvense, 141–142
Equisetum hyemale, 141–142
erectile dysfunction, 123
esophageal reflux, 223
estrogen, 271
eucalyptus, 164
Eupatorium perfoliatum, 81–82
Eupatorium purpureum, 134–135
Eupatorium sessilifolium, 81
European angelica, 41–42
European barberry, 51–53
European nettle, 168
Eutrochium maculatum, 134
Eutrochium purpureum, 134–135
expectorants, 48, 73, 156–157, 164, 185, 231, 246, 256, 260
eyebright, 193
eye pain, 287
eyewash, 35

F

fairy candles, 64–67
false goatsbeard, 65
false hellebore, 20
false Solomon's seal, 224
false unicorn root, 12
fennel, 41, 92, 118
ferns, 141
fever, 78, 89, 111–112, 140, 148, 179, 186, 227, 239, 280
fibrocystic breasts, 114, 201

fibromyalgia, 67
field horsetail, 141
figs, 114
figwort, 113–114
Filipendula ulmaria, 35
fire cherry, 259
first aid, 20, 214
flatulent dyspepsia, 191
flavonoids, 112, 122, 137–138,
    195, 236, 239, 279
flores de tilo, 152
flower identification, 19
flu, 81, 111, 140, 264
folding saw, 20
food allergies, 193, 204
food stagnation, 138
forgetfulness, 92
fragrant sumac, 237
Frances, Deborah, 258
frankincense, 47
French press, 26
fringe tree, 115–116
fungal infections, 73, 251
furanocoumarins, 42

G
Galium aparine, 95–97
gallbladder stimulation, 53, 116,
    118, 285
gallstones, 107, 116, 285
gangrene, 50
Ganoderma, 202–204
Ganoderma curtisii, 202–204
Ganoderma lucidum, 203
Ganoderma sessile, 202–204
Ganoderma tsugae, 202–204
Ganora, Lisa, 264
gastric ulcers, 154
gastritis, 258
gastrointestinal issues, 214

genital warts, 251
genitourinary tract
    inflammation, 135, 212,
    246, 258, 262
gentian, 41, 117–118
Gentiana saponaria, 117–118
Gentiana villosa, 117–118
Geranium carolinianum, 262
Geranium maculatum, 261–262
ghost pipe, 119–120
ghost plant, 119
giant hogweed, 102
ginger, 41, 94, 122, 191, 227,
    247, 263–264
gingivitis, 55
ginkgo, 91, 121–123, 151
Ginkgo biloba, 121–123
ginseng, 12, 16, 80, 124–126,
    230–231
glaucoma, 38
glycerin, 25–28
goatsbeard, 65
gobo, 89
goiters, 214
goldenrod, 15, 24, 60, 127–129
goldenseal, 12, 16, 52, 112,
    130–131, 246, 285
goosegrass, 95–97
Gossypium hirsutum, 100–101
gotu kola, 92, 123, 132–133,
    138, 225
gout, 97, 169, 216
grass, 170
gravel, 135, 266
gravel root, 97, 134–135, 181,
    236, 266
great angelica, 40
great ragweed, 192–193
greenbrier, 20
grief, 160

Gulf fritillary butterflies, 60
gum disease, 55, 214, 239, 253
gut flora, 89
gut infection, 53

H
hair, 142
hair conditions, 58, 142
hairy leafcup, 56
Hamamelis virginiana, 274–275
hand tools, 20–22, 31
hangover symptoms, 148
harvesting, 14–16
hawkweed, 106, 107
hawthorn, 136–138
hay fever, 169, 193
hazel, 236
head colds, 92, 94, 97, 140
heal all, 213–214
heart issues, 138, 148, 152,
    162, 204
heart rate, 86
heat, 179, 214, 264
Helicobacter pylori, 285
hemlock, 20, 39
hemlock reishi, 202–204
hemlock varnished shelf
    mushroom, 202–204
hemorrhoids, 84, 214, 236,
    253, 275
hemostatics, 279
hepatitis, 107
Heracleum lanatum, 102–103
Heracleum maximum, 102–103
herbicides, 16
Hericium erinaceus, 153–154
herpes, 162
Hexastylis, 263
Hoffmann, David, 168
hollyhocks, 100

honeysuckle, 139–140
hookworm, 71
hori hori, 21
hormone balance, 207, 271
Horne, Steven, 105
horse chestnut, 83–84
horsetail, 133, 138, 141–142,
    225
hot flashes, 67
hou tou gu, 154
human papillomavirus
    (HPV), 251
Hydrangea arborescens, 265–267
Hydrangea cinerea, 265–267
Hydrastis canadensis, 130–131
Hydrocotyle, 133
Hydrophyllum, 130
Hypericum, 232
Hypericum perforatum, 232–234
Hypericum punctatum, 233
hypertension, 152, 214
hyperthyroidism, 86, 162, 214
hypertonic tissue, 84

I

immune modulators, 204
immune system issues, 154,
    190, 200–201, 204,
    239, 264
incontinence, 35, 166, 251,
    262
Indian pink, 12
Indian pipe, 119
indigestion, 92, 94, 138,
    164, 285
infused oils, 29
infusions, 26
insect bites, 179
insect repellant, 20
insects, 20, 23

insomnia, 92, 160, 162, 176,
    179, 204, 219
interstitial cystitis, 97, 239,
    258, 267
inulin, 89
Iris pseudacorus, 90
iron, 169, 283
irritable bowel syndrome
    (IBS), 271

J

Jack in the pulpit, 124
Japanese barberry, 51–53
Japanese clematis, 99
Japanese honeysuckle, 139, 140
Japanese knotweed, 143–
    144, 148
jaundice, 107, 116
jimson weed, 20
Joe Pye weed, 134–135
joint inflammation, 146, 289
joint pain, 41–42, 47, 107, 146,
    206, 209, 216, 256, 273,
    275, 287, 289
Juglans cinerea, 70
Juglans nigra, 70–71
juniper, 145–146
Juniperus communis, 146
Juniperus sabina, 146
Juniperus virginiana, 145–146,
    250
Juniperus virginiana var.
    silicicola, 146

K

kidney cleansing, 89, 97,
    107–108, 129, 146, 169,
    207, 216, 280
kidney stones, 69, 97, 135, 181,
    236, 266–267

kidney yang tonic, 80
Klamath beetle, 233
Korean ginseng, 125
kudzu, 18, 147–148

L

labor, 114, 150
ladybug, 23
lamb's ear, 165
larkspur, 261
laryngitis, 212
late black cohosh, 65
leaf arrangement, 18–19
leaky gut syndrome, 207
lemon balm, 94, 234
lemons, 189
Leonurus cardiaca, 161–162
Leonurus sibiricus, 162
LeSassier, William, 122, 244
Lespedeza, 49
Letharia vulpina, 245–246
leukorrhea, 258
lichen, 245–246
liferoot, 149–150, 247
Light, Phyllis D., 81, 105, 179
Ligusticum canadense, 79–80
Ligusticum wallichii, 79
lily, 20
lily of the valley, 20
limbic system, 125–126
linden, 151–152
Lindera benzoin, 226–228
ling zhi, 204
"lion-hearted", 162
lion's mane, 45, 153–154
lipomas, 214
Liquidambar formosana, 242
Liquidambar styraciflua, 240–242
liver cleansing, 89, 107–
    109, 144

"liverish energy", 77

liver stimulation, 53, 58, 77, 116, 118, 131, 207, 214, 279–280, 282–283, 285

"liver wind", 219

lobelia, 155–157

Lobelia cardinalis, 155

Lobelia inflata, 155–157

Lobelia spicata, 155

lobeline, 157

Lonicera, 139

Lonicera japonica, 139–140

loosestrife, 76

loppers, 20–22

Lotti, Anna Claire, 28, 151

lu lu tong, 242

lung issues, 166, 185–186, 198, 211, 212, 230–231, 242, 249, 251, 256, 260

Lycopus virginicus, 85–86

Lyme disease, 144, 191, 206–207, 244

lymph cleansing, 89, 97

lymph movers, 50, 57, 97, 114, 188, 191, 198, 200–201, 248–249, 258

Lythrum salicaria, 76

M

mad-dog skullcap, 77, 217–219

magnesium, 169, 219

magnolia, 12

Maianthemum racemosum, 224

male pattern baldness, 58

Marano, Chris, 119

marshmallow, 100

mastitis, 188, 201, 249

mcdonald, jim, 166

meadow rue, 75

meadowsweet, 35

meat cleaver, 23

meditation, 45

Meesters, Dave, 60

Melilotus officinalis, 286–287

menopause, 67, 225

menses, 101, 150, 162, 228

menstrual cramps, 67, 75, 114, 162, 195–196

menstruum, 27, 29, 30

Mentha ×piperita, 26

Mexican wild yam, 271

migraine headaches, 38, 67, 77–78, 99, 123, 219

milkweed, 185–186

milky oat seed, 45, 154, 157, 170–172

mimosa, 18, 148, 158–160, 219

Mimosa, 158

mint, 19, 85, 113, 165, 217, 280

miscarriages, 69, 244

Mitchell, Bill, 246

Mitchella repens, 173–174

Monotropa hypopitys, 119

Monotropa uniflora, 119–120

Moore, Michael, 12, 38, 55, 103, 271, 275

Morella cerifera, 54

Morella pensylvanica, 55

Morris, Will, 242, 246

motherwort, 86, 161–162, 176

mountain angelica, 41–42

mountain cohosh, 65

mountain mint, 163–164

mouth bacteria, 73

mouth problems, 103, 214, 239, 256, 285

mucosa, 35, 60, 71, 128–129, 131, 169, 258

mullein, 67, 165–166, 185, 249, 281

multidrug resistance (MDR), 53

muscle pain/cramp, 47, 66–67, 69, 81, 148, 244, 275, 277

muscle relaxants, 156–157

muscular tension, 277

mushroom extraction, 30

mushrooms, 20, 119, 153

Myrica cerifera, 54

myrrh, 46, 47

N

nausea, 23, 50, 67, 156, 157, 188

nectar, 41

Nepeta cataria, 93–94

nerve growth factor synthesis, 154

nerve pain, 219, 234

nervines, 45, 78, 105, 157, 176, 242

nervous system issues, 45, 77, 103, 154, 162, 171–172, 219, 233–234

nettle, 24, 92, 94, 97, 142, 167–170, 193, 198, 216, 283

neuralgia, 191, 287

nicotine, 142

nitrates, 142

northern bayberry, 55

northern prickly ash, 189–191

northern white cedar, 250–251

nursery spade, 20–21

nutrient deficiency, 169

Nymphaea odorata, 257–258

O

oak, 153

oat, 170–172

oatstraw, 169, 198

obesity, 92

old man's beard, 245–246
oranges, 189
orchid, 19
orchitis, 75
oshá, 79–80
osteoarthritis, 207, 289
osteoporosis, 244
ovarian neuralgia, 287
oxytocin, 101

P

Packera, 247
Packera aurea, 149–150
pain relief, 119, 144, 148, 166, 191, 242, 244, 273, 287
palmately compound leaves, 18
Panax quinquefolius, 124
panic attacks, 37–38
parasites, 53, 71, 253
parsley, 19–20, 39, 79, 103
partridgeberry, 173–174
Passero, Lupo, 214
Passiflora edulis, 176
Passiflora incarnata, 175–177
Passiflora lutea, 176
passionflower, 78, 175–177
passionfruit, 176
pea, 19, 158, 199
peach, 178–179
Pedicularis, 276
Pedicularis canadensis, 276–277
Pedicularis groenlandica, 276
pelvic pain, 69, 135, 196
pelvic stimulant, 75, 84, 135, 150, 174, 212, 235–236, 258
pennyworts, 133
peony, 89
peppermint, 26, 41, 92, 94, 111, 164, 227

peptic ulcers, 131, 183, 223, 262
peripheral nervous system, 277
pesticides, 16
pet allergies, 169, 193
Phytolacca americana, 187–188
picão preto, 59
pinesap, 119
pink lady's slipper, 12
pinnately compound leaves, 18
Pinus strobus, 254–256
pinworm, 71
pipsissewa, 135, 180–181
Plantago major, 182–183
Plantago rugelii, 182–183
Plantago virginica, 182–183
plantain, 138, 146, 182–183
plant drying, 24
plant identification, 17–19
plant location, 16–17
plant processing, 22–24
platelet-activating factor (PAF), 123
pleurisy, 185
pleurisy root, 184–186
PMS, 37–38
pneumonia, 41, 166, 185, 186
pocketknife, 20
poison hemlock, 19, 39
poison ivy, 18, 19, 20, 58, 179, 193, 252–253
poison oak, 20
poisonous plants, 19–20
poison sumac, 20, 237–238
poke, 23, 187–188, 201, 249
pollinators, 14, 35, 41, 134, 152, 184, 185, 186, 277, 280
polycystic ovarian syndrome (PCOS), 212
Polygonatum biflorum, 224–225
Polygonum cuspidatum, 143–144

Polymnia uvedalia, 56
polysaccharides, 154, 204
Populus, 46–48
Populus balsamifera, 46
Populus ×jackii, 46
post traumatic stress disorder (PTSD), 119, 204
potassium, 108
prebiotic polysaccharide, 89
pregnancy
    use of baptisia, 50
    use of black cohosh, 67
    use of bloodroot, 73
    use of blue cohosh, 75
    use of cotton, 69, 101
    use of goldenseal, 131
    use of juniper, 146
    use of liferoot, 150
    use of lobelia, 157
    use of mimosa, 160
    use of motherwort, 162
    use of oat, 171
    use of raspberry, 196
    use of skunk cabbage, 221
    use of spicebush, 228
    use of white cedar, 251
    use of wild cherry, 260
    use of wild ginger, 264
    use of wild yam, 271
premenstrual syndrome (PMS), 45, 97, 162, 234
Presley, Elvis, 187
prickly ash, 118, 123, 189–191
prince's pine, 180
private land, 16–17
progesterone, 271
propolis tincture, 20
prostate issues, 150, 169, 174, 196, 201, 211, 236, 249, 251

prostatitis, 97, 135, 196, 251, 267
prunasin, 259–260
Prunella vulgaris, 213–214
pruners, 20–21
Prunus pensylvanica, 259
Prunus persica, 178–179
Prunus serotina, 259–260
prussic acid, 259–260
psoriasis, 97, 207, 282, 283
public land, 16
pukeweed, 156
purple cabbage, 225
purple loosestrife, 76
purple passionflower, 175–177
purplestem, 40
Pycnanthemum incanum, 163–164
pyrrolizidine alkaloids (PAs), 82

Q
qi, 230, 242, 269
Queen Anne's lace, 39, 110, 278
Quercus alba, 252–253

R
racing mind, 86, 179
ragweed, 92, 94, 192–193
raisins, 283
ramps, 20
raspberry, 18, 61, 194–196, 205
rat vein, 180
Raynaud's disease, 122, 191
red baneberry, 65–66
red bugs, 20
red clover, 18, 197–198, 248–249
red raspberry, 194–196
red root, 21, 23, 92, 97, 199–201, 249

reishi, 30, 154, 202–204, 219
"rescue remedy", 37–38
respiratory infections, 53, 60, 80, 86, 148, 225, 246, 251, 256, 264
respiratory system issues, 41, 128–129, 169, 193
respiratory tract tonifying, 60, 94
resveratrol, 144
Reynoutria japonica, 143–144
rheumatism, 66, 146
rheumatoid arthritis, 207, 289
Rhus copallinum, 237–239
Rhus glabra, 237–239
Rhus typhina, 237–239
ribwort, 183
ringworm, 71, 73, 251
romerillo, 59
root processing, 23
rose, 205
rose geranium essential oil, 20
rosemary, 214
rosmarinic acid, 214
Rubus allegheniensis, 61
Rubus idaeus, 194–196
Rubus occidentalis, 194–196
Rubus pensilvanicus, 61
rue, 189
Rumex crispus, 281–283
Rumex obtusifolius, 281–283
runny nose, 94, 200, 253

S
Sabal minor, 210
salicylates, 48
salicylic acid, 47, 273
salivation, 190–191
Salix, 272–273

Salix nigra, 272
salsify, 107
Sambucus nigra ssp. *canadensis*, 110–112
Sambucus racemosa, 110
Sanguinaria canadensis, 72–73
saponins, 154, 207, 271, 289
sarsaparilla, 105, 205–207, 269
sassafras, 105, 208–209
Sassafras albidum, 208–209
saw palmetto, 169, 210–212
sciatica, 191, 219, 234, 287
scouring rush horsetail, 141
scouting, 16
scrofula, 114
Scrophularia marilandica, 113–114
Scutellaria incana, 217–219
Scutellaria integrifolia, 218
Scutellaria lateriflora, 77, 217–219
seasonal affective disorder, 234
seasons, 15–16
sedatives, 38, 218, 219, 260
self heal, 213–214
Senecio aureus, 149–150
senega snakeroot, 12
senile dementia, 45, 123, 154
sepsis, 50
septicemia, 50
Serenoa repens, 210–212
7Song, 8, 38, 120
sexually transmitted infections (STIs), 191
sexual organs, 211
shelf mushroom, 202
shepherd's purse, 97, 169, 215–216
shrub yellowroot, 284–285
Siberian elm, 222

silica, 142
silktree, 158
sinus congestion, 92
sinus infections, 53, 55, 131, 140
sinusitis, 112
skin cancers, 73
skin conditions, 53, 89, 97, 114, 116, 140, 142, 169, 181, 206–207, 209, 251, 256, 282, 283
skin infections, 53, 131
skin ulcerations, 214
skullcap, 45, 77–78, 86, 120, 154, 157, 162, 176, 217–219
skunk cabbage, 220–221, 260
slippery elm, 186, 222–223
Smallanthus uvedalia, 56
Smilax, 205–207, 268, 270
Smilax bona-nox, 205
Smilax pumila, 205
Smilax rotundifolia, 205
smooth hydrangea, 265–267
smooth sumac, 237–239
snake bites, 50
snakes, 20, 50
"snow flower", 115
soil knife, 20–21
Solidago, 127–129
Solomon's plume, 224
Solomon's seal, 16, 133, 224–225
sore throat, 92, 140, 188, 200–201, 223, 242, 253, 256
southern bayberry, 54
southern juniper, 146
southern prickly ash, 189–191
sow thistle, 107
Spanish bayonet, 288–289

Spanish needles, 59
spicebush, 226–228
spider bites, 50
spider veins, 275
spikenard, 18, 186, 229–231, 256, 269
spinal pain, 219, 234
spleen enlargement, 201
spleen stimulation, 58
spotted Joe Pye weed, 134
spotted St. John's wort, 233
spotted wintergreen, 180
Stachys byzantina, 165
staghorn sumac, 237–239
staph infections, 60, 246
sticky willy, 95–97
stink bug, 23
St. John's wort, 28, 103, 162, 232–234
stone root, 22, 97, 135, 181, 235–236, 249, 266
stress, 152
stroke, 144, 154
sulphur powder, 20
sumac, 20, 237–239
sunburn, 42, 97, 103, 233
sun exposure, 103, 179
supplies, 31
sweating, 78, 81, 111–112, 179, 186, 191, 227, 280
sweet gum, 240–242
swollen glands, 97, 188, 200–201, 214
Symplocarpus foetidus, 220–221
syphilis, 207, 209
"systemic antibiotic" herbs, 60

T

tachycardia, 86
tall anemone, 36–37

Taraxacum officinale, 106–109
tea, 26, 30
teasel, 243–244
tea tree oil, 71
tendon issues, 225, 244
tendonitis, 225
tension headaches, 277
testosterone, 169, 207, 211
Thalictrum, 75
thiaminase, 142
thiamine, 142
thimbleweed, 36–37
thuja essential oil, 71
Thuja occidentalis, 146, 250–251
Thuja plicata, 250
thyroid issues, 86, 162, 214
ticks, 20
tics, 219
Tilia, 151
Tilia ×europaea, 151–152
tinctures, 25–29
Tinea corporis, 73
tobacco, 15, 157
tonsillitis, 50, 200–201
tools, 20–22, 31
toothache trees, 189
tooth mushroom, 153–154
tooth pain, 103, 190, 191
Toxicodendron radicans, 19
Toxicodendron vernix, 237
toxic roots, 23
trauma, 38, 160, 204, 219, 234
Treasure, Jonathan, 169
tree of collective happiness, 158
tremors, 219
trenching spade, 20–21
trifoliate leaves, 18
Trifolium incarnatum, 197

Trifolium pratense, 197–198

Trifolium repens, 197

trigeminal nerve pain, 103

trigone sphincter, 262

triterpenoid saponins, 271

trumpet creeper, 104

tuberculosis, 114

tulip poplar, 12

turmeric, 118, 138

Typha, 90

U

ulcers, 131, 183, 216, 223, 239, 262, 275, 285

Ulmus rubra, 222–223

upland boneset, 81

urethra, 35, 266–267, 280

uric acid, 97, 216

urinary tract infections, 53, 60, 97, 128–129, 131, 142, 146, 169, 181, 212, 223, 239, 242, 246, 258, 267, 279–280

urinary tract inflammation, 135, 142, 239, 258, 266–267, 289

urinary tract issues, 135, 211

urinary tract tonifying, 35, 60, 97, 166, 169, 239, 251, 262

urination pain, 223

Urtica chamaedryoides, 167, 168

Urtica dioica, 167, 168

Urtica gracilis, 167, 168

usnea, 245–246

Usnea, 245–246

usnic acid, 245

uterine fibroids, 75, 212, 236

uterine stimulant, 101

uterus, 174, 195–196, 258

V

vagina, 258

vaginitis, 131

vagus nerve, 157

valerian, 219, 277

varicose veins, 84, 236, 275

vasodilator, 99

Veratrum viride, 20

Verbascum thapsus, 165–166

Verbena, 77–78

Verbena brasiliensis, 77

Verbena hastata, 76–78

Verbena officinalis, 77

Verbena urticifolia, 77

Viburnum opulus, 69

Viburnum prunifolium, 68–69

vinegar, 13, 27, 78, 157, 169

Viola, 247–249

violet, 198, 201, 247–249

viral infections, 78, 81, 111, 148, 246, 278

viral pandemic, 82

Virginia creeper, 124

Virginia snakeroot, 12

virgin's bower, 99

vitamin B, 142

vitamin C, 112, 138, 169, 239

vitamin K, 169

W

warts, 73, 251

wasp stings, 183

water hemlock, 19, 39–42

waterleaf, 130

water retention, 97, 108, 129

wax myrtle, 54

Western herbal medicine, 12, 71, 89, 91, 148, 154, 159, 168, 179, 214, 219, 242, 256

what's-up dock, 87

white baneberry, 65–66

white cedar, 146, 250–251, 256

white clover, 197

white oak, 252–253

white pine, 48, 254–256

white pond lily, 257–258

white vervain, 77

Whitney, Alanna, 137

whooping cough, 67, 157, 198, 221

wild cherry, 67, 259–260

wildcrafting, 13–16

wild geranium, 261–262

wild ginger, 247, 263–264

wild hydrangea, 22, 23, 97, 135, 181, 236, 265–267

wild larkspur, 261

wild lettuce, 106

wild rose, 20

wild sarsaparilla, 268–269

wild yam, 67, 205, 270–271

willow, 47, 272–273

winged sumac, 237–239

Winston, David, 169

wintergreen, 277

witch hazel, 274–275

wolf lichen, 245–246

Wood, Matthew, 244

wood anemone, 36–37

wood betony, 276–277

worm infestation, 71

wounds, 35, 50, 97, 183, 198, 214, 234, 246, 253

X

Xanthorhiza simplicissima, 284–285

xu duan, 244

Y

yang, 225
Yarnell, Eric, 146, 207
yarrow, 81, 111, 135, 193,
    278–280
yeast infections, 251
yellow aster, 107
yellow buckeye, 83
yellow dock, 21, 41, 87,
    281–283
yellow iris, 90
yellow passionflower, 176

yellowroot, 52, 131, 284–285
yellow sweet clover, 286–287
yi mu cao ("herb to benefit the
    mother"), 162
yin, 225
yucca, 288–289
Yucca filamentosa, 288–289

Z

Zanthoxylum, 189
Zanthoxylum americanum,
    189–191

Zanthoxylum clava-herculis,
    189–191
Zheng Gu Shui, 144

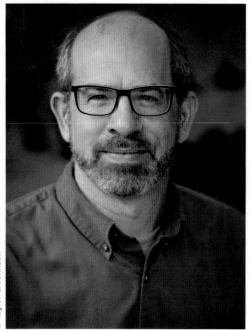

CoreyPine Shane, founder of the Blue Ridge School of Herbal Medicine in Asheville, North Carolina, has been seeing clients, teaching classes, and traveling for lectures for more than 25 years. He trained at the Northeast School of Botanical Medicine, the Southwest School of Botanical Medicine (under noted herbalist Michael Moore), and the Institute of Chinese Herbology. He has explored the Southeast extensively, identifying and harvesting plants from the wild for his herbal extract business, Pine's Herbals, and has led classes at many popular herb conferences, including multiple iterations of the International Herb Symposium, American Herbalists Guild (AHG) Symposium, Medicines from the Earth Symposium, and the Good Medicine Confluence. Visit him at blueridgeschool.org.